Endocrine Updates

Series Editor:
Shlomo Melmed
Cedars-Sinai Medical Center Div. Endocrinology,
Los Angeles, California, USA

More information about this series at http://www.springer.com/series/5917

Adrienne Youdim
Editor

The Clinician's Guide to the Treatment of Obesity

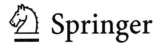 Springer

Editor
Adrienne Youdim, MD, FACP
Assistant Professor of Medicine
Cedars-Sinai Medical Center
Associate Professor of Medicine
David Geffen School of Medicine at University of California, Los Angeles
Los Angeles, CA, USA

ISSN 1566-0729
Endocrine Updates
ISBN 978-1-4939-2145-4   ISBN 978-1-4939-2146-1 (eBook)
DOI 10.1007/978-1-4939-2146-1

Library of Congress Control Number: 2015936279

Springer New York Heidelberg Dordrecht London

Springer is part of Springer Science+Business Media (www.springer.com)

Foreword

Recent epidemiologic studies have noted a plateauing of obesity rates in the USA following decades of steady escalation. Currently, 34.9% of the US adult population is considered obese, as defined by a body mass index of 30 or greater, which has been stable in the years 2011–2012 as compared to 2003–2004 [1]. However, these statistics belie that severe cases of obesity have escalated at a more dramatic rate than general obesity. Between the years 1986 and 2000, the prevalence of BMI 40 or greater quadrupled to one in 50 Americans and the prevalence of BMI of 50 or greater increased fivefold [2]. Currently, 6.4% of the US adults are classified as extremely obese (BMI 40 or greater), [1] having important implications for prognosis and treatment.

In 2013, the American Medical Association recognized obesity as a disease. This designation underscores the scientific literature that has linked obesity to appetite dysregulation, abnormal energy balance, endocrine dysfunction, and dysregulated signaling from adipocytes (fat cells) resulting in cardiometabolic morbidity [3]. In short, excess adipocity results in an aberrant physiology or *pathophysiology* that necessitates long-term treatment and prevention.

There have been significant advances in both the medical and surgical treatment of obesity. Recent years have seen the development of new pharmacologic agents approved for long-term treatment. Combination phentermine/topiramate, trade name Qsymia, is a combination of two well-established drugs. Phentermine, a commonly used appetite suppressant was coupled with topiramate, initially FDA approved as an anti-epileptic, but was found to result in weight loss and likely secondary gabaminergic appetite suppression in the brain. Combination phentermine/topiramate has been shown to result in up to 10.7% total weight loss [3] and improvement of cardiometabolic measures including blood pressure, glycemic abnormalities, and lipids including HDL and triglycerides [4]. A second agent, lorcaserin, selectively agonizes hypothalamic serotonin receptors specifically involved in appetite control. In contrast to historic nonselective serotonin agonists which resulted in valvulopathy and were subsequently removed from markets, lorcaserin does not result in statistically significant valvulopathy [6] and has proven a modest weight loss of 5% with improvement in cardiometabolic abnormalities [7]. Most recently, the FDA approved combination naltrexone/bupropion, trade name

Contrave, for the treatment of obesity with weight loss intermediate to that of lor-caserin and phentermine/topiramate. Bupropion reduces food intake by acting on hypothalamic anorectic pathways while naltrexone is believed to enhance satiety by blocking auto-inhibition of these pathways. [8] These drugs have all demonstrated successful weight losses of 5–10 %, the threshold at which improvements in obesity related comorbidities are achieved. Finally, liraglutide, a GLP-1 agonist currently approved for the treatment of type II diabetes, has demonstrated promising weight loss in obese, non-diabetic subjects. A study in Europe reported weight losses as high as 7.2 kg compared to 2.8 kg in the placebo arm [9]. This medication has been favorably reviewed by the FDA and is expected to become available later in 2015 as a pharmacologic treatment option for non-diabetic obese. Future strategies will likely capitalize on combination therapy and biologics as promising pharmacologic treatment options.

Surgical treatment of obesity has also evolved dramatically in recent years. The laparoscopic approach has proven not only feasible, but the mainstay owing to re-duced complication rates and quicker recovery time [10]. Sleeve gastrectomy, pre-viously considered a staged procedure, has demonstrated comparable efficacy to other bariatric procedures in regards to weight loss and comorbidity reduction, [11] and therefore has seen a dramatic increase in use while use of adjustable gastric banding has declined in the USA [12]. Clinical data has continued to emerge re-garding morbidity reduction in bariatric surgery patients, particularly in the area of diabetes [13–15], as has a greater understanding of potential mechanisms of weight loss and metabolic improvement including incretin effects of surgery [16]. Overall, the number of bariatric surgeries has increased in the USA over the last several decades leaving the long-term management of the bariatric surgery patient to the primary care practitioner.

Lifestyle modification remains the cornerstone of obesity therapy irrespective of adjunctive pharmacotherapy or surgery. Recent studies have supported the effi-cacy of lifestyle modification in reducing weight and improving comorbidities. The Look Ahead (Action for Health in Diabetes) trial, a multicentered trial completed in 2013, attempted to demonstrate the benefit of intensive lifestyle modification in the reduction of cardiovascular endpoints. While the primary endpoint was not accom-plished, this large cohort did confirm the favorable effects of lifestyle modification in weight reduction and reaffirmed behavioral predictors of weight loss such as at-tendance of group support and education [17].

It has been well established that obesity results in significant medical and psy-chosocial comorbidity as well as an increased hazard ratio for all-cause mortality [18]. Obesity also results in significant health-care costs [19] and collateral costs owing to absenteeism and reduced productivity [20]. As a result, numerous profes-sional societies and medical advisory boards have mandated that obesity be identi-fied, diagnosed, and treated. Despite this directive, obesity remains both under-diagnosed and undertreated. In one study of 845 million outpatient visits in the USA, only 29 % of visits by patients who were obese according to BMI had a docu-mented diagnosis of obesity [21]. Furthermore, recent studies have noted a decline in weight-related counseling by primary care practitioners. In one study, only 6.2 % of patients in a large sample of 32,519 adult primary care visits received counseling on diet, exercise, or weight-related issues. [22] Finally, in a survey of 5000 primary care physicians, less than half felt competent in prescribing weight loss programs and less than one fourth would refer a patient who met appropriate criteria for obesity surgery to a surgeon for evaluation [23]. Cited reasons in the literature by providers for lack of counseling and or treatment include lack of training in nutrition and obesity, perceived inability to change patient behaviors, lack of confidence in effectiveness of treatments, and the belief that patients are not motivated to undertake necessary treatments [24].

In response to these barriers to the treatment of obesity, we have collaborated to create a text aimed not only at educating practitioners about obesity, but also providing practical strategies in the comprehensive approach to treat this disease. There are inherent redundancies so that the busy clinician can use this text as a reference. However, the text is comprehensive enough to allow a thorough overview of obesity therapy for the clinician who wishes to read this text from start to finish. Despite recent reports heralding a leveling of obesity rates, it remains that one in three Americans are obese. These alarming statistics warrant aggressive diagnosis and treatment of obesity.

Adrienne Youdim, MD, FACP

References

1. Ogden CL, Carroll MD, Kit BK. Prevalence of childhood and adult obesity in the United States, 2011–2012. JAMA. 2014;311(8):806–14.
2. Sturm R. Increases in clinically severe obesity in the United States, 1986–2000. Arch Intern Med. 2003;163:2146–8.
3. *AMA Resolution* 420 (A-13) June 13 2013 downloaded http://media.npr.org/documents/2013/jun/ama-resolution-obesity.pdf.
4. Garvey WT, Ryan DH, Look M. Two-year sustained weight loss and metabolic benefits with controlled-release phentermine/topiramate in obese and overweight adults (SEQUEL): a randomized, placebo-controlled, phase 3 extension study. Am Jour of Clin Nutrition. 2012;95:297–308.
5. Gadde KM, Allison DB, Ryan DH. Effects of low-dose, controlled-release, phentermine plus topiramate combination on weight and associated comorbidities in overweight and obese adults (CONQUER): a randomized, placebo-controlled, phase 3 trial. Lancet. 2011;377(9774):1341–52.
6. Fidler MC, Sanchez M, Raether B. A one-year randomized trial of lorcaserin for weight loss in obese and overweight adults: the BLOSSOM trial. J Clin Endocrinol Metab. 2011;96(10):3067–77.
7. O'Neil PM, Smith SR, Weissman NJ. Randomized placebo-controlled clinical trial of lorcaserin for weight loss in type 2 diabetes mellitus: the BLOOM-DM study. Obesity (Silver Spring). 2012(7):1426–36.
8. Billes SK, Sinnayah P, Crowley MA. Naltrexone/bupropion for obesity: an investigational combination pharmacotherapy for weight loss. Pharmacol Res. 2014;84:1–11.
9. Astrup A, Rössner S, Van Gaal L, Rissanen A. Effects of liraglutide in the treatment of obesity: a randomised, double-blind, placebo-controlled study. Lancet. 2009;374:1606–16.

10. Reoch J, Mottillo S, Shimony A. Safety of laparoscopic vs open bariatric surgery: a systematic review and meta-analysis. Arch Surg. 2011;146:1314–22.

11. Hutter MM, Schirmer BD, Jones DB. First report from the American college of surgeons bariatric surgery center network: laparoscopic sleeve gastrectomy has morbidity and effectiveness positioned between the band and the bypass. Ann Surg. 2011;254(3):410–20.

12. Nguyen NT, Nguyen B, Gebhart A. Changes in the makeup of bariatric surgery: a national increase in use of laparoscopic sleeve gastrectomy.JACS. 2013;216(2):252–7.

13. Schauer PR, Kashyap SR, Wolski K. Bariatric surgery versus intensive medical therapy in obese patients with diabetes. NEJM. 2012;366(17):1567–76

14. Adams TD, Davidson LE, Litwin SE. Health benefits of gastric bypass surgery after 6 years. JAMA. 2012;308(11):1122–31.

15. Ikramuddin S, Korner J, Lee WJ. Roux-en-Y gastric bypass vs intensive medical management for the control of type 2 diabetes, hypertension, and hyperlipidemia: the Diabetes Surgery Study randomized clinical trial. JAMA. 2013;309(21):2240–9.

16. Bose M, Oliván B, Teixeira J. Do Incretins play a role in the remission of type 2 diabetes after gastric bypass surgery: What are the evidence? Obes Surg. 2009;19(2):217–29.

17. Wadden TA, West DS, Neiberg RH. One-year weight losses in the Look AHEAD study: factors associated with success. Obesity. 2009;17(4):713–22.

18. Berrington de Gonzalez A, Hartge P, Cerhan JR. Body-mass index and mortality among 1.46 million white adults. NEJM. 2010;363(23):2211–9.

19. Finkelstein EA, Trogdon JG, Cohen JW. Annual medical spending attributable to obesity: payer-and service-specific estimates. Health Aff. 2009;28(5):w822–31.

20. Finkelstein E, Fiebelkorn I, Wang G. The costs of obesity among full-time employees. Am J Health Promot. 2005;20(1): 45–51.

21. Ma J, Xiao L, Stafford RS. Underdiagnosis of obesity in adults in US outpatient settings. Arch Intern Med. 2009;169(3):312–31.

22. Kraschnewski JL, Sciamanna CN, Stuckey HL. A silent response to the obesity epidemic: decline in US physician weight counseling. Medical Care. 2013;52(2):186–92.

23. Foster GD, Wadden TA, Makris AP. Primary care physicians' attitudes about obesity and its treatment. Obes Res. 2003;11(10):1168–77.

24. Kushner RF. Barriers to providing nutrition counseling by physicians: a survey of primary care practitioners. Prev Med. 1995;24(6):546–52.

Contents

Contributors

Souheil W. Adra   Beth Israel Deaconess Medical Center, Harvard Medical School, Boston, MA, USA

Caroline M. Apovian   Department of Medicine, Section of Endocrinology, Diabetes and Nutrition, Boston University School of Medicine, Boston Medical Center, Boston, MA, USA

Jennifer Arussi   Change My Eating, Inc., Los Angeles, CA, USA

Gillian M. Barlow   Departments of Medicine and Obstetrics and Gynecology, Cedars-Sinai Medical Center, Los Angeles, CA, USA

Allison M. Barrett   Department of Surgery, North Shore-LIJ Hospital System, Manhasset, NY, USA

Richard N. Bergman   Diabetes and Obesity Research Institute, Cedars-Sinai Medical Center, Los Angeles, CA, USA

Patchaya Boonchaya-anant   King Chulalongkorn Memorial Hospital, Division of Endocrinology and Metabolism, Department of Medicine, Chulalongkorn University, Thai Red Cross Society, Bangkok, Thailand

George A. Bray   Pennington Biomedical Research Center, Baton Rouge, LA, USA

Miguel A. Burch   Minimally Invasive Surgery, Cedars-Sinai Medical Center, Los Angeles, CA, USA

Margaret E. Clark   Department of General Surgery, Tripler Army Medical Center, Honolulu, HI, USA

Scott Cunneen   Department of Surgery, Cedars-Sinai Medical Center, Los Angeles, CA, USA

Brandice Durkan   Department of Surgery, Cedars Sinai Medical Center, Los Angeles, CA, USA

Seth Felder   Surgery, Cedars-Sinai Medical Center, Los Angeles, CA, USA

Leslie J. Heinberg Cleveland Clinic Lerner College of Medicine, Bariatric and Metabolic Institute, Cleveland Clinic, Cleveland, OH, USA

Viorica Ionut Diabetes and Obesity Research Institute, Cedars-Sinai Medical Center, Los Angeles, CA, USA

Daniel B. Jones Department of Surgery, Harvard Medical School, Beth Israel Deaconess Medical Center, Boston, MA, USA

Robert B. Lim Department of Surgery, Tripler Army Medical Center, Honolulu, HI, USA

Eugenia A. Lin Department of Medicine, Cedars-Sinai Medical Center, Los Angeles, CA, USA

Ruchi Mathur Division of Endocrine Diabetes and Metabolism, Department of Medicine, Cedars-Sinai Medical Center, Los Angeles, CA, USA

Julie Merrell Rish Cleveland Clinic Lerner College of Medicine, Bariatric and Metabolic Institute, Cleveland Clinic, Cleveland, OH, USA

Monali Misra Department of Surgery, Cedars Sinai Medical Center, Los Angeles, CA, USA

Alexis Peraino Internal Medicine, California Health and Longevity Institute, Westlake Village, CA, USA

Amanda G. Powell Department of Medicine, Section of Endocrinology, Diabetes and Nutrition, Boston University School of Medicine, Boston Medical Center, Boston, MA, USA

Donna H. Ryan Pennington Biomedical Research Center, Louisiana State University System, Baton Rouge, LA, USA

List of Abbreviations

A

AAP	American Academy of Pediatrics
ACSM	American College of Sports Medicine
ADA	American Diabetes Association
AGB	Adjustable gastric band
AHA	American Heart Association
AHEAD	Action for Health in Diabetes
ALP	Alkaline phosphatase
APGARS	Acute post-gastric reduction surgery
ASBS	American Society of Bariatric Surgeons
ASMBS	American Society for Metabolic and Bariatric Surgery
AUDIT	Alcohol Use Disorders Identification Test
AgRP	agouti related protein

B

BAI	Body adiposity index
BDD	Balanced deficit diet
BDI	Beck Depression Inventory
BED	Binge eating disorder
BMI	Body mass index
BMP	Basic metabolic panel including kidney function
BOLD	Bariatric Outcomes Longitudinal Database
BP	Blood pressure
BPD/DS	Biliopancreatic diversion with duodenal switch
BRFSS	Behavioral Risk Factor Surveillance System
BPD	Biliopancreatic diversion
METs	Metabolic Equivalents

C

cAMP	Cylic AMP
CBP	cAMP response element binding binding protein (CBP)
CAD	Coronary artery disease
CDC	Centers for Disease Control and Prevention
CES-D	Centers for Epidemiological Studies-Depression Scale
CHD	Coronary heart disease
CMS	Center for Medicare Services
CPAP	Continuous positive airway pressure
CREB	cAMP-response element binding
CS	Cushing's syndrome
CT	Computed tomography
CART	cocaine and amphetamine regulating transcript
CCK	Cholecystokinin

D
DI	Disposition Index

E

ER	Extended release
EWL	Excess weight loss

G

GERD	Gastroesophageal reflux disease
GFR	Glomerular filtration rate
GGF	Gastro-gastric fistula
GI	Gastrointestinal
GJ	Gastojejunostomy
GLP-1	Glucagon-like Peptide-1 (GLP-1)
GIP	Gastric Inhibitory -Polypeptide
SI	Insulin Sensitivity Index

H

HBD	Hypo-energetic balanced diet
HDL	High-density lipoprotein
HR	Hazard ratio
HRQoL	Health-related quality of life

I

ICSI	Intracytoplasmic sperm injection
IL	Interleukin
IOM	Institute of Medicine
IOTF	International Obesity Task Force
iPTH	Intact parathyroid hormone
IV	Intravenous
IVC	Inferior vena cava

J

JJ	Jejunojejunostomy

L

LAGB	Laparoscopic adjustable gastric banding
LCM	Low carbohydrate Mediterranean
LDL	Low-density lipoprotein
LFTs	Liver function tests
LISA	Lifestyle Intervention Study for Adjuvant Treatment of Early Breast Cancer
LRYGB	Laparoscopic Roux-en-Y gastric bypass

M

MAOI	Monoamine oxidase inhibitor
MET	Metabolic equivalent
MR	Meal replacement
MRI	Magnetic resonance imaging

N

NAFLD	Nonalcoholic fatty liver disease
NB	Naltrexone/Bupropion
NIAAD	National Institute on Alcohol Abuse and Alcoholism
NIH	National Institutes of Health
NIPHS	Noninsulinoma pancreatogenous hypoglycemia syndrome
NSAID	Nonsteroidal anti-inflammatory drug
NPY	neuropeptide Y

O

OHS	Obesity hypoventilation syndrome
OR	Odds ratio
OSA	Obstructive sleep apnea
OS-MRS	Obesity Surgery Mortality Risk Score

P

$PaCO_2$	Arterial carbon dioxide tension
PCOS	Polycystic ovary syndrome
PCP	Primary-care physician
PDA	Personal Digital Assistant
PE	Pulmonary embolism
PHEN/TPM ER	Phentermine/topiramate-extended release
PHQ	Patient Health Questionnaire
PMR	Partial meal replacement
PTH	Parathyroid hormone
PTSD	Post-traumatic stress disorder
POUNDS LOST	Prevention of Obesity Using Novel Dietary Strategies
PCOS	Polycystic ovary Syndrome
POMC	Proopiomelanocortin
PYY	Peptide YY
PP	Pancreatic Polypeptide

R

RNYGB	Roux-en-Y gastric bypass
RR	Relative risk

S

SAGES	Society of Gastrointestinal Endoscopic Surgeons
SCD	Sequential compression devices
SCT	Social cognitive theory
SG	Sleeve gastrectomy
SILS	Single incision laparoscopic surgery
SSRI	Selective serotonin reuptake inhibitors
STAMPEDE	Surgical Treatment and Medications Potentially Eradicate Diabetes Efficiently
STOP	Study to Prevent Regain

T

TNFα	Tumor necrosis factor alpha
TG	Triglyceride

U

US FDA	United States Food and Drug Administration
UGI	Upper gastrointestinal

V

VLCD	Very low calorie diet
VLED	Very low energy diet
VTE	Venous thrombotic event

W

WLS	Weight loss surgery

Chapter 1
The Disease of Obesity

Viorica Ionut and Richard N. Bergman

Obesity is defined as "abnormal or excessive fat accumulation that may impair health" [1]. The extent to which obesity has impacted the USA and world population is astounding: More than one third of the US adults (35.7%) and approximately 17% (or 12.5 million) of children and adolescents aged 2–19 years are obese [1]. The alarming increase in obesity prevalence, the consequences on the personal health and on the health-care system (obesity contributes to over 112,000 deaths annually), and the relative lack of success in various interventions is undeniable. In June 2013, the American Medical Association recognized obesity as a disease requiring a range of medical interventions to advance obesity treatment and prevention.

Obesity has become an epidemic recently, but obesity is as old as humankind. We have evolved to defend our body mass, and to store excess energy as fat.

The concept that we are "wired" to store fat as a source of energy in times of abundance in order to be used in times of famine is called the "thrifty gene" hypothesis and seeks to explain the high rates of obesity and diabetes in modern populations, though its validity has been challenged lately [3]. A great example of the resources provided by stored fat is given by Spiegelman and Flier: An obese human of 250 lb. would in theory survive a fast of approximately 150 days, just using their fat stores (triglycerides have the highest energy content of all nutrients at 9 kcal/g and are stored in anhydrous form, increasing their efficiency as fuel) [4].

V. Ionut (✉) · R. N. Bergman
Diabetes and Obesity Research Institute, Cedars-Sinai Medical Center,
Los Angeles, CA, USA

© Springer Science+Business Media New York 2015
A. Youdim (ed.), *The Clinician's Guide to the Treatment of Obesity,*
Endocrine Updates, DOI 10.1007/978-1-4939-2146-1_1

Table 1.1 Factors contributing to obesity

Changes in diet
Hypercaloric (energy dense)
High fat
High saturated fat
Increased portion size
Less physical activity
Less manual/physical work
Increased use of cars
Sleep: less sleep, poor quality
Stress
Drug therapies that promote weight gain
Antipsychotics
Diabetes medication
Contraceptives
Steroids
Less smoking (nicotine promotes appetite suppression)
Maternal—gestational weight gain that favors obesity in offspring
Other putative factors
Plastics (endocrine disruptors)
Pollution (endocrine disruptors)
Less thermogenesis?
Genetics
FTO gene
Genetic syndromes (such as Prader-Willi)
Microbial and viral factors
Gut flora
Viruses associated with obesity

Etiology of Obesity

Though obesity was rare before the twentieth century, it was nevertheless known, and usually associated with wealth and prosperity. Thus, the cause appeared obvious: An excess of food intake, and in some cultures, such as classical Greek and Roman, obesity was considered largely the result of a lack of willpower, and associated with gluttony and other character flaws [5]. Until the advances of modern science, obesity was deemed to be simply the result of an imbalance between energy intake and energy expenditure resulting in energy accumulation as fat stores, and technically, it is so. However, we know now that obesity is the result of both genetic, environmental, and psychosocial factors, and has numerous contributors, some of which are summarized in Table 1.1, Fig. 1.1 [6, 7]

Obesity is defined by the World Health Organization using the body mass index (BMI): Obese refers to any person with a BMI greater than or equal to 30 [1]. BMI

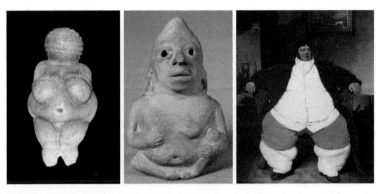

Fig. 1.1 Venus of Willendorf (c. 25,000 BC); Olmec figurine of an obese seated figure (c 400 BC); Daniel Lambert - portrait by Benjamin Marshall (c. 1806)

Table 1.2 Methods to assess adiposity and obesity

Indices
BMI
BAI
Waist circumference
Waist-to-hip ratio
Skinfold thickness
Underwater weighing (densitometry)
Air displacement plethysmography (BodPod)
Dilution method (hydrometry)
Bioelectrical impedance weighing scale
Dual energy X-ray absorptiometry (DEXA)
CT and MRI (percent fat, distribution)
Intra-organ fat quantification (MRS)

BMI body mass index, *BAI* body adiposity index, *CT* computerized tomography, *MRI* magnetic resonance imaging, *MRS* magnetic resonance spectroscopy

(a person's weight in kilograms divided by the square of his/her height in meters (kg/m^2)) is the most popular index, having the same reference values for both sexes and all ages. However, the BMI may not reflect most accurately a person's adiposity levels. Other measures and indices are needed to reflect the actual body fat percentage and, more importantly, fat distribution, as visceral fat (the so-called apple shape) appears to have more deleterious effects on health than subcutaneous fat, deposited preferentially around hips, and resulting in the "pear shape" pattern.

Assessment of obesity, adiposity, and fat distribution can be done through a variety of methods, from the simplest ones, requiring just a tape measure, such as body adiposity index (BAI, calculated as (hip circumference(cm)/(height(m))^1.5) − 18) [8] or waist-to-hip ratio, WHR; or requiring tape and scale (BMI) to the most sophisticated technology (e.g., magnetic resonance imaging, MRI; Table 1.2) [9].

But how do we get here? How is energy homeostasis regulated such that if chronically energy intake exceeds energy expenditure we end up obese?

Control of Energy Homeostasis

Food intake and energy expenditure are controlled by the brain, which integrates a large variety of signals and generates behavioral and physiological changes. The main area of the central nervous system (CNS) that regulates energy homeostasis is the hypothalamus, specifically the arcuate nucleus (ARC), paraventricular nucleus (PVN), the lateral hypothalamic area (LHA), the ventromedial hypothalamus (VMH), and the dorsomedial hypothalamus (DMH). In addition to the hypothalamus, neural systems in the brain stem, cerebral cortex, olfactory areas, and elsewhere are involved. There are two types of neurons that control food intake: the anorexigenic neurons that co-express proopiomelanocortin (POMC), cocaine- and amphetamine-regulating transcript (CART), and nesfatin and the orexigenic neuropeptide Y–agouti-related protein–gamma -aminobutyric acid (NPY/AgRP/GABA) neurons. Activation of the POMC neurons results in the release of α-melanocyte-stimulating hormone (α-MSH) from POMC axon terminals, leading to inhibition of food intake and increase in energy expenditure. Conversely, the activation of NPY/AgRP/GABA neurons leads to increases in AgRP, which inhibits melanocortin cells, and has the opposite effect: stimulation of food intake [10]. It is important to mention that the reverse is not true; the unidirectionality of NPY–POMC neurons inhibition thus reflects the wiring of the system towards favoring positive energy balance, which in turn provides an explanation why gaining weight is easy but losing it is hard [11].

The presence of a meal results in nutrient-activated signals: the nutrients themselves (glucose, free fatty acids, and amino acids), hormonal release, or generation of neural signals. But unlike, for example, glucose homeostasis or sodium balance regulation, food intake, and energy balance regulation have an important hedonic and cultural aspect. Thus, one has to distinguish between physiologic and reward-driven circuits of energy homeostatic regulation. In addition, the signals for short-term (meal-related) and long-term (related to adiposity) regulation are sometimes overlapping, but certainly not identical.

The synthesis and release of these brain peptides involved in energy homeostasis are regulated by neural, hormonal, and metabolic-regulated signals related to meals, and control hunger and satiety: mostly gastrointestinal (hormones like cholecystokinin (CCK), glucagon-like peptide 1 (GLP-1), peptide YY (PYY)) as well as plasma glucose and amino acids but also others such as body temperature. The long-term circuits signal adiposity stores via leptin and insulin and are involved in regulating energy expenditure as well (Table 1.3) [12].

Table 1.3 Signals that regulate food intake and energy balance. (Adapted from refs [12–14])

Positive energy balance	Negative energy balance
Proximal NPY AgRP Orexin A and B MCH Norepinephrine (α2, β-adrenergic) Endocannabinoids	Proximal POMC/ α-MSH CART Norepinephrine (a1 agonists)
Distal Ghrelin	Distal CCK GLP-1 Oxyntomodulin PYY Amylin Adiponectin (increases energy expenditure) Pancreatic polypeptide PP Serotonin Insulin Leptin

AgRP agouti-related peptide, *NPY* neuropeptide Y, *MCH* melanin-concentrating hormone, *POMC* proopiomelanocortin, *MSH* melanocyte-stimulating hormone, *CART* cocaine- and amphetamine-regulating transcript, *GLP-1* glucagon-like peptide 1, *PYY* peptide YY, *CCK* cholecystokinin

Gut Hormones

The gut secretes over 40 hormones with diverse cell localization and clustering. As expected, a large number of these hormones are related to nutrient sensing, relaying of information about nutrient amount and type, and to orchestration of energy balance and glucose, lipid, and protein.

CCK is a duodenal peptide released after high lipid and protein meals. It stimulates gall bladder contraction, exocrine pancreatic secretion, and inhibits gastric emptying and food intake through stimulation of vagal nerve endings. Moreover, there are recent data that CCK interacts with long-term signals of energy balance: CCK1R expressing neurons of the vagus also express receptors for ghrelin, orexin, cannabinoids (CB1), and leptin. CKK appears to control the expression of G-protein-coupled receptors and neurotransmitters involved in the control of food intake, further contributing to this regulation [15, 16].

Ghrelin, secreted by the P/D1 stomach cells, is a potent orexigenic hormone. Ghrelin levels increase before meals and decrease after meal ingestion, suggesting that ghrelin acts on the hypothalamic centers to promote meal initiation. Ghrelin infusion promotes food intake in humans, and it appears to change respiratory quotient, suggesting a role in energy expenditure. Ghrelin promotes food intake and adiposity by acting on brain centers, and is a weight regulator. In addition, ghrelin acts on vagal afferents in the gastrointestinal area to inhibit the effects of CCK and leptin [17, 18]. Ghrelin concentration in plasma is inversely related to fat mass; obese people have lower levels of ghrelin, but post-meal ghrelin levels remain higher than in lean people. Patients with Prader–Willi syndrome have high ghrelin levels, and consequently suffer from increased appetite, hyperphagia, and obesity. A disturbed gut–brain ghrelin axis has been suggested as one of the causes of anorexia nervosa [19].

GLP-1 is a 30-amino-acid peptide released from L cells in response to meal ingestion. L-cell stimulation increases not only GLP-1 but also GLP-1-related peptides, all derived from the same proglucagon molecule (glicentin, oxyntomodulin, intervening peptide-2, and GLP-2), as well as PYY. GLP-1 is a major insulinotropic hormone, but it also inhibits food and water intake and promotes satiety [20]. A meta-analysis of studies investigating the effect of GLP-1 on food intake found that GLP-1 reduced ad libitum caloric intake by 12% in normal or obese humans [21]; subcutaneous administration of recombinant GLP-1 to obese humans reduced caloric intake by 15% and produced weight loss [22]. A number of drugs based on GLP-1 and currently used for diabetes therapy (GLP-1 agonists and dipeptidyl peptidase IV (DPP-IV) inhibitors) have taken advantage of these effects and are currently investigated as obesity treatments. The GLP-1 agonists exenatide and liraglutide, which have longer half-life than the native compound, have been shown to inhibit food intake and promote weight loss (2.8–3.2 kg in one meta-analysis) [23]. The other group of GLP-1-based drugs, the DPP-IV inhibitors (sitagliptin, vildagliptin, linagliptin, saxagliptin, alogliptin), are weight neutral, a significant advantage in treating type 2 diabetes, since many anti-diabetes therapies result in weight gain [24].

PYY is a 36-amino-acid member of the polypeptide family that also includes NPY and pancreatic polypeptide. Though part of a different peptide family, PYY has many similarities with GLP-1. Like GLP-1, it is released by the L cells of the gastrointestinal tract, mainly in the ileum and colon, as well as by the brain. PYY is co-secreted from L cells with GLP-1 in response to meal stimulation (probably by both direct contact with luminal nutrients and via neural and endocrine mechanisms). PYY inhibits gastric emptying and intestinal motility, being part of the "ileal brake" together with GLP-1. Its active form PYY 3-36 inhibits food intake by binding to Y-2 neuronal receptors and inhibiting the release of NPY [25, 26].

Other Hormones

Leptin is an adipocyte-derived hormone, an adipokine. Plasma leptin concentration correlates with body fat content and signals the adipose reserves: High leptin reduces food intake by inhibiting NPY/AgRP neurons and stimulating the α-MSH neurons. Leptin is an important signal for starvation: Low leptin increases food intake and suppresses energy expenditure; conversely, leptin is usually increased in obese subjects. Mice deficient in the leptin gene (*ob/ob* mice) or in the leptin receptor gene (*db/db*) mice are examples of genetically induced obesity, since the absence of the hormone or its receptor drives increased food intake and low energy expenditure resulting in obesity. Several medical conditions are associated with low leptin: lipodystrophy, hypothalamic amenorrhea, and anorexia nervosa. In contrast, obese patients have high leptin levels; diet-induced weight loss results in a decrease in plasma leptin concentration, which could contribute to the difficulty of weight loss maintenance, since it will promote hunger. In spite of the increased leptin levels, obese humans do not have abnormal appetite suppression. This is because most obese patients are leptin resistant, limiting the ability to treat obesity with leptin. The precise mechanism of this resistance is not known, though it is believed to include both impaired leptin transport into the brain and impaired signaling in the hypothalamus (ER (endoplasmic reticulum) stress; hypothalamic inflammation; and defective autophagy)[13, 27, 28].

Insulin, well known for its fundamental role in controlling blood glucose levels and glucose homeostasis, insulin plays an equally important role in controlling energy balance. Insulin receptors are abundant in CNS, and early work by Woods and Porte showed that intraventricular administration of insulin in laboratory animals inhibits food intake [29]. A large amount of research has been devoted since to understanding the role played by insulin in the CNS. Though the exact mechanisms are not completely understood, it is generally accepted that insulin crosses the blood–brain barrier in the hypothalamic area and inhibits the NPY/AgRP neurons (that stimulate food intake) via the insulin receptor substrate–phosphatidylinositol-3-OH kinase (IRS–PI3K) pathway. Moreover, insulin acts on nonhypothalamic areas, such as the midbrain areas (ventral tegmental area and substantia nigra), populated by dopaminergic neurons involved in reward pathways. The insulin inhibition of food intake is greatly decreased in obese patients. Recent research in preclinical models has shown that in cases of consumption of high-fat food and overweight (but not in lean controls) insulin release from the pancreas triggers a signaling cascade in steroidogenic factor 1 (SF-1)-expressing neurons of the VMH, resulting in inhibition of POMC neurons, which promotes food intake and perpetuates obesity [30, 31]. The action of insulin on the reward pathway dopaminergic neurons is thought to additionally contribute to development of obesity, since signaling of these higher neuronal circuits can override hypothalamic signaling. Wang et al. have proposed that reward-driven overconsumption of high-fat, high-sugar, and energy-dense foods leads to neuronal insulin resistance, dysregulation of dopamine homeostasis, and hypodopaminergic reward deficiency syndrome [32].

Afferent Pathways

Vagal neural afferents, which are abundant in the gastrointestinal area, integrate a variety of signals: hormonal (CCK, gastric leptin, GLP-1, ghrelin) or mechanical (gastric distension). The merging of multiple signals on the same vagal neuron allows integration of a large amount of information and rapid response and adaptability of the digestive system to the metabolic needs. Vagal afferents project to the nucleus of the solitary tract in the caudal brain stem; neurons in this area further project to the specific regions of hypothalamus involved in food intake and adiposity regulation [18].

Effector Signals

The brain modulates the activity of organs and systems involved in energy homeostasis (adipose tissue, pancreas, gut, liver, stomach, brain itself) via sympathetic and parasympathetic signals. Efferent pathways from hypothalamic energy expenditure network (EEN) and fat accrual network (FAN) transmit signals leading to effects on neuroendocrine systems (hormones), autonomic nervous system, and behavior, including feeding and physical activity [4]. Some of these effects favor weight loss: fatty acid oxidation and a reduction in adipose tissue mass, increased energy expenditure, decrease in food intake, and increased sympathetic activity to brown adipose tissue. Others favor fat accumulation and obesity: increased fat deposition, reduction in energy expenditure, and increased food intake. The sympathetic nervous system promotes a negative energy balance by increasing energy expenditure (movement and thermogenesis, while the parasympathetic system promotes energy storage by increasing alimentary tract digestion and absorption, adipose tissue insulin sensitivity, and insulin secretion [14].

Health Consequences of Obesity

There is no doubt that obesity affects all organs and systems, from the well-established effects on the cardiovascular system, to less predictable ones, such as circadian rhythm and gut microflora (Table 1.4) [33–35].

An area that has gained a lot of attention in the past decades is the impact of obesity on inter-organ communication. Metabolic regulation, by its very nature, affects virtually all tissues and organs in the body and most importantly, it affects inter-organ communication. Regulation of glucose homeostasis in health and obesity is one such example. Because the brain is acutely dependent upon glucose availability for its energy, it is generally assumed that the metabolic regulating system evolved to guarantee an adequate supply of glucose to the CNS for energy. Glucose uptake by the brain in the short term is not dependent upon hormonal factors such as insulin; therefore, it is necessary for life to maintain an appropriate level of glucose in the blood. Various tissues orchestrate a beautifully designed regulating system to guarantee energy delivery to the brain [36]. Additional interconnected systems provide energy for other systems which may be called upon for organismal protection—for example, lipid moieties (free fatty acids) to provide energy for heart and liver, for example. How is the blood sugar level regulated? The simplest regulation is based upon the propensity of glucose itself to activate its own utilization (mostly by brain) or storage (by liver), or to suppress the endogenous production of glucose

Table 1.4 Health consequences of obesity

Cardiovascular
Cardiomyopathy, coronary artery disease
Atherosclerosis
High blood pressure
Dyslipidemia
Stroke
Type 2 diabetes
Cancers
Reproductive: breast, uterus, cervix, prostate
Colon, pancreas
Liver—NAFLD
Steatosis
Steatohepatitis
Cirrhosis
Gallbladder disease
Reproductive
Menstrual abnormalities
Infertility
PCOS
Pulmonary
Obstructive sleep apnea
Abnormal function
Kidney
Adipose tissue
Inflammation (proliferation of macrophages)
Release of adipokines and cytokines
Hypoxia
Brown adipose tissue—hypoactivity
Gut
Changes in gut hormone secretion
Changes in gut microflora
Osteoarticular
Bone architecture
Bone mass
Muscle
Systemic
Inflammation
Circadian rhythm
Inter-organ communication
Fat accumulation in heart, liver, pancreas, and skeletal muscle

Table 1.4 (continued)

Psychosocial
Eating disorders
Poor self-esteem
Depression

NAFLD nonalcoholic fatty liver disease, *PCOS* polycystic ovary syndrome

by the liver and kidneys from other noncarbohydrate precursors (lactate, amino acids). An additional regulating system which synergizes glucose effectiveness to guarantee the availability of fuel utilizes the ubiquitous hormone insulin. Insulin has varied molecular effects, but its primary action is to magnify or synergize glucose's ability to regulate itself. Thus, for a given increase in glucose concentration in the blood, adding insulin will further activate glucose uptake (and storage as a carbo-hydrate or lipid macromolecule, glycogen, or triglyceride), and suppress glucose production (mediated directly or indirectly via free fatty acids) [37]. Insulin under fasting conditions is not zero as one might expect, but is maintained at a low level to support the expression of important transcription factors and enzymes. After food intake, plasma insulin increases markedly (as much as eightfold). The increased insulin after nutrient intake limits the increases in glucose itself and other blood-borne nutrient compounds, and guarantees rapid recovery of the blood sugar to the postprandially regulated value (about 5.5 mM in humans). The increase in insulin is due primarily to glucose itself; however, proteins released by the L cells of the gastrointestinal tract (GLP-1 and GIP (gastric inhibitory polypeptide)) play a very significant synergistic role [38].

It is now known that obesity has a substantial effect on insulin's ability to regulate metabolism. Obesity interferes with the ability of insulin to enhance carbohydrate utilization and suppress glucose utilization. This interference is generally referred to as insulin resistance, and it means that the ability of a specifically enhanced insu-lin increase has a reduced effect on glucose production and uptake. Originally, the concept of insulin resistance was nonquantitative, recognized as enhanced insulin levels in the face of normal glucose levels. Eventually, methods were introduced to quantify insulin's effects using methods such as the "euglycemic glucose clamp" [39]; ours was the first to introduce the "insulin sensitivity index (SI)" which as-sociated insulin resistance with an actual number which could be compared among different individuals or even different species. (In normal individuals, SI averages about 5 min^{-1} per µU/ml which measures the ability of a single increase in insulin units (1 µU/ml) to enhance glucose clearance from plasma (in terms of fraction of the blood volume). In SI units, moderate obesity reduces SI to about 2 min^{-1} per µU/ml; in severe obesity, this value is less than 1.

How does a normal (if obese) insulin-resistant person regulate the blood glucose concentration in the face of insulin resistance? In such a condition, the release of in-sulin from the pancreatic islets is increased; additionally the propensity of the liver to destroy insulin is reduced. Together, what is observed in the insulin-resistant situ-

Fig. 1.2 The hyperbolic sensitivity/secretion curve. Curves of "normal" individuals (○) versus individuals with a β-cell defect (⊕). (Adapted from [5])

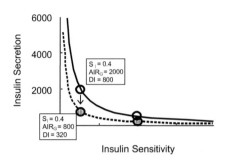

ation is elevated insulin in the blood (hyperinsulinemia). In fact, hyperinsulinemia is often regarded as a surrogate for insulin resistance, although the latter assumes normal function of the pancreatic islets and liver [40]. For many years, confusion reigned regarding how to understand the quantitative relationship between insulin sensitivity and secretion. Some years ago, we hypothesized that in a healthy individual any reduction in insulin sensitivity (insulin resistance) would be compensated by an equal and opposite increase in insulin release (or decrease in clearance). We expressed this in an equation:

Insulin secretion × Insulin sensitivity = the disposition index (DI), and we hypothesized that the DI would be characteristic for a given individual. An elevated DI reflects very healthy pancreatic β cells, as the response to resistance is robust; a diminished DI would be reflective of an islet defect. This latter hypothesis has proven correct [41]. The DI equation above is tantamount to a hyperbola; this is illustrated in Fig. 1.2.

Thus, any decrease in insulin sensitivity (due to obesity, for example) would be compensated by an increase in secretion and DI should remain normal. But, with an islet defect, resistance due to obesity would be undercompensated, such an individual (Fig. 1.1) would lie on a "lower" DI curve (nearer the origin), and would be an indicator of a latent pancreatic β-cell dysfunction. In fact, reduced DI is the strongest predictor known for conversion from normal glucose tolerance to type 2 diabetes mellitus [42]. Also, genetic variants related to DI have been identified from genome-wide association studies (GWAS) studies [43].

Therefore, obesity is related to a reduced insulin sensitivity which is normally compensated by increased insulin. If compensation results in a reduced DI value, this is indicative that the obese subject may be at risk for type 2 diabetes mellitus.

Bariatric Surgery and its Beneficial Effects on Body Weight

To date, bariatric surgery remains the most successful treatment for obesity. Compared with behavioral intervention and pharmacological treatment, which produce modest outcomes of 5–10 % weight loss [44], bariatric surgery results in weight loss that is rapid (immediately after surgery), substantial (12–39 % of presurgical body weight or 40–71 % excess weight loss), and sustained (as long as 10 years or more post surgery) [45].

As the term "bariatric surgery" encompasses a large and diverse group of surgical interventions (adjustable gastric banding, AGB; sleeve gastrectomy, SG; Roux-en-Y gastric bypass, RYGB; and biliopancreatic diversion, BPD) the mechanisms by which bariatric surgery results in weight loss are diverse. All procedures have a restrictive component (reduction in stomach size) and result in weight loss, at least in the period immediately following the surgery, due to caloric restriction. Caloric intake is dramatically reduced after bariatric surgery to 200–300 kcal/day, and it has been shown that obese subjects placed on an identical diet lose substantial amounts of weight [46]. Bariatric surgery results not only in decreased food intake but also in changes in frequency of food intake (fewer snacks, less food per meal) and in food preference: reduced preference for sweet and fat taste and for high-calorie and high-fat food, though no difference appears to exist between different procedures [47]. Research shows that patients find sweet and fatty meals less pleasant through changes in the sense of taste, with an increased perception of sweetness [48]. Besides caloric restriction, some bariatric surgery procedures have an additional component of bypassing large portions of the upper intestinal tract (such as the duodenum and part of the jejunum), resulting in decreased absorption and even malnutrition [49].

Last, but not least, procedures with intestinal rearrangement are likely to result in changes in the profile of gut hormones secreted, and in changes in neuroendocrine communication between different parts of the gastrointestinal tract, or between the gut and other organs, such as liver, pancreas, adipose tissue, and brain. It has been shown that RYGB and BPD, and, to a certain extent, SG, result in increased levels of GLP-1 and PYY [50, 51]. GLP-1 is an excellent candidate as the mediator of bariatric surgery effects via actions on satiety and food intake. Plasma GLP-1 levels are higher after bariatric surgery than after equivalent diet-induced weight loss [46]. Moreover, it has been shown that increases in postprandial plasma GLP-1 correlate with reduction of hunger and increases in satiety [52]. However, a recent study in rodents challenged the role of GLP-1 in bariatric surgery-induced weight loss [53]. PYY increases after bariatric surgery but not after nonsurgical weight loss, indicating that increases in PYY are related to the surgical procedure and not to weight loss per se. Infusion of PYY 3-36 in humans has been shown to decrease hunger score and food intake [54]. There is convincing evidence that PYY (together with GLP-1) is one of the major hormonal contributors to post-bariatric surgery weight loss. Increased PYY resulting from bariatric surgery (via increased direct delivery of nutrients to the L cells, decreased transit time, or high pH of undigested chyme) results in satiety, decreased food intake, and possibly changes in energy expenditure, leading to weight loss in both the early phase and over long term [55, 56]. It is possible that other hormones such as oyntomodulin, GIP, ghrelin, and others might play a role in bariatric surgery-induced weight loss, but their role remains yet to be demonstrated. Most likely, synergistic action of increased PYY and GLP-1 and possible other L cells products, combined with reductions in GIP and ghrelin, the trophic role of GLP-2, all may contribute to a negative energy balance and consequent weight loss.

Table 1.5 Obesity therapy

Dietary modification
Behavior modification
Exercise
Weight loss drugs:
Long term:
Orlistat
Lorcaserin
Phentermine/topiramate
Short-term/off-label
Phentermine
Benzphetamine
Diethylpropion
Phendimetrazine
Methylphenidate
Zonisamide
Octreotide
Metformin
GLP-1 agonists (exenatide, liraglutide)
Antidepressants (SSRI)
Ephedrine and caffeine
Investigative strategies
Cannabinoid receptor antagonists
Ghrelin antagonists
α-MSH antagonists
NPY antagonists
β-3 adrenergic agonists
PYY agonists
Amylin
Targeting L cells: (several hormones involved in energy homeostasis: GLP-1, PY, oxyntomodulin)
Combination hormones
Modulation of adipose tissue thermogenesis—brownification of white fat ("beige fat")
increased brown fat thermogenesis using chenodeoxycholic acid
Less conventional strategies
Acupuncture
Homeopathic
Herbal supplements
Nutritional supplements (most non-FDA approved, sometimes harmful)

GLP-1 glucagon-like peptide 1, *PYY* peptide YY, *α-MSH* α-melanocyte-stimulating hormone, *NPY* neuropeptide Y, *SSRI* selective serotonin reuptake inhibitors

In addition, modified neural signaling from the enteric nervous system and to various organs and tissues can contribute to hormonal changes directly or via enhancing or inhibiting hormonal actions [57]. An interesting, though yet little explored, area of research is the potential role of hormonal response to bariatric surgery as predictor of weight loss and of maintenance of weight loss post surgery.

Nonsurgical Therapy of Obesity

Nonsurgical therapy of obesity is based on dieting, behavior modification therapy, and exercise (Table 1.5). Dietary modification has a long history but usually with limited success. There are a variety of options centered either on reduced portions and low-calorie diets or different nutrient alterations (low fat, low carbohydrate, etc.). Dietary intervention should be done under the supervision of a health-care professional who can customize it to the patient and combine it with weight loss drugs and exercise to optimize the results. Behavior modification therapy aims at changes in eating and lifestyle habits and encourages strategies such as developing realistic goals, recording diet and exercise, improvement in quantity and quality of sleep, developing a support network, and others [58–61].

Quo Vadis?

The global switch from diseases of nutritional deficiency to conditions of overnutrition has occurred, and continues to occur over a remarkably short time span. Not only does this provide a great challenge relative to diabetes risk but also for a large variety of pathologies. Ironically, the availability of the Internet and tremendously enhanced global communication can make it possible for at least the information regarding the negative effects of obesity to be widely disseminated. Yet, it remains a great challenge to imagine how to get a significant number of individuals in first and second world countries to alter their lifestyle in terms of reducing caloric intake, as well as increasing physical activity (although that will probably have less effect). There are a variety of interventions that have involved local or federal regulations (nutritional labeling, calorie labeling, taxing the soda, etc.) or incentivizing healthy eating and exercising (insurance companies or employers can reward individuals that maintain a healthy body weight or exercise regularly). The Look Ahead Trial in the USA has demonstrated that reduced weight can be maintained, but at a great cost of personal intervention [62]. Possibly, research related to informational transfer via the Internet will eventually reveal effective approaches. Certain particularly offensive foodstuffs will have to be reduced, despite the possible costs in terms of industrial interests—thus, there will need to be international cooperation such that the cost to benefit ratio for international industrial interests will be on the side of restricting calories and maximizing quality. It is certainly in the interest of the international problem to expand our understanding of the causes of obesity, the role of the CNS, and addiction pathways, and the possibility of discovering more potent molecules to regulate food intake. However, it is unlikely that a global problem will be dealt with at the pharmaceutical level, and international cooperation and policy will no doubt be at the center of diminishing the negative consequences of overnutrition, overweight, and obesity.

References

1. World Health Organization. Obesity and overweight. Fact sheet no.311. 2013. http://www.who.int/mediacentre/factsheets/fs311/en/2013. Accessed: 25 Jan 2014.
2. Prevention CDC. Overweight and obesity 2013. http://www.cdc.gov/obesity/data/facts.html2012. Accessed: 2 Feb 2014.
3. Neel JV. The "thrifty genotype" in 1998. Nutr Rev. 1999;57(5 Pt 2):S2–9. PubMed PMID: 10391020.
4. Spiegelman BM, Flier JS. Obesity and the regulation of energy balance. Cell. 2001;104(4):531–43. PubMed PMID: 11239410.
5. Hill SE. Eating to excess: the meaning of gluttony and the fat body in the ancient world. Santa Barbara: Praeger; 2011.
6. McAllister EJ, Dhurandhar NV, Keith SW, Aronne LJ, Barger J, Baskin M, et al. Ten putative contributors to the obesity epidemic. Crit Rev Food Sci Nutr. 2009;49(10):868–913. doi:10.1080/10408390903372599. PubMed PMID: 19960394; PubMed Central PMCID: PMCPMC2932668.
7. Wright SM, Aronne LJ. Causes of obesity. Abdom Imaging. 2012;37(5):730–2. doi:10.1007/s00261-012-9862-x. PubMed PMID: 22426851.
8. Bergman RN. A better index of body adiposity. Obesity (Silver Spring). 2012;20(6):1135. doi:10.1038/oby.2012.99. PubMed PMID: 22627975.
9. Heymsfield SB. Development of imaging methods to assess adiposity and metabolism. Int J Obes (Lond). 2008;32(Suppl 7):S76–82. doi:10.1038/ijo.2008.242. PubMed PMID: 19136995.
10. Xu Y, Elmquist JK, Fukuda M. Central nervous control of energy and glucose balance: focus on the central melanocortin system. Ann N Y Acad Sci. 2011;1243:1–14. doi:10.1111/j.1749-6632.2011.06248.x. PubMed PMID: 22211889; PubMed Central PMCID: PMCPMC3467098.
11. Dietrich MO, Horvath TL. Hypothalamic control of energy balance: insights into the role of synaptic plasticity. Trends Neurosci. 2013;36(2):65–73. doi:10.1016/j.tins.2012.12.005. PubMed PMID: 23318157.
12. Woods SC. The control of food intake: behavioral versus molecular perspectives. Cell Metab. 2009;9(6):489–98. doi:10.1016/j.cmet.2009.04.007. PubMed PMID: 19490904; PubMed Central PMCID: PMCPMC3090647.
13. Flier JS. Obesity wars: molecular progress confronts an expanding epidemic. Cell. 2004;116(2):337–50. PubMed PMID: 14744442.
14. Lustig RH. The neuroendocrine control of energy balance. In: Freemark M, editor. Contemporary endocrinology: Pediatric obesity: etiology, pathogenesis, and treatment. New York: Springer 2010. pp. 15–32.
15. Raybould HE. Mechanisms of CCK signaling from gut to brain. Curr Opin Pharmacol. 2007;7(6):570–4. doi:10.1016/j.coph.2007.09.006. PubMed PMID: 17954038; PubMed Central PMCID: PMCPMC2692370.
16. Dockray GJ. Cholecystokinin and gut-brain signalling. Regul Pept. 2009;155(1–3):6–10. doi:10.1016/j.regpep.2009.03.015. PubMed PMID: 19345244.

17. Cummings DE, Foster-Schubert KE, Overduin J. Ghrelin and energy balance: focus on current controversies. Curr Drug Targets. 2005;6(2):153–69. PubMed PMID: 15777186.
18. Chambers AP, Sandoval DA, Seeley RJ. Integration of satiety signals by the central nervous system. Curr Biol. 2013;23(9):R379–88. doi:10.1016/j.cub.2013.03.020. PubMed PMID: 23660361; PubMed Central PMCID: PMCPMC3688053.
19. Cardona Cano S, Merkestein M, Skibicka KP, Dickson SL, Adan RA. Role of ghrelin in the pathophysiology of eating disorders: implications for pharmacotherapy. CNS Drugs. 2012;26(4):281–96. doi:10.2165/11599890-000000000-00000. PubMed PMID: 22452525.
20. Torekov SS, Madsbad S, Holst JJ. Obesity—an indication for GLP-1 treatment? Obesity pathophysiology and GLP-1 treatment potential. Obes Rev. 2011;12(8):593–601. doi:10.1111/j.1467-789X.2011.00860.x. PubMed PMID: 21401851.
21. Verdich C, Flint A, Gutzwiller JP, Näslund E, Beglinger C, Hellström PM, et al. A meta-analysis of the effect of glucagon-like peptide-1 (7–36) amide on ad libitum energy intake in humans. J Clin Endocrinol Metab. 2001;86(9):4382–9. PubMed PMID: 11549680.
22. Näslund E, King N, Mansten S, Adner N, Holst JJ, Gutniak M, et al. Prandial subcutaneous injections of glucagon-like peptide-1 cause weight loss in obese human subjects. Br J Nutr. 2004;91(3):439–46. doi:10.1079/BJN20031064. PubMed PMID: 15005830.
23. Vilsbøll T, Christensen M, Junker AE, Knop FK, Gluud LL. Effects of glucagon-like peptide-1 receptor agonists on weight loss: systematic review and meta-analyses of randomised controlled trials. BMJ. 2012;344:d7771. PubMed PMID: 22236411; PubMed Central PMCID: PMCPMC3256253.
24. Foley JE, Jordan J. Weight neutrality with the DPP-4 inhibitor, vildagliptin: mechanistic basis and clinical experience. Vasc Health Risk Manag. 2010;6:541–8. PubMed PMID: 20730070; PubMed Central PMCID: PMCPMC2922315.
25. De Silva A, Salem V, Long CJ, Makwana A, Newbould RD, Rabiner EA, et al. The gut hormones PYY 3-36 and GLP-1 7-36 amide reduce food intake and modulate brain activity in appetite centers in humans. Cell Metab. 2011;14(5):700–6. doi:S1550–4131(11)00356–1 [pii]10.1016/j.cmet.2011.09.010. PubMed PMID: 22000927; PubMed Central PMCID: PMCPMC3267038.
26. Ballantyne GH. Peptide YY(1-36) and peptide YY(3-36): Part I. Distribution, release and actions. Obes Surg. 2006;16(5):651–8. doi:10.1381/096089206776944959. PubMed PMID: 16687037.
27. Friedman JM. Leptin at 14 y of age: an ongoing story. Am J Clin Nutr. 2009;89(3):973S-9S. doi: 10.3945/ajcn.2008.26788B. PubMed PMID: 19190071; PubMed Central PMCID: PMCPMC2667654.
28. Jung CH, Kim MS. Molecular mechanisms of central leptin resistance in obesity. Arch Pharm Res. 2013;36(2):201–7. doi:10.1007/s12272-013-0020-y. PubMed PMID: 23359004.
29. Woods SC, Lotter EC, McKay LD, Porte D. Chronic intracerebroventricular infusion of insulin reduces food intake and body weight of baboons. Nature. 1979;282(5738):503–5. PubMed PMID: 116135.
30. Vogt MC, Brüning JC. CNS insulin signaling in the control of energy homeostasis and glucose metabolism—from embryo to old age. Trends Endocrinol Metab. 2013;24(2):76–84. doi:10.1016/j.tem.2012.11.004. PubMed PMID: 23265947.
31. Sisley S, Sandoval D. Hypothalamic control of energy and glucose metabolism. Rev Endocr Metab Disord. 2011;12(3):219–33. doi:10.1007/s11154-011-9189-x. PubMed PMID: 21695389.
32. Wang GJ, Volkow ND, Logan J, Pappas NR, Wong CT, Zhu W, et al. Brain dopamine and obesity. Lancet. 2001;357(9253):354–7. PubMed PMID: 11210998.
33. Bray GA. Medical consequences of obesity. J Clin Endocrinol Metab. 2004;89(6):2583–9. doi:10.1210/jc.2004-0535. PubMed PMID: 15181027.
34. Sweeney TE, Morton JM. The human gut microbiome: a review of the effect of obesity and surgically induced weight loss. JAMA Surg. 2013;148(6):563–9. doi:10.1001/jamasurg.2013.5. PubMed PMID: 23571517.

35. Drager LF, Togeiro SM, Polotsky VY, Lorenzi-Filho G. Obstructive sleep apnea: a cardio-metabolic risk in obesity and the metabolic syndrome. J Am Coll Cardiol. 2013;62(7):569–76. doi:10.1016/j.jacc.2013.05.045. PubMed PMID: 23770180.

36. Bergman RN. Orchestration of glucose homeostasis: from a small acorn to the California oak. Diabetes. 2007;56(6):1489–501. doi:10.2337/db07–9903. PubMed PMID: 17526912.

37. Bergman RN. New concepts in extracellular signaling for insulin action: the single gateway hypothesis. Recent Prog Horm Res. 1997;52:359–85; discussion 85–7. PubMed PMID: 9238859.

38. Holst JJ, Vilsbøll T, Deacon CF. The incretin system and its role in type 2 diabetes mellitus. Mol Cell Endocrinol. 2009;297(1–2):127–36. doi:S0303–7207(08)00362–6 [pii]10.1016/j.mce.2008.08.012. PubMed PMID: 18786605.

39. DeFronzo RA, Tobin JD, Andres R. Glucose clamp technique: a method for quantifying insulin secretion and resistance. Am J Physiol. 1979;237(3):E214–23. PubMed PMID: 382871.

40. Bergman RN, Ader M, Huecking K, Van Citters G. Accurate assessment of beta-cell function: the hyperbolic correction. Diabetes. 2002;51(Suppl 1):S212–20. PubMed PMID: 11815482.

41. Kodama K, Tojjar D, Yamada S, Toda K, Patel CJ, Butte AJ. Ethnic differences in the relationship between insulin sensitivity and insulin response: a systematic review and meta-analysis. Diabetes Care. 2013;36(6):1789–96. doi:10.2337/dc12-1235. PubMed PMID: 23704681; PubMed Central PMCID: PMCPMC3661854.

42. Lorenzo C, Wagenknecht LE, Rewers MJ, Karter AJ, Bergman RN, Hanley AJ, et al. Disposition index, glucose effectiveness, and conversion to type 2 diabetes: the Insulin Resistance Atherosclerosis Study (IRAS). Diabetes Care. 2010;33(9):2098–103. doi:10.2337/dc10-0165. PubMed PMID: 20805282; PubMed Central PMCID: PMCPMC2928371.

43. McCarthy MI. Genomics, type 2 diabetes, and obesity. N Engl J Med. 2010;363(24):2339–50. doi:10.1056/NEJMra0906948. PubMed PMID: 21142536.

44. Brown T, Avenell A, Edmunds LD, Moore H, Whittaker V, Avery L, et al. Systematic review of long-term lifestyle interventions to prevent weight gain and morbidity in adults. Obes Rev. 2009;10(6):627–38. doi:OBR641 [pii]10.1111/j.1467–789X.2009.00641.x. PubMed PMID: 19754634.

45. Garb J, Welch G, Zagarins S, Kuhn J, Romanelli J. Bariatric surgery for the treatment of morbid obesity: a meta-analysis of weight loss outcomes for laparoscopic adjustable gastric banding and laparoscopic gastric bypass. Obes Surg. 2009;19(10):1447–55. doi:10.1007/s11695-009-9927-2. PubMed PMID: 19655209.

46. Isbell JM, Tamboli RA, Hansen EN, Saliba J, Dunn JP, Phillips SE, et al. The importance of caloric restriction in the early improvements in insulin sensitivity after Roux-en-Y gastric bypass surgery. Diabetes Care. 2010;33(7):1438–42. doi:dc09-2107 [pii]10.2337/dc09-2107. PubMed PMID: 20368410; PubMed Central PMCID: PMCPMC2890335.

47. Pepino MY, Bradley D, Eagon JC, Sullivan S, Abumrad NA, Klein S. Changes in taste perception and eating behavior after bariatric surgery-induced weight loss in women. Obesity (Silver Spring). 2013. doi:10.1002/oby.20649. PubMed PMID: 24167016.

48. Miras AD, le Roux CW. Bariatric surgery and taste: novel mechanisms of weight loss. Curr Opin Gastroenterol. 2010;26(2):140–5. doi:10.1097/MOG.0b013e328333e94a. PubMed PMID: 19901832.

49. Crookes PF. Surgical treatment of morbid obesity. Annu Rev Med. 2006;57:243–64. doi:10.1146/annurev.med.56.062904.144928. PubMed PMID: 16409148.

50. Stefater MA, Wilson-Pérez HE, Chambers AP, Sandoval DA, Seeley RJ. All bariatric surgeries are not created equal: insights from mechanistic comparisons. Endocr Rev. 2012;33(4):595–622. doi:10.1210/er.2011-1044. PubMed PMID: 22550271; PubMed Central PMCID: PMCPMC3410227.

51. Michalakis K, le Roux C. Gut hormones and leptin: impact on energy control and changes after bariatric surgery–what the future holds. Obes Surg. 2012;22(10):1648–57. doi:10.1007/s11695-012-0698-9. PubMed PMID: 22692670.

52. Borg CM, le Roux CW, Ghatei MA, Bloom SR, Patel AG, Aylwin SJ. Progressive rise in gut hormone levels after Roux-en-Y gastric bypass suggests gut adaptation and explains altered satiety. Br J Surg. 2006;93(2):210–5. doi:10.1002/bjs.5227. PubMed PMID: 16392104.

53. Ye J, Hao Z, Mumphrey MB, Townsend RL, Patterson LM, Stylopoulos N, et al. GLP-1 receptor signaling is not required for reduced body weight after RYGB in rodents. Am J Physiol Regul Integr Comp Physiol. 2014. doi:10.1152/ajpregu.00491.2013. PubMed PMID: 24430883.

54. Batterham RL, Cowley MA, Small CJ, Herzog H, Cohen MA, Dakin CL, et al. Gut hormone PYY(3-36) physiologically inhibits food intake. Nature. 2002;418(6898):650–4. doi:10.1038/nature02666. PubMed PMID: 12167864.

55. Evans S, Pamuklar Z, Rosko J, Mahaney P, Jiang N, Park C, et al. Gastric bypass surgery restores meal stimulation of the anorexigenic gut hormones glucagon-like peptide-1 and peptide YY independently of caloric restriction. Surg Endosc. 2012;26(4):1086–94. doi:10.1007/s00464-011-2004-7. PubMed PMID: 22044971; PubMed Central PMCID: PMCPMC3302936.

56. Valderas JP, Irribarra V, Boza C, de la Cruz R, Liberona Y, Acosta AM, et al. Medical and surgical treatments for obesity have opposite effects on peptide YY and appetite: a prospective study controlled for weight loss. J Clin Endocrinol Metab. 2010;95(3):1069–75. doi:jc.2009-0983 [pii]10.1210/jc.2009-0983. PubMed PMID: 20097707.

57. Ionut V, Burch M, Youdim A, Bergman RN. Gastrointestinal hormones and bariatric surgery-induced weight loss. Obesity (Silver Spring). 2013;21(6):1093–103. doi: 10.1002/oby.20364. PubMed PMID: 23512841.

58. NIDDK. Prescriptions medications for the tretament of obesity 2013. http://win.niddk.nih.gov/publications/prescription.htm. Accessed: 2 Feb 2014.

59. Jensen MD, Ryan DH, Apovian CM, Ard JD, Comuzzie AG, Donato KA, et al. 2013 AHA/ACC/TOS Guideline for the Management of Overweight and Obesity in Adults: A Report of the American College of Cardiology/American Heart Association Task Force on Practice Guidelines and The Obesity Society. Circulation. 2013. doi:10.1161/01.cir.0000437739.71477.ee. PubMed PMID: 24222017.

60. Igel LI, Powell AG, Apovian CM, Aronne LJ. Advances in medical therapy for weight loss and the weight-centric management of type 2 diabetes mellitus. Curr Atheroscler Rep. 2012;14(1):60–9. doi:10.1007/s11883-011-0221-0. PubMed PMID: 22113707.

61. Aronne LJ, Powell AG, Apovian CM. Emerging pharmacotherapy for obesity. Expert Opin Emerg Drugs. 2011;16(3):587–96. doi:10.1517/14728214.2011.609168. PubMed PMID: 21834735.

62. Perri MG. Effects of behavioral treatment on long-term weight loss: Lessons learned from the look AHEAD trial. Obesity (Silver Spring). 2014;22(1):3–4. doi:10.1002/oby.20672. PubMed PMID: 24415676.

Chapter 2
The Health Burden of Obesity

Eugenia A. Lin, Gillian M. Barlow and Ruchi Mathur

"Corpulence is not only a disease itself but a harbinger of others." Hippocrates

Obesity: Definitions

The obesity epidemic affects people of all ages, socioeconomic levels, geographic regions, and ethnicities, and causes significant medical consequences. Obesity has been defined as a medical condition in which excess body fat accumulates to an extent that may have short- and long-term consequences on morbidity and mortality [1, 2]. Globally, in an analysis of 199 countries, 1.46 billion adults worldwide are estimated as being overweight, and 502 million are estimated as being obese [3]. In the USA, the prevalence of obesity (2009–2010) has been reported as 35.7% [4]. "Overweight" technically refers to an excess of body weight, whereas "obesity" refers to an excess of fat. However, the methods used to directly measure body fat are not available in daily practice. For this reason, obesity is often assessed by means

R. Mathur (✉)
Division of Endocrine Diabetes and Metabolism, Department of Medicine,
Cedars-Sinai Medical Center, Los Angeles, CA, USA
e-mail: ruchi.mathur@cshs.org

E. A. Lin
Department of Medicine, Cedars-Sinai Medical Center, Los Angeles, CA, USA
e-mail: eames.lin@gmail.com

G. M. Barlow
Departments of Medicine and Ob/Gyn, Cedars-Sinai Medical Center,
Los Angeles, CA, USA
e-mail: Gillian.Barlow@cshs.org

© Springer Science+Business Media New York 2015
A. Youdim (ed.), *The Clinician's Guide to the Treatment of Obesity,*
Endocrine Updates, DOI 10.1007/978-1-4939-2146-1_2

of indirect estimates of body fat (i.e., anthropometrics). In the clinical setting, adult obesity is most often defined by the use of body mass index (BMI), which is a calculation based on the weight of a person in kilograms over their height in meters squared (kg/m^2). Though widely used, there are fundamental concerns with this method of classification. While easy to calculate, and routinely used as a population measurement of overweight and obesity, BMI does not take into account body composition. We are well aware that a person with a percent body fat of 8% who is a body builder may have the same weight as someone with a body fat of 35% who is inactive. Herein lies the flaw of simply measuring BMI. While there are more accurate means of measuring body composition, such as skin-fold thickness, waist circumference, and techniques such as ultrasound, computed tomography, and magnetic resonance imaging (MRI), many of these are not possible in the routine office setting. More recently, a newer model of measurement, the body adiposity index (BAI), has been proposed. The BAI mathematical model takes into account hip circumference and appears to better measure percent adiposity [5]. However, as BMI is still the most commonly used model for calculating obesity, we focus our discussion on this criterion.

The BMI criteria for adult obesity in Western societies are accepted as noted in Table 2.1 [6], whereas in Asian populations, the criteria are more stringent. This difference is based on the observations of investigators [7–9], along with health policy-making organizations [10, 11], which have shown that cardiovascular risk and diabetes in some Asian countries increase significantly in those with weight parameters that are only modestly elevated by American standards. Thus, the current proposal is that definitions and thresholds of overweight and obesity should be lower in Asian countries. It should be noted that there is considerable debate on this point, and over whether BMI criteria should be country-specific, or ethnicity-based [12]. At present, the Japanese define obesity as a BMI greater than $25 kg/m^2$ [13], while the Chinese use a cut off of $28 kg/m^2$ [14].

Table 2.1 Weight categories for adults and youth

Category	Adults (20+ years)	Youth (2–19 years) CDC, AAP, IOM, ES, IOTF
Underweight	BMI < 18.5	BMI < 5th percentile for age
Normal weight	BMI 18.5–24.9	BMI ≥ 5th to < 85th percentile
Overweight	BMI 25–29.9	BMI ≥ 85th to < 95th percentile
Obesity	BMI ≥ 30	BMI ≥ 95th percentile
Class III obesity (super obesity)	BMI ≥ 40	Not used[a]

AAP American Academy of Pediatrics, *IOM* Institute of Medicine, *ES* Endocrine Society, *CDC* Centers for Disease Control, *IOTF* International obesity task force, *BMI* body mass index
[a] In children, proposed definitions of severe obesity are BMI > 120% of the 95th percentile, or BMI > 99th percentile

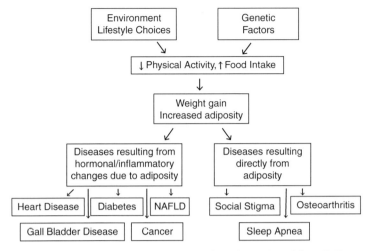

Fig. 2.1 Heath problems related to the development of obesity. (Adapted from [26])

In children, defining criteria for obesity is more complex, as the age, sex, expected growth curves, and body composition must all be factored in. A child's weight status is determined using an age- and sex-specific percentile for BMI rather than the BMI categories. The Centers for Disease Control growth charts are used to determine the corresponding BMI-for-age and sex percentile. For children and adolescents (aged 2–19 years), overweight is defined as a BMI at or above the 85th percentile and lower than the 95th percentile for children of the same age and sex, while obesity is defined as a BMI at or above the 95th percentile for children of the same age and sex [15]. Figure 2.1 shows the classification of obesity for children based on the American Academy of Pediatrics, the Institute of Medicine, the Centers for Disease Control, and the International Obesity Task Force.

The Economic Burden of Obesity

Globally, in an analysis of 199 countries, 1.46 billion adults worldwide were estimated as overweight, with 502 million estimated as obese [3]. The global economic burden of obesity accounts for an average of 0.7–2.8% of a country's total health-care costs [16]. These costs represent the monetary value of health-care resources devoted to managing obesity-related disorders. This includes such costs as those incurred through the use of outpatient clinics and visits, hospitalizations, pharmaceutical therapy, laboratory testing, and chronic care. Obese individuals have, on average worldwide, medical costs 30% higher than those with normal weight [16]. Interestingly, in the USA specifically, the medical economic burden of obesity is higher: an estimated US$ 75 billion in 2003 [17], accounting for 4–7% of total health-care expenditure. The increase in costs seen in obese individuals tends to be largely driven by the increased incidence of type 2 diabetes, the increased cardio-vascular burden, and obesity-related cancers [18].

Overweight/obesity in middle age appears to have long-term adverse conse-quences for health-care costs as one ages. A review of US Medicare data collected from 1984 to 2002 showed that after multivariate analysis, Medicare health charges were significantly higher by baseline BMI in both men and women [19]. This held true for overall costs, and costs specifically related to diabetes and cardiovascu-lar disease. After adjusting for variables such as baseline age, race, education, and smoking, the total average annual medical-related charges for overweight, obese, and severely obese men were US$ 8390, $ 10,128, and $ 13,674, respectively. This is a significant trend over normal-weight men who, as a group, averaged an annual health-care cost of $ 7205. Other US data show that compared to normal-weight in-dividuals, obese patients incur 27 % more outpatient visits, and 80 % more prescrip-tion costs [20]. In addition, in the inpatient setting, obese patients have an increased cost of 46 % over nonobese patients. Similar trends have been reported in the UK, France, and the Netherlands.

The Health Burden of Obesity

The World Health Organization describes obesity as one of the most neglected pub-lic health problems we face today [21]. The health implications of obesity are not geographically limited. Sequelae of obesity include commonly thought of condi-tions, such as hypertension, heart disease, fatty liver, and diabetes, [22] to more esoteric associations such as infertility [22], idiopathic intracranial hypertension [23], and gout [24]. The incidences of certain cancers also increase with obesity, including cancers of the breast, ovaries, esophagus, colon, liver, pancreas, endome-trium, and prostate [25].

The health conditions associated with obesity are thought to arise as either a direct consequence of adiposity—such as with social stigmatization, sleep apnea, and osteoarthritis; or via the various changes associated with the increase in adipose cell hypertrophy and/or hyperplasia (Fig. 2.1) [26]. It is important to remember that adipose tissue is a functional endocrine organ, with secretory products such as cyto-kines (interleukin (IL)-1 and 6) and tumor necrosis factor alpha (TNF-α). These cy-tokines have further effects, including suppression of adiponectin—which worsens insulin resistance. Diabetes, cancer, cardiovascular disease, and non-alcoholic liver disease are a few examples of disease states attributed in part to these hormonal and metabolic alterations. Having abdominal obesity seems to worsen these associated conditions, in part because of the high influx of free fatty acids, adipokines, and cytokines into the portal circulation by virtue of approximation. Subsequent hepatic production of very-low-density lipoprotein (VLDL) and dysregulation of insulin release set off a cascade of metabolic derangements [22].

Social Stigmatization

Many societies tend to chastise those who are overweight, and many consider those with weight issues as being unable or unwilling to control impulsive/compulsive behaviors. There is often public disapproval expressed openly by colleagues, neighbors, family members, and acquaintances. Such reproach often results in measurable changes in the quality of life parameters reported by obese subjects [26, 27]. These changes are more profound in women, and tend to reverse with intentional weight loss [28, 29]. Children and adolescents also tend to suffer the psychosocial consequences of obesity, including alienation [30], distorted peer relationships, poor self-esteem [31, 32], anxiety [33], and depression [34, 35]. The risk of psychosocial morbidity increases with increasing age during childhood, and is greater among girls than boys [36–38].

The distorted and negative self-images that develop in adolescence often persist into adulthood, especially in women. Data from the National Longitudinal Survey of Youth indicate that women who were obese in late adolescence and early adulthood completed fewer years of advanced education, and had lower rates of marriage and higher rates of poverty compared to their *non-obese* peers [39]. Interestingly, these long-term social repercussions were not nearly as profound in obese men.

Sleep Apnea

In the absence of underlying pulmonary disease, obese patients are noted as having pulmonary-related issues only in the presence of significant obesity. The main obesity-related change in pulmonary function testing is an increase in residual lung volume associated with an increase in intra-abdominal pressure [40, 41]. While these pulmonary function changes may be mild, the other effects of obesity on the respiratory system can be quite significant. Obstructive sleep apnea (OSA) is a syndrome characterized by episodic hypopnea or apnea due to recurrent partial or complete upper airway obstruction during sleep. Obesity is the most documented risk factor for OSA. Significant sleep apnea is present in approximately 40 % of obese individuals, and the prevalence of OSA progressively increases as the BMI increases [42].

OSA frequently coexists with, and may be one of the causes of obesity hypoventilation syndrome (OHS). OHS is defined as obesity and chronic alveolar hypoventilation (arterial carbon dioxide tension [$PaCO_2$] >45 mmHg) during wakefulness, which occur in the absence of other conditions that cause hypoventilation [43].

Osteoarthritis

Diseases of the bone including osteoarthritis and other joint issues are directly related to the weight placed on the joints by obesity [44]. For example, the incidence of knee osteoarthritis was found to be increased in men in heaviest quintile of weight compared with those in the lightest three quintiles (age-adjusted relative risk, 1.51; 95% confidence interval (CI), 1.14–1.98), and was further increased in women in the heaviest quintile versus those in the lightest three quintiles (relative risk 2.07; 95% CI, 1.67–2.55) [44]. There is some suggestion that non-weight-bearing joints also suffer changes in the obese; however, the mechanism underlying these changes is not known.

Nonalcoholic Fatty Liver Disease (NAFLD)

NAFLD is a term describing a collection of liver abnormalities including hepatomegaly, elevated liver enzymes, and changes in histology which include (in progressive order) steatosis, non-alcoholic steatohepatitis, fibrosis, and cirrhosis [45]. Once NAFLD has progressed to cirrhosis, liver failure may ensue. Obesity is associated with this clinical spectrum of liver damage and disease [45, 46]. The pathogenesis of NAFLD in overweight and obese individuals is not fully understood, but insulin resistance appears to be an important component [47]. A retrospective analysis of liver biopsies in individuals who were overweight and obese without any other underlying contributors to liver disease showed the presence of fibrosis in 30% of samples, and cirrhosis in a further 10% [48]. Other authors have performed cross-sectional analysis of liver biopsies and suggest that the prevalence of steatosis is 75% in the obese population [49]. In another study, metabolic syndrome (of which obesity and insulin resistance are components) was associated with an odds ratio (OR) of 3.5 for the development of severe liver fibrosis [50].

Hypertension

Obesity is associated with hypertension. The relation between obesity and hypertension is clinically important because weight loss may lead to a significant fall in systemic blood pressure (BP) [51, 52]. The impact of obesity on the presence of hypertension may have ethnic differences. It is estimated that weight control would eliminate hypertension in 28% of the Black population. This is almost doubled to an estimated 48% in the White population [53].

The mechanism by which obesity raises the BP is not well understood. One postulate is that hyperinsulinemia is the cornerstone of this relationship [54], and many mechanisms have been proposed to explain the resultant increase in BP including increased sympathetic activity [55], volume expansion due to increased renal sodium reabsorption [56], endothelial dysfunction [57], upregulation of angiotensin II receptors [57], and decreased cardiac natriuretic peptide [58]. The risk of hypertension appears to be greatest in people who have predominantly upper body and abdominal obesity. The mechanism by which upper body obesity raises BP remains unclear. Insulin resistance is thought to be a central component, leading to impaired glucose tolerance and hyperinsulinemia. Hyperinsulinemia may then raise the BP by the mechanisms noted above. Despite these observations, insulin resistance or hyperinsulinemia as a cause of hypertension remains controversial. There is also mounting evidence that leptin may have a role in obesity-related hypertension, via increased sympathetic activity [54].

The sleep apnea syndrome associated with obesity is an additional contributing factor to the development of hypertension [59]. It is thought that activation of the sympathetic nervous system, elevated aldosterone levels, and increased levels of endothelin by repeated episodes of hypoxia are responsible for the associated hypertension [60].

The presence of sustained weight loss has a beneficial effect on hypertension. The long-term effect of weight loss was evaluated over an 8-year period among overweight 30- to 49-year-olds and overweight 50- to 65-year-olds [61]. A sustained reduction in weight of 6.8 kg or more was associated with a 22% reduction in relative risk for developing hypertension (defined by 140/90 mmHg) in the younger age group and 26% reduction in relative risk in the older overweight population. A simple relationship to remember is that for each 1 kg of weight loss, systolic and diastolic pressures fall by approximately 1 mmHg [62].

Cardiovascular Disease and Stroke

Overweight and obesity are associated with multiple cardiovascular abnormalities. In addition to an association with coronary artery disease, there is an increase in cardiac volume, cardiac work increases, and this may produce cardiomyopathy and heart failure.

Heart Failure

It is often forgotten that obesity can be an independent etiology of heart failure that is just as significant as hypertension, coronary disease, and diabetes. Evidence from the Framingham Heart Study showed that obesity doubled the risk of heart failure. In the 6000 subjects studied, multivariate analysis showed a 5–7% increase in risk for every 1 kg/m^2 increase in BMI [63]. The physiologic processes responsible for this increase are likely multifactorial, and include an increase in cardiac work, an association with insulin resistance, subclinical right ventricular dysfunction, and association with diabetes, sleep apnea, and hypertension.

Cardiac Rhythm Abnormalities

Patients with a BMI of greater than 30 kg/m^2 are significantly more likely to develop atrial fibrillation than individuals of normal weight. [64]. This increased risk has also been shown in many studies, and appears to be particularly associated with sustained atrial fibrillation as compared to transient or intermittent atrial fibrillation [65]. There does not appear to be an increased risk in ventricular dysrhythmias associated directly with increasing BMI or weight gain.

Coronary Heart Disease (CHD)

The Nurses' Health Study has shown a 3.3-fold higher risk of developing coronary artery disease in women with a BMI greater than 29 when compared to lean women [66]. When followed longitudinally, there is also an associated increase in heart disease with weight gain in women over time. This finding was highest in women who gained over 20 kg, and was independent of starting BMI. The association between obesity and CHD has also been observed in many other large-scale population-based studies [67–69]. The distribution of body fat again appears to play a role, with those subjects having predominantly abdominal or central fat being the group at greatest risk. Using the waist-to-hip ratio as a measurement for abdominal obesity in a female cohort, researchers have shown that a value of >0.88 provides a three-fold higher risk of CHD when compared to women with a ratio of <0.72 [70]. Others have shown that the risk appears to increase sharply once the ratio is >0.8 [71].

It is well known that dyslipidemia is an important risk factor for the development of atherosclerosis. The classic dyslipidemic pattern of obesity consists of an elevated triglyceride (TG) level and a decreased level of high-density lipoprotein (HDL). While the decrease in HDL may be an important contributor to the development of heart disease in obesity, perhaps more suspect is the changes associated with the character and quality of low-density lipoprotein (LDL) seen in obesity. Central fat distribution is associated with an increase in small, dense LDL. This form of LDL is more atherogenic than the alternate large fluffy LDL [72]. It has also been postulated that obesity poses an increased CHD risk because of associated low concentrations of adiponectin, which has antiathrogenic properties and lowers insulin resistance [73].

Stroke

The data linking obesity to stroke risk are not as clear as the data linking obesity to CHD. The Emerging Risk Factors Collaboration reviewed data on over 85,000 subjects and found that the risk of ischemic stroke increased by 20 % for every 1 standard deviation increase in BMI [74]. However, this risk was dramatically attenuated once adjusted for age, smoking, hypertension, diabetes, and cholesterol status. Some studies have shown an increased risk of both ischemic and hemorrhagic stroke in obese patients [75]. Most other studies have not seen this association with hemorrhagic stroke [76]. The Nurses' Health Study indicates that both a BMI of greater than 27 kg/m^2 and accelerated weight gain after age 18 are associated with increased ischemic stroke risk. The relative risk reported was 2.4 for a BMI of 32 kg/m^2 or greater when compared to a BMI of 21 kg/m^2 or less [77]. The Women's Health Study also reported similar findings [78].

Insulin Resistance and Diabetes

Insulin Resistance

Insulin resistance and type 2 diabetes are significant health risks well known to be associated with obesity, such that even mild detriment to insulin release has been shown to have profound effects on metabolic processes, and thus regulation of weight and obesity [79]. Insulin resistance is stimulated by fat deposited within cells and cytokines (IL1, IL6, TNF-α) secreted by adipocytes that actively suppresses insulin sensitizers. Insulin resistance is only one part of the pathophysiology of type 2 diabetes, with B cell dysfunction in the pancreas also playing a role. Notably, the connection between insulin resistance and inflammatory pathways provides an explanation for the comorbid association between type 2 diabetes and obesity, examined further in clinical studies associating weight loss with an increase in insulin sensitivity in adults ($P < 0.002$) [80, 81]. Environmental, genetic, and societal factors contribute to the development and repercussions of obesity and insulin resistance, as well as differences in ethnicity and gender. Men and African Americans exhibit a greater prevalence for insulin resistance, with African Americans constituting the highest rate of diagnosed diabetes among all the races at 11.2% [82].

Diabetes

Data from the Behavioral Risk Factor Surveillance System (BRFSS) from 2001 of 195,005 adults in the USA showed that obese adults (BMI ≥40) have greater than a sevenfold OR for a diagnosis of diabetes than the average adult [82]. This figure may be a staggering underestimation of the true presence of diabetes in the population due to various survey constraints within the survey population and the criterion that only doctor-diagnosed diabetes was tabulated, though an estimated 27% of those affected by diabetes remain undiagnosed [83]. The link is irrefutable when the converse association is considered: 64% of men and 77% of women with type 2 diabetes are overweight or obese. There is also sufficient evidence linking obesity to the development of gestational diabetes mellitus. Using a regression analysis between prepregnancy BMI and presence of gestational diabetes, researchers calculated the percentage of gestational diabetes attributed to obesity and found a statistically significant higher risk of gestational diabetes correlated to higher BMI and 46.2 % of gestational diabetes occurrences ascribed to being overweight, obese, or extremely obese (95 % CI = 26.1, 56.3) [84]. With an estimated $ 174 billion spent annually on the treatment of diabetes and a projected number of one in three Americans with diabetes by 2050, the health burden of obesity and its connection to insulin resistance and type 2 diabetes poses as an immense public health problem for worldwide populations [85].

Cancers

In 2008, there were an estimated 12.7 million cancer cases and 7.6 million cancer deaths worldwide [86, 87]. Together, modifiable risks such as tobacco use, excess weight, poor diet, and inactivity are thought to account for almost 70 % of all cancers in the USA [88]. Obesity as a sole risk factor is estimated to cause 20 % of all cancers [89]. Excess weight and obesity are associated with an increased risk of developing multiple cancers including colorectal, postmenopausal breast, endometrial, renal, and esophageal cancer. The attributable risk of excess weight ranges from 9 % (postmenopausal breast cancer) to 39 % (endometrial cancer) [90]. Newer data suggest that excess body weight and increased body fat also have a direct association with additional cancers including pancreas, thyroid, non-Hodgkin lymphoma, leukemia, and myeloma [91].

Weight gain itself is also associated with cancer risk. For example in a Canadian report, men who gained ≥ 21 kg after age 20 had a 60 % higher risk of colorectal cancer than men who gained only 1–5 kg [92]. In another study, women who lost ≥ 10 kg after menopause and kept it off saw a 50 % reduction in breast cancer risk [93].

The exact mechanism behind the association of weight with cancer development is not clear—and is likely multiple. One contributing factor is thought to be related to the increased aromatization that occurs in fat tissue, resulting in higher levels of estrogen. This may be a factor in endometrial cancer and breast cancer risk. Other proposed mechanisms include the influence of obesity and weight gain on insulin resistance and subsequent effects on inflammation. The latter may be particularly important in colon cancer [89].

A recent report suggests that bariatric surgery is associated with a 60 % reduction in overall cancer mortality (5.5 vs. 13.3 per 10,000 person-years). The follow-up for this study was 7 years, however, more data of this sort are needed to confirm this observation [94]. In addition, this benefit seen with bariatric surgery may not be the case with every cancer (see *colon cancer*).

While the above refers directly to excess body weight as a contributor to cancer risk, it is important to remember that physical inactivity and poor dietary intake are also contributors to cancer risk. While often intertwined with obesity, these two factors are independent and carry with them their own cancer risks that are beyond the scope of this chapter's discussion.

What about the role of weight after the diagnosis of cancer is made? The relative impact of weight on the prognosis and recurrence rates of cancer is dependent on the type of cancer being discussed.

Breast Cancer

Women who are obese at the time of breast cancer diagnosis have a 30% higher risk of breast-cancer-related mortality as compared to leaner women [95]. The reasons for this remain unclear and causality versus association remains debated. The authors who reported this finding also noted that the association holds true in both pre-menopausal and postmenopausal women, with the relative risk of death from breast cancer in obese versus nonobese individuals being 1.47 in premenopausal and 1.22 in postmenopausal women, respectively. It has also been reported that women with a BMI of greater than 35 kg/m^2 have a 60% higher risk of breast cancer recurrence as compared to women with BMIs of less than 25 kg/m^2 [96, 97].

In addition to weight at the time of diagnosis, weight gain after the diagnosis of breast cancer may also be associated with an increased risk of recurrence, although the data are inconsistent. In the Nurses' Health Study, women previously treated for breast cancer who gained 0.5–2 kg/m^2 and those who gained more than 2 kg/m^2 had risks of breast cancer death of 35–64% compared to women who maintained a stable weight [98]. However, other analyses have not supported these findings [99].

There are relatively few studies evaluating the efficacy and potential benefits of weight loss interventions in breast cancer survivors. The largest weight loss study to date in breast cancer survivors has been the Lifestyle Intervention Study for Adjuvant Treatment of Early Breast Cancer (LISA) [100]. In this study, more than 300 postmenopausal women with hormone receptor-positive breast cancer were randomly assigned to a weight loss intervention arm (including counseling by regular phone calls) or to usual care. The authors found that women randomized to the intervention lost approximately 4.5 kg more than the control. More importantly, there were significant improvements in physical functioning scores in those who lost weight. There is also evidence to suggest that the incidence of breast cancer may be decreased in women following bariatric surgery—although the results did not reach significance, a large-scale study in Utah found a lower incidence of breast cancer in gastric bypass patients compared with severely obese controls (hazard ratio (HR) of 0.91; 95% CI, 0.67–1.24; $P = 0.54$) [101]. Other studies have also suggested that cancer rates are reduced following bariatric surgery, particularly in women, although the group sizes in most cases prevented statistical analysis of site-specific cancers [102–105].

Prostate Cancer

Obesity is associated with worse outcomes among men with prostate cancer. However, whether changes in weight following a diagnosis of prostate cancer can modify prognosis is currently unknown. A study of almost 2000 men undergoing prostate biopsy showed that the risk of a high-grade prostate cancer (i.e., Gleason score ≥ 7) increased with an increasing BMI [106]. Similarly, there appears to be an association with obesity and advanced disease. A 2012 meta-analysis demonstrated a relative risk increase of 9% for each 5 kg/m^2 increase, and an inverse relationship between BMI and the development of localized prostate cancer [107]. Prostate-specific mortality appears to increase by 20% for each 5 kg/m^2 increase in BMI [108].

Colorectal Cancer

Studies have shown that patients diagnosed with nonmetastatic colorectal cancer with a high pre-diagnosis BMI (BMI ≥ 30 kg/m^2) have significantly poorer cancer-specific survival when compared to those within the normal BMI range [109]. The authors of this study did not see an association with post-diagnosis BMI and outcomes. In contrast, another study demonstrated that stage II and III colon cancer patients with BMI > 35 kg/m^2 after surgery had less disease-free survival compared to normal-weight patients [110]. There are little data on weight loss and survival benefit in patients with colon cancer.

Endometrial Cancer

Unlike prostate cancer, there appears to be an association of a less aggressive type of endometrial cancer with obesity [111]. It is thought that there is a greater likelihood of developing an estrogen-responsive tumor in women with a higher level of circulating estrogen. Accordingly, severely obese women were also more likely to present with stage I disease (77 vs. 61%) or low-grade tumors (44 vs. 24%). Despite this, among women with endometrial carcinoma, obesity is associated with an increased risk of death [112]. The risk of dying from endometrial carcinoma among those with the highest BMI (≥ 40 kg/m^2) was 6.25-fold higher than that of normal-weight women [25]. Unfortunately, the benefits of weight loss on outcome and recurrence are not well studied in endometrial cancer.

Reproductive Issues

Obesity affects ovulation, response to fertility treatment, pregnancy rates, and outcome. The National Health and Nutrition Examination Survey found that 32% of women between the ages of 20 and 39 were obese [113]. The prevalence varied with ethnicity, and was the highest (56%) in non-Hispanic blacks. Adipose tissue is an endocrine organ, and women with obesity have elevations in leptin and reductions in adiponectin, both of which may lead to insulin resistance. Obesity can also be associated with changes in estrogen and androgen levels. All of these factors can impact fertility.

Polycystic ovary syndrome (PCOS) is the most common reproductive disorder in women. PCOS is associated with obesity and ovulatory dysfunction along with hyperandrogenemia and insulin resistance. Restoration of ovulation often occurs with weight loss. One study reports that after a weight loss ranging from 4.8 to 15.2 kg (mean 9.7 kg), significant reductions in the concentration of luteinizing hormone (LH), fasting insulin, and testosterone were noted, and most of the women ovulated after weight reduction [114]. Similar results have been reported by other researchers [115].

In women without a cause of ovulatory dysfunction, obesity is associated with a decrease in spontaneous pregnancies and also with an increased length of time to achieving conception [116–118]. Obesity appears to be associated with subfertility and poor reproductive outcome regardless of the mode of conception, but the exact physiological mechanisms linking obesity to decreased fertility are not known. While some studies have shown weight loss results in higher live birthrates [119, 120], other authors have not shown this benefit in outcome. Large-scale studies have yet to be performed.

In women undergoing fertility treatment, some studies have shown that obesity is associated with insufficient follicular development, and lower oocyte counts during treatment [121–123]. Other studies have shown that ovulation-inducing medical regimens must be given in higher doses to allow for success of treatment in the obese female patients [124, 125]. In a recent meta-analysis including 33 studies and almost 48,000 in vitro fertilization (IVF)/intracytoplasmic sperm injection (ICSI) treatment cycles, women who were overweight or obese had reductions in clinical pregnancy rates and live birthrates that were marginal but significant when compared to normal-weight women. Overweight and obese women in this analysis also had significantly higher miscarriage rates (RR = 1.31) than normal-weight women [126].

While the data appear compelling in associating obesity with suboptimal fertility, many questions remain. Much of the literature thus far has been suboptimal, with poor patient selection for many trials and lack of viable controls. In addition, many of the studies conducted have been retrospective in nature. Thus, while an association can be seen, there is no clear conclusion or consensus on the mechanism of obesity on fertility.

Life Expectancy

While in the past two centuries life expectancy has lengthened due to factors such as lifesaving scientific discoveries, medical progress, and enhanced hygiene, the negative impact of obesity may end this trend. As a result, the current generation may be the first in evolution which has a lower life expectancy than their parents [127]. An analysis of data from the Framingham study confirmed that obesity is related to a reduction in life expectancy—for subjects who were 40 years old, obese men and women both had reductions in life expectancy of 6–7 years when compared to non-overweight cohorts [128]. The Prospective Studies Collaboration analysis [129] found that each 5 kg/m^2 incremental increase in BMI over 25 is associated with increased risks for CHD (39%), stroke (39%), diabetes (216%), cancer (10%), and respiratory disease (20%).

Effect of Fitness

Fitness level is also an important factor in obese individuals. In one study, higher levels of fitness appeared to negate some of the excess cardiovascular mortality risk associated with obesity in men [130]. In contrast, in the Lipids Research Clinics and the Nurses' Health Studies, both physical fitness and adiposity were independent predictors of mortality, and higher levels of fitness did not negate the association between obesity and mortality [131, 132]. Recently, there has been a considerable debate as to whether or not it is possible to be "fat but fit," with earlier studies seeming to suggest that individuals who were overweight or even obese but who were also physically fit and metabolically healthy had no greater risk of mortality as a result from heart disease or cancer than their normal-weight counterparts [133–135]. However, a recent meta-analysis has challenged these findings, indicating that metabolically healthy obese individuals had increased risk for all-cause mortality and/or cardiovascular events (relative risk (RR), 1.24; 95% CI, 1.02–1.55) when compared to metabolically healthy normal-weight individuals, and also found that all metabolically unhealthy groups (normal weight, overweight, and obese) exhibited similarly increased risks [136].

The Burden of Obesity in Children

Disease Burdens on Obese Children

The prevalence of obesity has increased dramatically across all countries, races, and social factors, with an estimated global prevalence of childhood obesity reaching 170 million children under the age of 18, such that life expectancy for younger generations is projected to be shorter for the first time in the modern era [127, 137] (see *Life Expectancy*). The childhood obesity epidemic is the result of a culmination of factors that include biological factors such as genetic factors and family histories of obesity, diabetes mellitus and hypertension, social determinants, and the newer factor of technological advancements that are associated with obesogenic behaviors and which promote sedentary lifestyles [138, 139]. Comorbidities significantly associated with childhood obesity include diabetes, sleep apnea, fatty liver disease, and cardiovascular disease [140]. Childhood obesity also adversely affects lipid profiles [141], and is associated with elevated systolic and diastolic BP, high risks of hypertension, and adverse total cholesterol to HDL ratios, which can persist throughout childhood and adolescence and into adulthood [142–144]. Childhood obesity has also been shown to increase the risk for menstrual problems later in life—for example, one study found that obesity at 7 years of age was associated with an increased risk of menstrual problems by age 33 (OR = 1.59) [145].

Social Burdens on Obese Children

The biological underpinnings and pathophysiology of obesity have been extensively researched, and more recently the psychosocial factors are also being determined to have a pronounced effect on child development and the quality of life [146]. Social determinants such as socioeconomic status affect children, in that lower-income children are more likely to be more obese than their higher-income counterparts, though there is no consistency across race or ethnicity. Children living in a household where the head of the household was not educated with a college degree were also found to be more likely to be obese than their counterparts living in a household where the head of the household was educated with a college degree [147]. Childhood obesity causes an overall negative impact on the physical health of children, both directly and indirectly. Much of the research on the psychosocial effects in children focus on adolescents, but recent studies using logistic regression using data from a "Be Active, Eat Right" Study of 2372 5-year-old children over the course of 2 years found through parent report that overweight and obese children have OR of 5.70 (95 % CI: 4.10 to 7.92), and 35.34 (95 % CI: 19.16; 65.17), respectively for adverse treatment (such as being teased, left behind, or ignored) in comparison to normal-weight children [148]. Body weight is a contributing factor to mental issues that overweight and obese children face, such as self-esteem, self-worth, body image, and mental health disorders [149]. The lack of research on the long-term effects of the psychosocial factors associated with the childhood obesity epidemic renders an unquantifiable negative impact. Researchers have begun to establish other social implications, specifically the associations between academic differences and increased BMI in children. Severe school absenteeism was found to be a more likely occurrence at an OR of 2.27 (95 % CI = 0.64–8.03) and 3.93 (1.55–9.95) for overweight and obese children, respectively [150]. According to 2009–2010 data, 17 % of all children were overweight or obese, leading to serious health consequences including premature mortality and adult morbidity, and imposing the childhood obesity epidemic as a prominent public health problem [4].

Where Do We Go from Here?

Historical Overview

The immeasurable health burden of obesity has pushed the epidemic into the limelight as a significant public health issue of modern times, and its unprecedented growth in recent decades has prompted various legislative acts and calls to action by public health leaders [151]. Figure 2.2 shows the most recent obesity statistics by

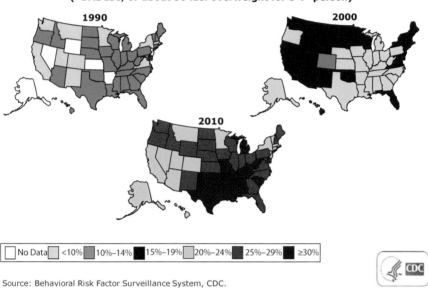

Fig. 2.2 Obesity trends among adults in the USA from 1990 to 2010. (Maps generated by the Centers for Disease Control and Prevention (CDC), Atlanta Georgia)

state in the USA. Recently, obesity rates in the USA have slowed down and leveled off for the first time in decades [4].

The question remains as to whether the rate of obesity has merely reached a satu-ration threshold in the population of the USA, or whether policy, community health initiatives, nutritional education, or growing health-conscious culture has dictated a halt in the epidemic. Obesity first became a dominant issue as significant changes occurred to the state of food supplies, transportation, physical activity, and commu-nity infrastructures [152]. The food industry began substituting healthy ingredients for unhealthy, processed counterparts and increased portion sizes, while making "faster" foods more readily accessible and more affordable. Simultaneously, as technological advancements progressed, for example, in the automobile industry, and a drastic flight to suburban life ensued, Americans engaged in less unstructured physical activity to supplement a more sedentary lifestyle [153]. In the most recent two decades, as health-care costs associated with being overweight and obese in-creased immensely, the government responded with implementation of regulations in the food and beverage industry such as nutritional information labeling, educa-tion and awareness campaigns, and subsidies for farm-fresh food [154–156]. In ad-dition, a general shift to "green" culture occurred in higher socioeconomic classes, as consumers directly demanded more transparency from the food industry by the

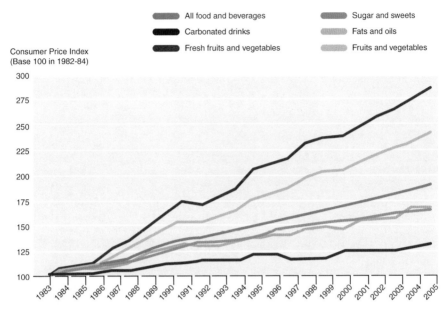

Fig. 2.3 Development of relative prices for various foods in the USA from 1983 to 2005. (Reproduced with permission from: Popkin, BM. Agricultural policies, food and public health. EMBO reports (2011) 12, 11–18. Illustration used with the permission of Nature Publishing Group. All rights reserved)

increased consumer interest in organic, sustainable, and unprocessed foods. However, obesity remains ingrained in the societal normalcy, as environmental factors and accessibility to healthy foods and time to dedicate to healthy living is compromised, especially for lower socioeconomic status individuals and communities [157] (Fig. 2.3).

Future Directions

The stagnant obesity rate may reflect a variety of the initiatives taken by different levels of societal infrastructure, including government, community, family, and individual, and is a hopeful statistic elucidating the impact of the intrinsically collaborative nature of the four different levels on population health. At the onset of the obesity epidemic, a discussion on a person's increase in weight was a segregating topic, but with the increasing shift in BMI of an entire global population, the epidemic prompted and continues to prompt an investigation of the many upstream and downstream constraints that affect worldwide health [158]. The upstream factors, such as information asymmetry about the foods we eat, the neighborhoods in which we live and the environmental constraints they pose, the budget and time constraints we face, and even the social reinforcement from those around us, have powerful effects on the choices we make in terms of our health [159]. Moving forward to address the issue of obesity, policy makers must utilize a population approach that focuses on the gradual shift of the average adult and child BMI through even more transparency from the food and beverage industry, preventative efforts through nutritional education in primary schooling, and incentivizing individuals to establish trusting relationships between primary care providers to better their health [160, 161].

References

1. Physical status: the use and interpretation of anthropometry. Report of a WHO Expert Committee. WHO Technical Report Series No. 854. Geneva:World Health Organization; 1995.
2. Obesity: preventing and managing the global epidemic. Report of a WHO Consultation on Obesity, 3–5 June 1997. WHO Technical Report Series No. 894. Geneva: World Health Organization, 1998:p. 1–276.
3. Finucane MM, Stevens GA, Cowan MJ, et al. National, regional, and global trends in body-mass index since 1980: systematic analysis of health examination surveys and epidemiological studies with 960 country-years and 9.1 million participants. Lancet. 2011;377:557–67.
4. Ogden CL, Carroll MD, Kit BK, et al. Prevalence of obesity in the United States, 2009–2010. NCHS Data Brief. 2012:1–8.
5. Bergman RN. A better index of body adiposity. Obesity (Silver Spring). 2012;20:1135.
6. Obesity and overweight. Fact sheet No. 311, Updated March 2013. Geneva: World Health Organization, 2013.
7. Moon OR, Kim NS, Jang SM, et al. The relationship between body mass index and the prevalence of obesity-related diseases based on the 1995 National Health Interview Survey in Korea. Obes Rev. 2002;3:191–6.
8. Ko GT, Tang J, Chan JC, et al. Lower BMI cut-off value to define obesity in Hong Kong Chinese: an analysis based on body fat assessment by bioelectrical impedance. Br J Nutr. 2001;85:239–42.
9. Deurenberg P, Yap M, van Staveren WA. Body mass index and percent body fat: a meta analysis among different ethnic groups. Int J Obes Relat Metab Disord. 1998;22:1164–71.
10. The Asia-Pacific perspective: redefining obesity and its treatment Geneva: World Health Organization; 2000. p. 1–55.
11. WHO expert consultation. Appropriate body-mass index for Asian populations and its implications for policy and intervention strategies. Lancet. 2004;363:157–63.
12. Stevens J. Ethnic-specific cutpoints for obesity vs country-specific guidelines for action. Int J Obes Relat Metab Disord. 2003;27:287–8.
13. Kanazawa M, Yoshiike N, Osaka T, et al. Criteria and classification of obesity in Japan and Asia-Oceania. Asia Pac J Clin Nutr. 2002;11(Suppl 8):S732–7.
14. Bei-Fan Z. Predictive values of body mass index and waist circumference for risk factors of certain related diseases in Chinese adults: study on optimal cut-off points of body mass index and waist circumference in Chinese adults. Asia Pac J Clin Nutr. 2002;11(Suppl 8):S685–93.
15. Barlow SE. Expert committee recommendations regarding the prevention, assessment, and treatment of child and adolescent overweight and obesity: summary report. Pediatrics. 2007;120(Suppl 4):S164–92.
16. Withrow D, Alter DA. The economic burden of obesity worldwide: a systematic review of the direct costs of obesity. Obes Rev. 2011;12:131–41.
17. Finkelstein EA, Fiebelkorn IC, Wang G. State-level estimates of annual medical expenditures attributable to obesity. Obes Res. 2004;12:18–24.

18. Wang YC, McPherson K, Marsh T, et al. Health and economic burden of the projected obesity trends in the USA and the UK. Lancet. 2011;378:815–25.
19. Daviglus ML, Liu K, Yan LL, et al. Relation of body mass index in young adulthood and middle age to Medicare expenditures in older age. Jama. 2004;292:2743–9.
20. Finkelstein EA, Trogdon JG, Cohen JW, et al. Annual medical spending attributable to obesity: payer-and service-specific estimates. Health Aff (Millwood). 2009;28:w822–31.
21. Obesity: preventing and managing the global epidemic. Report of a WHO consultation. World Health Organ Tech Rep Ser 2000;894:i–xii, 1–253.
22. Haslam DW, James WP. Obesity. Lancet. 2005;366:1197–209.
23. Wall M. Idiopathic intracranial hypertension (pseudotumor cerebri). Curr Neurol Neurosci Rep. 2008;8:87–93.
24. Choi HK, Atkinson K, Karlson EW, et al. Obesity, weight change, hypertension, diuretic use, and risk of gout in men: the health professionals follow-up study. Arch Intern Med. 2005;165:742–8.
25. Calle EE, Rodriguez C, Walker-Thurmond K, et al. Overweight, obesity, and mortality from cancer in a prospectively studied cohort of U.S. adults. N Engl J Med. 2003;348:1625–38.
26. Bray GA. Medical consequences of obesity. J Clin Endocrinol Metab. 2004;89:2583–9.
27. Fontaine KR, Cheskin LJ, Barofsky I. Health-related quality of life in obese persons seeking treatment. J Fam Pract. 1996;43:265–70.
28. Williamson DA, O'Neil PM. Obesity and quality of life. In: Bray GA, Bouchard C, editors. Handbook of obesity: etiology and pathophsiology. 2nd ed. New York: Marcel Dekker; 2004. pp. 1005–23.
29. Sarwer DB, Moore RH, Diewald LK, et al. The impact of a primary care-based weight loss intervention on the quality of life. Int J Obes (Lond). 2013;37(Suppl 1):S25–S30.
30. Eisenberg ME, Neumark-Sztainer D, Story M. Associations of weight-based teasing and emotional well-being among adolescents. Arch Pediatr Adolesc Med. 2003;157:733–8.
31. Strauss RS. Childhood obesity and self-esteem. Pediatrics. 2000;105:e15.
32. French SA, Story M, Perry CL. Self-esteem and obesity in children and adolescents: a literature review. Obes Res. 1995;3:479–90.
33. Becker ES, Margraf J, Turke V, et al. Obesity and mental illness in a representative sample of young women. Int J Obes Relat Metab Disord. 2001;25(Suppl 1):S5–S9.
34. Sjoberg RL, Nilsson KW, Leppert J. Obesity, shame, and depression in school-aged children: a population-based study. Pediatrics. 2005;116:e389–92.
35. Zeller MH, Roehrig HR, Modi AC, et al. Health-related quality of life and depressive symptoms in adolescents with extreme obesity presenting for bariatric surgery. Pediatrics. 2006;117:1155–61.
36. Erickson SJ, Robinson TN, Haydel KF, et al. Are overweight children unhappy?: Body mass index, depressive symptoms, and overweight concerns in elementary school children. Arch Pediatr Adolesc Med. 2000;154:931–5.
37. Falkner NH, Neumark-Sztainer D, Story M, et al. Social, educational, and psychological correlates of weight status in adolescents. Obes Res. 2001;9:32–42.
38. Lawlor DA, Mamun AA, O'Callaghan MJ, et al. Is being overweight associated with behavioural problems in childhood and adolescence? Findings from the Mater-University study of pregnancy and its outcomes. Arch Dis Child. 2005;90:692–7.
39. Gortmaker SL, Must A, Perrin JM, et al. Social and economic consequences of overweight in adolescence and young adulthood. N Engl J Med. 1993;329:1008–12.
40. Strohl KP, Strobel RJ, Parisi RA. Obesity and pulmonary function. In: Bray GA, Bouchard C, editors. Handbook of obesity: etiology and pathophsiology. 2nd ed. New York: Marcel Dekker; 2004. p. 725–239.
41. Thyagarajan B, Jacobs DR Jr, Apostol GG, et al. Longitudinal association of body mass index with lung function: the CARDIA study. Respir Res. 2008;9:31.
42. Young T, Skatrud J, Peppard PE. Risk factors for obstructive sleep apnea in adults. JAMA. 2004;291:2013–6.

43. Piper AJ, Grunstein RR. Obesity hypoventilation syndrome: mechanisms and management. Am J Respir Crit Care Med. 2011;183:292–8.
44. Felson DT, Anderson JJ, Naimark A, et al. Obesity and knee osteoarthritis. The Framingham study. Ann Intern Med. 1988;109:18–24.
45. Matteoni CA, Younossi ZM, Gramlich T, et al. Nonalcoholic fatty liver disease: a spectrum of clinical and pathological severity. Gastroenterology. 1999;116:1413–9.
46. Speiser PW, Rudolf MC, Anhalt H, et al. Childhood obesity. J Clin Endocrinol Metab. 2005;90:1871–87.
47. Mandato C, Lucariello S, Licenziati MR, et al. Metabolic, hormonal, oxidative, and inflammatory factors in pediatric obesity-related liver disease. J Pediatr. 2005;147:62–6.
48. Ratziu V, Giral P, Charlotte F, et al. Liver fibrosis in overweight patients. Gastroenterology. 2000;118:1117–23.
49. Bellentani S, Saccoccio G, Masutti F, et al. Prevalence of and risk factors for hepatic steatosis in Northern Italy. Ann Intern Med. 2000;132:112–7.
50. Marchesini G, Bugianesi E, Forlani G, et al. Nonalcoholic fatty liver, steatohepatitis, and the metabolic syndrome. Hepatology. 2003;37:917–23.
51. Aucott L, Rothnie H, McIntyre L, et al. Long-term weight loss from lifestyle intervention benefits blood pressure?: a systematic review. Hypertension. 2009;54:756–62.
52. Straznicky N, Grassi G, Esler M, et al. European Society of Hypertension Working Group on Obesity Antihypertensive effects of weight loss: myth or reality? J Hypertens. 2010;28:637–43.
53. Rocchini AP. Obesity and blood pressure regulation. In: Bray GA, Bouchard C, editors. Handbook of obesity: etiology and pathophsiology. 2nd ed. New York: Marcel Dekker; 2004. p. 873–97.
54. Rahmouni K, Correia ML, Haynes WG, et al. Obesity-associated hypertension: new insights into mechanisms. Hypertension. 2005;45:9–14.
55. Reaven GM, Lithell H, Landsberg L. Hypertension and associated metabolic abnormalities-the role of insulin resistance and the sympathoadrenal system. N Engl J Med. 1996;334:374–81.
56. Rocchini AP, Katch V, Kveselis D, et al. Insulin and renal sodium retention in obese adolescents. Hypertension. 1989;14:367–74.
57. Steinberg HO, Chaker H, Leaming R, et al. Obesity/insulin resistance is associated with endothelial dysfunction. Implications for the syndrome of insulin resistance. J Clin Invest. 1996;97:2601–10.
58. Sarzani R, Salvi F, Dessi-Fulgheri P, et al. Renin-angiotensin system, natriuretic peptides, obesity, metabolic syndrome, and hypertension: an integrated view in humans. J Hypertens. 2008;26:831–43.
59. Pedrosa RP, Drager LF, Gonzaga CC, et al. Obstructive sleep apnea: the most common secondary cause of hypertension associated with resistant hypertension. Hypertension. 2011;58:811–7.
60. Goodfriend TL, Calhoun DA. Resistant hypertension, obesity, sleep apnea, and aldosterone: theory and therapy. Hypertension. 2004;43:518–24.
61. Moore LL, Visioni AJ, Qureshi MM, et al. Weight loss in overweight adults and the long-term risk of hypertension: the Framingham study. Arch Intern Med. 2005;165:1298–303.
62. Neter JE, Stam BE, Kok FJ, et al. Influence of weight reduction on blood pressure: a meta-analysis of randomized controlled trials. Hypertension. 2003;42:878–84.
63. Kenchaiah S, Evans JC, Levy D, et al. Obesity and the risk of heart failure. N Engl J Med. 2002;347:305–13.
64. Wang TJ, Parise H, Levy D, et al. Obesity and the risk of new-onset atrial fibrillation. Jama. 2004;292:2471–7.
65. Dublin S, French B, Glazer NL, et al. Risk of new-onset atrial fibrillation in relation to body mass index. Arch Intern Med. 2006;166:2322–8.
66. Manson JE, Willett WC, Stampfer MJ, et al. Body weight and mortality among women. N Engl J Med. 1995;333:677–85.
67. Willett WC, Dietz WH, Colditz GA. Guidelines for healthy weight. N Engl J Med. 1999;341:427–34.

68. Wilson PW, D'Agostino RB, Sullivan L, et al. Overweight and obesity as determinants of cardiovascular risk: the Framingham experience. Arch Intern Med. 2002;162:1867–72.
69. Poirier P, Giles TD, Bray GA, et al. Obesity and cardiovascular disease: pathophysiology, evaluation, and effect of weight loss. Arterioscler Thromb Vasc Biol. 2006;26:968–76.
70. Rexrode KM, Carey VJ, Hennekens CH, et al. Abdominal adiposity and coronary heart disease in women. JAMA. 1998;280:1843–8.
71. Bjorntorp P. Regional patterns of fat distribution. Ann Intern Med. 1985;103:994–5.
72. Despres JP, Krauss RM. Obesity and lipoprotein metabolism. In: Bray GA, Bouchard C, editors. Handbook of obesity: etiology and pathophsiology. 2nd ed. New York: Marcel Dekker; 2004. p. 845–71.
73. Arita Y, Kihara S, Ouchi N, et al. Paradoxical decrease of an adipose-specific protein, adiponectin, in obesity. Biochem Biophys Res Commun. 1999;257:79–83.
74. Wormser D, Kaptoge S, Di Angelantonio E, et al. Separate and combined associations of body-mass index and abdominal adiposity with cardiovascular disease: collaborative analysis of 58 prospective studies. Lancet. 2011;377:1085–95.
75. Kurth T, Gaziano JM, Berger K, et al. Body mass index and the risk of stroke in men. Arch Intern Med. 2002;162:2557–62.
76. Hu G, Tuomilehto J, Silventoinen K, et al. Body mass index, waist circumference, and waist-hip ratio on the risk of total and type-specific stroke. Arch Intern Med. 2007;167:1420–7.
77. Rexrode KM, Hennekens CH, Willett WC, et al. A prospective study of body mass index, weight change, and risk of stroke in women. JAMA. 1997;277:1539–45.
78. Kurth T, Gaziano JM, Rexrode KM, et al. Prospective study of body mass index and risk of stroke in apparently healthy women. Circulation. 2005;111:1992–8.
79. Bonadonna RC, Groop L, Kraemer N, et al. Obesity and insulin resistance in humans: a dose-response study. Metabolism. 1990;39:452–9.
80. Garber AJ. Obesity and type 2 diabetes: which patients are at risk? Diabetes Obes Metab. 2012;14:399–408.
81. McLaughlin T, Schweitzer P, Carter S, et al. Persistence of improvement in insulin sensitivity following a dietary weight loss programme. Diabetes Obes Metab. 2008;10:1186–94.
82. Mokdad AH, Ford ES, Bowman BA, et al. Prevalence of obesity, diabetes, and obesity-related health risk factors, 2001. JAMA. 2003;289:76–9.
83. National diabetes fact sheet: general information and national estimates on diabetes in the United States, 2011. Atlanta, GA: Centers for Disease Control and Prevention, 2013.
84. Kim SY, England L, Wilson HG, et al. Percentage of gestational diabetes mellitus attributable to overweight and obesity. Am J Public Health. 2010;100:1047–52.
85. Number of Americans with diabetes projected to double or triple by 2050. Atlanta, GA Centers for Disease Control and Prevention, 2011.
86. Siegel R, Ward E, Brawley O, Jemal A. Cancer statistics, 2011. CA: A Cancer Journal for Clinicians. 2011;61(4):212–36.
87. Brawley OW. Avoidable cancer deaths globally. CA Cancer J Clin. 2011;61:67–8.
88. Harvard report on cancer prevention volume 2: prevention of human cancer. Cancer Causes Control. 1997;8(Suppl 1):S5.
89. Wolin KY, Carson K, Colditz GA. Obesity and cancer. Oncologist. 2010;15:556–65.
90. Wolin KY, Yan Y, Colditz GA, et al. Physical activity and colon cancer prevention: a meta-analysis. Br J Cancer. 2009;100:611–6.
91. Renehan AG, Tyson M, Egger M, et al. Body-mass index and incidence of cancer: a systematic review and meta-analysis of prospective observational studies. Lancet. 2008;371:569–78.
92. Campbell PT, Cotterchio M, Dicks E, et al. Excess body weight and colorectal cancer risk in Canada: associations in subgroups of clinically defined familial risk of cancer. Cancer Epidemiol Biomarkers Prev. 2007;16:1735–44.
93. Eliassen AH, Colditz GA, Rosner B, et al. Adult weight change and risk of postmenopausal breast cancer. JAMA. 2006;296:193–201.

94. Adams TD, Gress RE, Smith SC, et al. Long-term mortality after gastric bypass surgery. N Engl J Med. 2007;357:753–61.
95. Protani M, Coory M, Martin JH. Effect of obesity on survival of women with breast cancer: systematic review and meta-analysis. Breast Cancer Res Treat. 2010;123:627–35.
96. Sestak I, Distler W, Forbes JF, et al. Effect of body mass index on recurrences in tamoxifen and anastrozole treated women: an exploratory analysis from the ATAC trial. J Clin Oncol. 2010;28:3411–5.
97. Pfeiler G, Konigsberg R, Fesl C, et al. Impact of body mass index on the efficacy of endocrine therapy in premenopausal patients with breast cancer: an analysis of the prospective ABCSG-12 trial. J Clin Oncol. 2011;29:2653–9.
98. Kroenke CH, Chen WY, Rosner B, et al. Weight, weight gain, and survival after breast cancer diagnosis. J Clin Oncol. 2005;23:1370–8.
99. Caan BJ, Emond JA, Natarajan L, et al. Post-diagnosis weight gain and breast cancer recurrence in women with early stage breast cancer. Breast Cancer Res Treat. 2006;99:47–57.
100. Segal R, Pond GR, Vallis M, et al. Randomized trial of a lifestyle intervention for women with early-stage breast cancer (BC) receiving adjuvant hormone therapy: Initial results. J Clin Oncol. 2011;29:512.
101. Adams TD, Stroup AM, Gress RE, et al. Cancer incidence and mortality after gastric bypass surgery. Obesity (Silver Spring). 2009;17:796–802.
102. Sjostrom L, Narbro K, Sjostrom CD, et al. Effects of bariatric surgery on mortality in Swedish obese subjects. N Engl J Med. 2007;357:741–52.
103. Sjostrom L, Gummesson A, Sjostrom CD, et al. Effects of bariatric surgery on cancer incidence in obese patients in Sweden (Swedish obese subjects study): a prospective, controlled intervention trial. Lancet Oncol. 2009;10:653–62.
104. McCawley GM, Ferriss JS, Geffel D, et al. Cancer in obese women: potential protective impact of bariatric surgery. J Am Coll Surg. 2009;208:1093–8.
105. Christou NV, Lieberman M, Sampalis F, et al. Bariatric surgery reduces cancer risk in morbidly obese patients. Surg Obes Relat Dis. 2008;4:691–5.
106. Fowke JH, Motley SS, Concepcion RS, et al. Obesity, body composition, and prostate cancer. BMC Cancer. 2012;12:23.
107. Discacciati A, Orsini N, Wolk A. Body mass index and incidence of localized and advanced prostate cancer-a dose-response meta-analysis of prospective studies. Ann Oncol. 2012;23:1665–71.
108. Cao Y, Ma J. Body mass index, prostate cancer-specific mortality, and biochemical recurrence: a systematic review and meta-analysis. Cancer Prev Res (Phila). 2011;4:486–501.
109. Campbell PT, Newton CC, Dehal AN, et al. Impact of body mass index on survival after colorectal cancer diagnosis: the Cancer Prevention Study-II Nutrition Cohort. J Clin Oncol. 2012;30:42–52.
110. Dignam JJ, Polite BN, Yothers G, et al. Body mass index and outcomes in patients who receive adjuvant chemotherapy for colon cancer. J Natl Cancer Inst. 2006;98:1647–54.
111. Everett E, Tamimi H, Greer B, et al. The effect of body mass index on clinical/pathologic features, surgical morbidity, and outcome in patients with endometrial cancer. Gynecol Oncol. 2003;90:150–7.
112. Fader AN, Arriba LN, Frasure HE, et al. Endometrial cancer and obesity: epidemiology, biomarkers, prevention and survivorship. Gynecol Oncol. 2009;114:121–7.
113. Flegal KM, Carroll MD, Kit BK, et al. Prevalence of obesity and trends in the distribution of body mass index among US adults, 1999-2010. JAMA. 2012;307:491–7.
114. Bates GW, Whitworth NS. Effect of body weight reduction on plasma androgens in obese, infertile women. Fertil Steril. 1982;38:406–9.
115. Guzick DS, Wing R, Smith D, et al. Endocrine consequences of weight loss in obese, hyperandrogenic, anovulatory women. Fertil Steril. 1994;61:598–604.
116. van der Steeg JW, Steures P, Eijkemans MJ, et al. Obesity affects spontaneous pregnancy chances in subfertile, ovulatory women. Hum Reprod. 2008;23:324–8.

117. Gesink Law DC Maclehose RF Longnecker MP. Obesity and time to pregnancy. Hum Reprod. 2007;22:414–20.
118. Ramlau-Hansen CH, Thulstrup AM, Nohr EA, et al. Subfecundity in overweight and obese couples. Hum Reprod. 2007;22:1634–7.
119. Clark AM, Thornley B, Tomlinson L, et al. Weight loss in obese infertile women results in improvement in reproductive outcome for all forms of fertility treatment. Hum Reprod. 1998;13:1502–5.
120. Maggard MA, Yermilov I, Li Z, et al. Pregnancy and fertility following bariatric surgery: a systematic review. JAMA. 2008;300:2286–96.
121. Wang JX, Davies M, Norman RJ. Body mass and probability of pregnancy during assisted reproduction treatment: retrospective study. BMJ. 2000;321:1320–1.
122. Crosignani PG, Ragni G, Parazzini F, et al. Anthropometric indicators and response to gonadotrophin for ovulation induction. Hum Reprod. 1994;9:420–3.
123. Petersen GL, Schmidt L, Pinborg A, et al. The influence of female and male body mass index on live births after assisted reproductive technology treatment: a nationwide register-based cohort study. Fertil Steril. 2013;99:1654–62.
124. Souter I, Baltagi LM, Kuleta D, et al. Women, weight, and fertility: the effect of body mass index on the outcome of superovulation/intrauterine insemination cycles. Fertil Steril. 2011;95:1042–7.
125. Balen AH, Platteau P, Andersen AN, et al. The influence of body weight on response to ovulation induction with gonadotrophins in 335 women with World Health Organization group II anovulatory infertility. BJOG. 2006;113:1195–202.
126. Rittenberg V, Seshadri S, Sunkara SK, et al. Effect of body mass index on IVF treatment outcome: an updated systematic review and meta-analysis. Reprod Biomed Online. 2011;23:421–39.
127. Olshansky SJ, Passaro DJ, Hershow RC, et al. A potential decline in life expectancy in the United States in the 21st century. N Engl J Med. 2005;352:1138–45.
128. Peeters A, Bonneux L, Barendregt J, et al. Methods of estimating years of life lost due to obesity. JAMA. 2003;289:2941; author reply 2941–2.
129. Whitlock G, Lewington S, Sherliker P, et al. Body-mass index and cause-specific mortality in 900 000 adults: collaborative analyses of 57 prospective studies. Lancet. 2009;373:1083–96.
130. Calle EE, Teras LR, Thun MJ. Obesity and mortality. N Engl J Med. 2005;353:2197–9.
131. Lee CD, Blair SN, Jackson AS. Cardiorespiratory fitness, body composition, and all-cause and cardiovascular disease mortality in men. Am J Clin Nutr. 1999;69:373–80.
132. Stevens J, Cai J, Evenson KR, et al. Fitness and fatness as predictors of mortality from all causes and from cardiovascular disease in men and women in the lipid research clinics study. Am J Epidemiol. 2002;156:832–41.
133. Moore SC, Patel AV, Matthews CE, et al. Leisure time physical activity of moderate to vigorous intensity and mortality: a large pooled cohort analysis. PLoS Med. 2012;9:e1001335.
134. Ortega FB, Lee DC, Katzmarzyk PT, et al. The intriguing metabolically healthy but obese phenotype: cardiovascular prognosis and role of fitness. Eur Heart J. 2013;34:389–97.
135. Hamer M, Stamatakis E. Metabolically healthy obesity and risk of all-cause and cardiovascular disease mortality. J Clin Endocrinol Metab. 2012;97:2482–8.
136. Kramer CK, Zinman B, Retnakaran R. Are metabolically healthy overweight and obesity benign conditions?: A systematic review and meta-analysis. Ann Intern Med. 2013;159:758–69.
137. Population-based approaches to childhood obesity prevention. In: World Health Organization, Geneva, Switzerland, 2012.
138. Han JC, Lawlor DA, Kimm SY. Childhood obesity. Lancet. 2010;375:1737–48.
139. Patrick H, Hennessy E, McSpadden K, et al. Parenting styles and practices in children's obesogenic behaviors: scientific gaps and future research directions. Child Obes. 2013;9(Suppl):S73–86.

140. Wake M, Clifford SA, Patton GC, et al. Morbidity patterns among the underweight, overweight and obese between 2 and 18 years: population-based cross-sectional analyses. Int J Obes (Lond). 2013;37:86–93.

141. Freedman DS, Dietz WH, Srinivasan SR, et al. The relation of overweight to cardiovascular risk factors among children and adolescents: the Bogalusa Heart Study. Pediatrics. 1999;103:1175–82.

142. Lauer RM, Clarke WR. Childhood risk factors for high adult blood pressure: the Muscatine Study. Pediatrics. 1989;84:633–41.

143. Srinivasan SR, Bao W, Wattigney WA, et al. Adolescent overweight is associated with adult overweight and related multiple cardiovascular risk factors: the Bogalusa Heart Study. Metabolism. 1996;45:235–40.

144. Must A, Strauss RS. Risks and consequences of childhood and adolescent obesity. Int J Obes Relat Metab Disord. 1999;23(Suppl 2):S2–11.

145. Lake JK, Power C, Cole TJ. Women's reproductive health: the role of body mass index in early and adult life. Int J Obes Relat Metab Disord. 1997;21:432–8.

146. Griffiths LJ, Parsons TJ, Hill AJ. Self-esteem and quality of life in obese children and adolescents: a systematic review. Int J Pediatr Obes. 2010;5:282–304.

147. Ogden CL, Lamb MM, Carroll MD, et al. Obesity and socioeconomic status in children and adolescents: United States, 2005-2008. NCHS Data Brief. 2010:1–8.

148. van Grieken A, Renders CM, Wijtzes AI, et al. Overweight, obesity and underweight is associated with adverse psychosocial and physical health outcomes among 7-year-old children: the 'Be active, eat right' study. PLoS ONE. 2013;8:e67383.

149. Talen MR, Mann MM. Obesity and mental health. Prim Care. 2009;36:287–305.

150. Li Y, Raychowdhury S, Tedders SH, et al. Association between increased BMI and severe school absenteeism among US children and adolescents: findings from a national survey, 2005–2008. Int J Obes (Lond). 2012;36:517–23.

151. The surgeon general's call to action to prevent and decrease overweight and obesity. Publications and Reports of the Surgeon General. Rockville (MD): Office of the Surgeon General (US), 2001.

152. Wang Y, Baker JL, Hill JO, et al. Controversies regarding reported trends: has the obesity epidemic leveled off in the United States? Adv Nutr. 2012;3:751–2.

153. Eknoyan G. A history of obesity, or how what was good became ugly and then bad. Adv Chronic Kidney Dis. 2006;13:421–7.

154. Gortmaker SL, Swinburn BA, Levy D, et al. Changing the future of obesity: science, policy, and action. Lancet. 2011;378:838–47.

155. Brownell KD, Warner KE. The perils of ignoring history: big tobacco played dirty and millions died. How similar is big food? Milbank Q. 2009;87:259–94.

156. Novak NL, Brownell KD. Role of policy and government in the obesity epidemic. Circulation. 2012;126:2345–52.

157. Prevention andP. Atlanta, GA Centers for Disease Control and Prevention, 2009.

158. McKinlay JB. A case for refocusing upstream: the political economy of illness. In: Conrad P, Kern R, editors. The Sociology of health and illness: Critical perspectives. New York: St Martin's Press; 1990.

159. Feng J, Glass TA, Curriero FC, et al. The built environment and obesity: a systematic review of the epidemiologic evidence. Health Place. 2010;16:175–90.

160. Vos T, Carter R, Barendregt J, et al. Assessing cost-effectiveness in prevention (ACE-Prevention): Final Report. Melbourne: University of Queensland, Brisbane and Deakin University; 2010.

161. Rose G. The strategy of preventive medicine. USA: Oxford University Press; 1994.

Chapter 3
Psychosocial Morbidity and the Effect of Weight Loss

Julie Merrell Rish and Leslie J. Heinberg

Overview/Introduction

There currently is an obesity epidemic that threatens the population of the USA and that of the world. Currently, two thirds of the US population is overweight or obese. As a result, a large proportion of the population is at risk for a number of short- and long-term health consequences. These have been well described in preceding chapters. However, obesity is also associated with a number of significant psychiatric and psychosocial consequences. This chapter will review the most common psychiatric comorbidities of obesity with a focus on depression, anxiety, eating disorders, and substance use. These sections will include strategies for assessment and the impact of these disorders on outcome as well as the impact of weight loss on these disorders. Next, psychosocial consequences of obesity such as stigma, quality of life, and body image will be reviewed. Similarly, the bidirectional impact of these factors on weight loss will be discussed. Finally, conclusions will include future directions for the examination of the complex relationship between obesity and psychological factors.

L. J. Heinberg (✉) · J. Merrell Rish
Cleveland Clinic Lerner College of Medicine, Bariatric and Metabolic Institute, Cleveland
Clinic, 9500 Euclid Avenue/M61, Cleveland, OH 44195, USA
e-mail: heinbel@ccf.org

J. Merrell Rish
e-mail: merrelj@ccf.org

© Springer Science+Business Media New York 2015
A. Youdim (ed.), *The Clinician's Guide to the Treatment of Obesity,*
Endocrine Updates, DOI 10.1007/978-1-4939-2146-1_3

Psychological Comorbidities

Depression

A total of 20.9 million American adults or 9% of the population have a mood disorder, the most common of which is major depression. Major depression is characterized by a depressed or irritable mood and/or a loss of interest in previously pleasurable activities lasting at least 2 weeks that represents a change from the person's baseline. Additionally, symptoms often include problems with eating and sleeping, guilt, energy disturbance (e.g., fatigue and loss of energy), difficulty concentrating, negative self-evaluation, and thoughts about death or suicide [9, 10]. In population-based studies, women are twice as likely to have depression as men [100]. A number of brief measures are frequently utilized to assess depression in medical populations and include clinical cutoffs for making diagnostic determinations. Such measures include the Centers for Epidemiological Studies-Depression Scale (CES-D) [96], the Patient Health Questionnaire (PHQ-9) [72], and the Beck Depression Inventory (BDI) [14].

There is a positive association between obesity and depression in women—one in seven obese women meets criteria for depression, a rate that is 37% higher than normal-weight women [33]. In contrast, there is either a negative or no association between obesity and depression in men with 1 in 14 obese men meeting criteria for depression [6]. However, the relationship changes with more severe obesity. Both men and women with body mass index (BMI)$\geq$40 are more likely to have major depression. Population-based studies demonstrate five times as many severely obese individuals have had depressive episode in the last year [88]. Further, in women seeking treatment for obesity, 37% have clinical depression [89]. In severely obese individuals who are seeking weight loss surgery, research has documented significant psychiatric vulnerability with depression, the most frequent comorbid psychiatric condition [62, 85]. For example, approximately 25–30% of surgical candidates report depression at the time of evaluation with 50% reporting a lifetime prevalence of mood disorder or an anxiety disorder [60]. Further, 72.5% report a lifetime history of psychotropic medication use—87.7% of which were antidepressants. Even after controlling for BMI, depression predicts greater prevalence of certain medical comorbidities among depressed bariatric surgery patients including: dyslipidemia, gastroesophageal reflux disease (GERD), back pain, joint pain, sleep apnea, stress incontinence, and hernias [3].

The relationship between depression and obesity is likely bidirectional. Depression may be a maintaining or exacerbating factor of obesity. For example, appetite disturbance is a key feature of depression and there is a close association between binge eating disorder (BED) and depression (~50%; [57]). Depression often includes symptoms of avolition and loss of energy which may affect motivation for dietary change and physical activity. Additionally, the majority of mood stabilizers and antidepressants have weight gain side effects [123, 129]. Further, obesity may be a maintaining or exacerbating factor of depression. Body image disturbance (see below for further discussion of body image) increases as BMI escalates and body image disturbance is a risk factor for depression [99]. In addition, as BMI increases, individuals are more likely to experience stigmatization, discrimination, and prejudice. Finally, obesity is associated with a number of medical comorbidities and chronic pain conditions which may exacerbate depressive symptoms. Studies have suggested shared genetic and pathophysiological pathways that put patients at risk for both obesity and depression including inflammation, structural, and functional abnormalities in various brain regions, metabolic, and hormonal factors [112, 117]. Meta-analyses examining the relationship between depression and obesity endorse bidirectionality. In reviewing longitudinal studies [75], Luppino et al. (2010) found that obese persons had a 55 % increased risk of developing depression over time and depressed persons had a 58 % increased risk of obesity over time.

Treatment of obesity often leads to a decrease in depression [17] and improvements in depression have been reported after weight loss via lifestyle modification [18, 34, 35], pharmacotherapies [31, 45, 67, 101], and weight loss surgery [30, 39, 85]. The impact of weight loss on depression is most strikingly demonstrated in weight loss surgery patients. Hayden and colleagues [47] demonstrated reductions of more than 50 % in BDI total scores from baseline to 1-year post adjustable gastric banding. In a prospective study following patients up to 3 years after Roux-en-Y gastric bypass, the point prevalence of depressive disorders as measured by structured clinical interviews dropped from 33 % preoperatively to 16.5 % between 6 and 12 months postoperatively and to 14 % between years 2 and 3 [26]. Prospective studies have also demonstrated reductions in antidepressant usage and dosage following weight loss surgery [22, 47, 102]. However, depression may result in poorer weight loss outcomes in behavioral weight loss interventions [73, 89] and following weight loss surgery [61, 110]; and has been associated with poorer treatment adherence [40]. Of significant concern are studies indicating a higher rate of suicide and accidental death post-bariatric surgery in comparison to population base rates and obesity-matched controls. However, it is unclear what risk is conferred from surgery versus baseline differences in psychopathology and suicide history (see [51] for a review of obesity and suicide).

Overall, the impact of weight loss on mood-related improvement is highly encouraging. However, patients with symptoms of mood disorders should be followed closely to minimize any negative effects on weight loss. Some evidence suggests that adding behavior therapy to lifestyle weight loss interventions results in greater depression remission rates although weight loss is equivalent [90] .

Anxiety

Anxiety disorders are the most common psychiatric disorders, affecting approximately 25 % of individuals at some point in their lifetime [64]. Anxiety disorders cross a large spectrum of psychological symptoms but include disorders such as generalized anxiety disorder, panic disorder, specific phobias, social phobias, post-traumatic stress disorder, among others [10]. Anxiety disorders are often marked by both psychological symptoms (e.g., excessive worry, fear, rumination) and physical symptoms (e.g., tension, fatigue, agitation). Unfortunately, these symptoms are often chronic in nature and may co-occur with other psychiatric symptoms such as depression. Thus, anxiety is often screened with both broad-based measures of psychopathology such as the Symptom Checklist-90–Revised [27] or PRIME-MD [115] as well as specific instruments such as the Beck Anxiety Inventory (BAI; [15]).

Anxiety is markedly prevalent in obese populations. The pooled odds ratio from cross-sectional studies suggests an increased risk of 1.4 when compared to normal-weight populations and specific and social phobias are particularly prevalent [39]. Although mood disorders are the most common lifetime diagnosis in bariatric patients, anxiety disorders are the most common current diagnosis, affecting approximately 18 % of those who present for weight loss surgery [26].

Like depression, the relationship between obesity and anxiety is stronger in higher BMI categories [16, 109] and may be reciprocal. For example, the negative impact of obesity on health and quality of life may be highly stressful and the stigmatization experienced by patients may exacerbate certain anxiety disorders (e.g., social phobia; [39]). Conversely, anxiety disorders have been hypothesized to lead to weight gain due to hypothalamic–pituitary–adrenal axis dysregulation in stressed populations [23] or due to increased appetite and cravings due to anxiety symptoms [120]. However, the overall association between anxiety and obesity appears to be only moderate, and is based upon less rigorous studies in the empirical literature [39].

Far fewer studies have examined the impact of weight loss on anxiety with most focusing on anxiety following bariatric procedures. Unlike the impact of postsurgical weight loss on depression described above, no significant declines have been noted on point prevalence of anxiety disorders after massive weight loss post-bariatric surgery [26]. Interestingly, individuals with both depression and anxiety disorders—either currently or in their past—at baseline assessment had poorer weight loss outcomes [26]. Similarly, a lifetime history of an anxiety disorder was associated with poorer outcomes in surgical populations. Given the prevalence of anxiety in obese populations and its potential impact, continued monitoring and possible treatment are recommended in obese populations.

Binge Eating Disorder

BED has been defined as eating a larger quantity of food than normal in a discrete period of time (i.e., within 2 hours) and having a subjective sense of loss of control over eating (i.e., feeling as though one cannot stop eating; [10]). Binge eating episodes are associated with at least three of the following associated symptoms: eating past the point of fullness (i.e., uncomfortably full), eating large amounts of food when not physically hungry, eating rapidly, eating alone or hiding eating due to embarrassment, and experiencing distress/guilt after overeating [10]. Diagnostic criteria are met when binge episodes occur one time per week for a period of 3 months [10]. Importantly, the diagnosis of BED was only recently added to the *Diagnostic and Statistical Manual of Mental Disorders* (DSM; [10]). Previously, such symptoms were considered an eating disorder not otherwise specified with suggested diagnosis when binge episodes occurred a minimum of two times per week for a period of 6 months [10]. The following literature review is from studies using the latter criterion for the proposed diagnosis of BED as per the DSM and may be underrepresentative as the threshold for meeting diagnostic criteria has been lowered.

BED is differentiated from other eating disorders, in that it does not include compensatory behaviors (i.e.; vomiting, laxative/diuretic abuse, overexercise) as in bulimia nervosa or restricting calories as in anorexia nervosa [10]. Additionally, binge eating is differentiated from night eating and graze eating disorders. Although not formally recognized as a diagnosis in the DSM·[10], night eating may be clinically present in a subset of patients presenting for weight loss interventions [4, 87] [5]. Night eating is characterized by consuming at least 25 % of one's daily caloric intake after the evening meal and/or nocturnal ingestions at least two times per week with subsequent distress related to the night eating episode [7]. Night eating episodes are associated with three of the following symptoms: no desire to eat in the morning and/or skipping breakfast four or more mornings per week, a strong urge to eat after dinner and/or during the night, sleep onset and/or sleep maintenance insomnia four or more times per week, perception of needing to eat to fall asleep, or worsening mood in the evening hours. A less researched maladaptive eating pattern is graze eating described as continuously snacking throughout the day often resulting in an irregular meal pattern and increased caloric intake, and is associated with a sense of loss of control over eating [25].

Researchers estimate that approximately 1 % (1.2 % 12-month prevalence, 2.8 % lifetime prevalence) of the population meets criteria for BED [54]. However, higher prevalence rates of BED are seen in obese patients seeking treatment in weight loss programs (ranging from 18 to 46 %) [24]. Additionally, lifetime prevalence rates for BED amongst obese patients seeking weight loss surgery utilizing a structured interview range from 13.1 [85], 14 [103], and 27.1 % [60]. Current prevalence rates of BED amongst those seeking weight loss surgery range from 10.1 [85], 16.0 [60], and 23.3 % [103].

Research indicates that BED is associated with higher rates of psychopathology [54, 121]. Specifically, BED has been associated with comorbid depression, anxiety, impulse control, substance abuse [44, 54, 114] [57], bulimia, and personality traits [114]. Amongst patients seeking weight loss surgery, BED has been associated with higher rates of a current and lifetime mood disorder, current and lifetime anxiety disorder, as well as greater symptoms of reported depression and lower self-esteem [57].

The impact of BED on weight loss outcomes has been examined in a weight loss surgery population with variable results. Specifically, the majority of the literature indicates a lack of relationship between presurgical binge eating and weight loss outcomes, with only some studies indicating a negative or positive impact on weight loss [74]. However, postoperative loss of control eating has been associated with poorer weight loss and psychological functioning (i.e., depressive symptoms, eating disturbance, and quality of life) at 12 and 24 months [128]. Due to the restrictive nature of bariatric surgery, there is a question as to whether patients could meet the "large amount of food" criteria for BED postoperatively [107]. However, when this behavioral criterion is omitted and the focus turns to "loss of control" eating, there are higher rates of BED found postoperatively [21, 58, 59, 80]. Despite a lack of association found between preoperative binge eating and postoperative weight loss, preoperative eating disorder treatment has been shown efficacious. Ashton and colleagues [11] found that patients diagnosed with BED who completed a psycho-educational group for binge eating treatment and had a positive response to this intervention lost significantly more weight postoperatively than nonresponders.

Best practices in evaluating binge eating point to the utilization of standardized, empirically validated assessments of BED based on the DSM in addition to a brief, standardized DSM-based clinical interview [42] (Allison et al. 2006), with the most commonly used self-report screening questionnaire being the binge eating scale (BES; [13, 41]). Unfortunately, the methodology for assessing BED varies considerably across studies [42] [5], making it difficult to draw conclusions, leading to a large prevalence of discrepancy and emphasizing the need for empirically validated measures of binge eating. The recent addition of BED to the DSM may facilitate standardization across future studies and direct validated measures of associated symptoms. However, with a lowered threshold for meeting diagnostic criteria (i.e., one binge episode per week for 3 months compared to two binge episodes per week for 6 months), previous literature may have underrepresented BED.

Substance Abuse/Dependence

According to the DSM [10], substance use disorders are the abuse or dependence of any substance including alcohol, tobacco, illicit drugs, or prescription medication(s). Substance abuse is defined as the recurrent use of a substance despite a negative and recurrent impact on social or occupational functioning, recurrent interaction with the legal system, and continuing to use in situations in which it is physically hazardous [10]. Substance dependence is defined when a minimum of three of the following associated symptoms are met: tolerance (i.e., needing more of the substance in order to achieve the same effect), withdrawal, inability to reduce use despite attempts to do so, using more than intended, increased time spent in activities to obtain substances, withdrawal from other activities due to substance use, and continual use despite physical or psychological consequences [10].

The lifetime prevalence rate for any substance use disorder in the general population is 15.3 % [65] with current prevalence rates for any substance use disorder of 8.5–8.9 % in the general population [46, 65]. Interestingly, the lifetime prevalence rate for any substance use disorder is significantly higher amongst obese patients seeking weight loss surgery (35.7 % compared to 15.3 %; [85]) in comparison to population norms. However, current rates of substance use disorder are lower than the population amongst obese patients seeking weight loss surgery [46, 65] (1 % compared to 8.5–8.9%; [85]). The prevalence of current alcohol abuse or dependence is less than 1 % in preoperative bariatric patients [60, 85]; however, a study examining alcohol use disorders based on a measure rather than clinical interview reported a prevalence rate of 7.6% [66] which is similar to the general population rate of 8.5–8.9% [46, 65]. It is unclear why current rates of abuse or dependence are lower in weight loss surgery populations; however, perhaps they are related to presurgical intervention or education as active alcohol and/or substance abuse or dependence is a contraindication for weight loss surgery [79].

Recent literature has examined increased rates of alcohol use disorders after weight loss surgery. Studies have found that 8.6–12.8% of patients reported an alcohol use disorder prior to gastric bypass surgery and 7.7–10% reported an alcohol use disorder after surgery [32, 80]. Another study found that amongst patients who had gastric bypass surgery within the past 2 years and who had reported an alcohol use disorder preoperatively in remission (83.3 % of patients), 21.4% reported a current alcohol use disorder [118]. Additionally, a study examined substance abuse treatment admissions and found that 2–6% of admissions consisted of patients who had previously had weight loss surgery [106]. In a prospective study examining alcohol use in the year prior and 2 years post-weight loss surgery, higher rates of hazardous drinking as measured by the Alcohol Use Disorders Identification Test (AUDIT; [12]) were demonstrated prior to versus after weight loss surgery [66]. However, the rate of hazardous drinking increased significantly between the first and second year after gastric bypass surgery [66]. Specifically, the prevalence rate of alcohol use disorders was 7.6% prior to surgery and 9.6% after 2 years postoperative gastric bypass surgery [66]; a higher percentage than the population prevalence rate [46]. Risk factors identified include male gender, younger age, smoking, recreational drug use, regular consumption of alcohol prior to surgery, lower sense of belonging, and worse postoperative mental health and treatment [66]. Interestingly, these findings are not replicated amongst patients who underwent alternate surgical procedures (i.e., adjustable gastric banding, sleeve gastrectomy) likely due to pharmacokinetic changes in the absorption of alcohol after gastric bypass surgery [66].

Despite literature indicating that gastric bypass patients are a particularly vulnerable population for concerns regarding alcohol use, a few studies have demonstrated improved weight loss outcomes in patients with a history of substance abuse in remission [20, 48]. In particular, these studies found that patients with substance abuse in remission had better weight loss outcomes than patients without this history [20, 48]. The authors suggest that this history and subsequent remission of symptoms resulted in an increased ability to make major lifestyle changes similar to those required by weight loss surgery [20, 48].

The literature above indicating increased rates of lifetime substance use disorders [85] in obese patients emphasizes the importance of careful screening of substance use disorders, particularly screening for alcohol abuse in those seeking weight loss surgery [66]. Best practices in evaluating alcohol use disorders amongst weight loss surgery candidates follow the screening guidelines from the National Institute on Alcohol Abuse and Alcoholism [50, 83] and include screening for at-risk or heavy drinking (i.e., five or greater drinks in a day for a man and four or greater drinks in a day for a woman; [83]) in addition to lifetime and/or current abuse or dependence [50] defined by the DSM-V; [10]. In addition to a brief, standardized DSM-based clinical interview, patient may be administered an AUDIT [12] to screen for at-risk drinking behaviors [50]. Other studies indicated screening for alcohol abuse using the CAGE [83]. CAGE items include the following: C—Have you ever felt you should cut down on your drinking? A—Have people annoyed you by criticizing your drinking? G—Have you ever felt bad or guilty about your drinking? E—Have you ever had a drink first thing in the morning to steady your nerves or to get rid of a hangover? [83].

For additional information on assessing and treating alcohol use disorders, visit http://pubs.niaaa.nih.gov/publications/AssessingAlcohol/index.htm [83]. For additional information on assessing and treating alcohol in a weight loss surgery population read suggested recommendations by [50].

Psychosocial Consequences

Stigma

Persons with obesity are highly stigmatized and face prejudice and discrimination due to their weight. Although the majority of the population is overweight or obese, the prevalence of weight discrimination is comparable to rates of racial discrimination, especially among women [94]. Indeed, [38] Friedman et al. (2008) found 100 % of bariatric patients reported a stigmatizing experience in the last month. In a review of the obesity stigma literature, [92] Puhl and Heuer (2009) noted empirical support for discrimination against the obese in a wide variety of domains including hiring, placement, and discharge prejudice in employment; wages and promotions; education; public accommodations (e.g., airlines, restaurants, theaters, buses, etc.); jury selection; rental housing; media; interpersonal relationships; and in adoption. Sources of stigmatization are varied. Puhl and Brownell (2006) [91] queried obese individuals about most common and frequent sources of stigmatization and found that family members were most frequent followed by doctors, classmates, coworkers, spouses, and employers/supervisors. Commonly held stereotypes include that obese individuals are: lazy, overeat, or binge; unintelligent, lack willpower, and have poor hygiene; and are unattractive/ugly [91].

Unfortunately, there is little public attention to the issue of weight bias. Thus, obese individuals must endure, confront, and cope with these injustices largely on their own [92]. Stigmatization experiences have been associated with psychological distress as well as health behaviors. Weight stigmatization and weight-based teasing have been frequently suggested as mediators between obesity and depression [37] and weight-related teasing has been associated with depression in bariatric samples even after controlling for BMI [19]. Weight bias may also mediate the relationship between obesity and self-esteem and poor body image that is often present in obese individuals [92]. When patients are queried regarding coping strategies for managing stigmatizing experiences, 80% of women and 79% of men endorsed eating. This was the second most utilized strategy after coping self-statements [91] suggesting that stigmatization may make obesity worse. Similarly, a survey of obese women found that those who had internalized negative weight-based stereotypes had more frequent binge eating behaviors [93]. Experience with stigma has also been associated with avoidance of physical activity even after controlling for BMI and body image dissatisfaction [129]

Stigmatization of obese persons by physicians and other health-care professionals have been well documented. These include more explicit attitudes that are held in conscious awareness as well as implicit attitudes which occur automatically and are outside of conscious awareness. Physician's explicit attitudes towards obese patients have been reported to include that they are: noncompliant, lazy, lacking in self-control, awkward, weak-willed, sloppy, unsuccessful, unintelligent, dishonest, and a "waste of physicians' time" [92]. Higher BMI is significantly and negatively associated with physician perceptions that their patients will be non-adherent to medication (Prevalence risk ratio (PrR)$=0.76$ per 10 kg/m^2 increase in BMI) and is independent of actual medical adherence [55] and a higher BMI is significantly and negatively associated with physicians' reported "respect" for their patients (PrR$=0.83$ per 10 kg/m^2 increase in BMI; [55]). Physicians too may be stigmatized due to their weight. Individuals report more mistrust of overweight and/or obese physicians are less likely to follow their medical advice and more likely to switch providers and these attitudes are independent of the respondents' weight status [95].

Obese patients experiencing stigmatizing encounters in health care have been shown to delay or forgo a variety of preventative health-care services (e.g., mammography, cervical and colorectal cancer screenings; [92]. Patients often report negative attitudes of their providers, disrespect, and embarrassment about weighing procedures, unsolicited advice about their weight, and lack of weight-appropriate equipment [10]. Like cultural sensitivity, health-care professionals can increase skills and their environment to make all patients more comfortable and welcome. Language is an important component to this sensitivity [126]. Wadden and Didie (2003) queried obese men and women about what term they would like their physician to use when discussing their obesity. "Fatness," "excess weight," "large size," and "obesity" were the lowest rated, most negative terms while "weight" and "BMI" were most favorable. Interestingly, when queried about attitudes about terms "obese people" or "fat people," obese evoked stronger negative reactions in both genders [125]. To make patients of all sizes more comfortable, individuals should be weighed in a private setting, away from other patients and personnel. Further, weight should be recorded silently without commentary or negative body language (e.g., expression of shock or disgust). Finally, appropriate, wide-based scales that measure>350 pounds are recommended for all health-care settings. More information on setting up an appropriate physical environment is offered by the Yale Rudd Center for Food Policy and Obesity (http://www.yaleruddcenter.org/resources/

bias_toolkit/index.html). To combat bias and stigma, providers should strive to re-member that: (1) obesity is a chronic disease that results from a complex interplay between biological, genetic, psychosocial, and environmental factors; (2) obese patients come in all shapes and sizes as well as personality profiles, physical and psychological strengths, and weaknesses; (3) there is benefit and merit in all human diversity including the diversity of size, shape, and weight; and (4) obese patients have the right to be treated as a unique individual.

Impact on Outcome

Quality of Life

Health- and weight-related quality of life are negatively impacted by obesity [69]. Numerous studies have indicated that patients seeking weight loss surgery have more impaired health-related quality of life (HRQoL) than patients seeking non-surgical weight loss intervention [62, 68], obese patients not seeking weight loss intervention [68], and those in normative samples [28]. Additionally, several studies have shown improved health-related quality of life (HQRoL) after weight loss via weight loss surgery [70, 71, 105, 111]. Compared to individuals treated nonsurgi-cally, those who underwent weight loss surgery showed better outcomes on several measures of HRQoL over a 10-year period [66]. Improvements in the quality of life related to postoperative phases of weight loss, weight regain, and weight mainte-nance with most improvements noted in the first year of weight loss [63]. Between years 1 and 6, the authors noted a decline in HRQoL due to weight regain and then between years 6 and 10 noted stabilized HRQoL due to weight maintenance with 10-year data suggesting improved HRQoL over baseline [63]. Similarly, other stud-ies indicated improved HRQoL in surgical patients over nonsurgical patients at 2 years [70] and 3–6 years [71, 86].

Body Image

Body image is an important aspect of the quality of life [105] and one of the most prevalent motivators for weight loss amongst weight loss surgery candidates [127]. Severe obesity is associated with body image dissatisfaction [36, 116]. Specifically, body image dissatisfaction has been positively associated with BMI, indicating worsening body image with increasing obesity [36, 103]. Obese individuals seeking weight loss surgery have been shown to have higher body image dissatisfaction than normative samples even after weight loss [119]. Risk factors for poor body image including the degree of obesity, female gender, younger age, Caucasian race, history of childhood onset obesity, and a history of BED or weight cycling [108]. Amongst obese women, body image dissatisfaction is also associated with increased depressive symptoms, lower self-esteem, and a history of teasing [43, 78, 103].

Much of the literature indicates that body image improves with weight loss [1, 29, 36] and after weight loss via weight loss surgery [2, 53, 76, 84, 104, 105, 119, 122]. Additionally, reductions in body image dissatisfaction has been associated with increased weight loss [29, 105] and improved quality of life [105]. However, some literature indicates persistent negative body image after weight loss via weight loss surgery [52]. This may be related to decreasing ideal body size with weight loss [82, 113]. Improvements or lack thereof in body image may also be related to continual depressive symptoms rather than excess weight loss [77]. Additionally, persistent negative body image may be related to excess skin, continual overweight/ obese status despite weight loss, traits such as perfectionism or low self-esteem [119] [102], size estimations [108], or unrealistic weight loss expectations [49].

Conclusions/Future Directions

Obesity is associated with significant psychiatric and psychosocial impairment including higher rates of depression, anxiety, substance abuse or dependence, as well as impaired quality of life, negative body image, and experiencing negative social stigma. Escalating rates of obesity amongst both adults and children emphasize the need to comprehensively assess and treat obesity and its comorbid medical and psychological conditions. Given the potential impact of and bidirectional relationship between obesity, mood, substance use disorders, eating disorders, and quality of life, all must be taken into account in determining an appropriate patient-centered treatment plan. The complexity of obesity points to the utilization of a multidisciplinary treatment team including medicine, psychology, nutrition, exercise physiology, and when appropriate surgery, when assessing and treating this condition.

Future research should further examine the impact of obesity on psychological and psychosocial factors with sustained weight loss as well as duration of weight maintenance. Future research should also begin to explore preventative strategies for obesity and its medical and psychological comorbidities.

References

1. Adami GF, Gandolfo P, Campostano A. Body image and body weight in obese patients. Int J Eat Disord. 1998;24:229–306.
2. Adami GF, Meneghelli A, Bressani A, et al. Body image in obese patients before and after stable weight reductions following bariatric surgery. J Psychosom Res. 1999;46:275–81.
3. Ali MR, Rasmussen JJ, Monash JB, Fuller WD. Depression is associated with increased severity of co-morbidities in bariatric surgical candidates. Surg Obes Relat Dis. 2009;5(5):559–64.

4. Allison KC, Stunkard AJ. Obesity and eating disorders. Psychiatr Clin North Am. 2005;28:55–67.

5. Allison K, Wadden T, Sarwer D, et al. Night eating syndrome and binge eating disorder among persons seeking bariatric surgery: prevalence and related features. Obesity. 2006a;14(Suppl 2):S77–S82.

6. Allison DB, Newcomer JW, Dunn AL, Blumenthal JA, Fabricatore AN, Daumit GL, Cope MB, Riley WT, Vreeland B, Hibbeln JR, Alpert JE. Obesity among those with mental disorders: a National Institute of Mental Health meeting report. Am J Prev Med. 2009;36(4):341–50.

7. Allison KC, Lundgren JD, O'Reardon JP, et al. Proposed diagnostic criteria for night eating syndrome. In J Eat Disord. 2010;43:241–7.

8. American Psychiatric Association. Diagnostic and statistical manual of mental disorders (4th ed., text rev.). Washington, DC:Author; 2000.

9. American Psychiatric Association. Diagnostic and statistical manual of mental health disorders: DSM-V. 5th ed. Washington, DC:American Psychiatric Publishing; 2013.

10. Amy NK, Aalborg A, Lyons P, Keranen L. Barriers to routine gynecological cancer screening for White and African-American obese women. Int J Obes. 2006;30:147–55.

11. Ashton K, Heinberg L, Windover A, Merrell J. Positive response to binge eating intervention enhances postoperative weight loss. Surg Obes Relat Dis. 2011;7:315–20.

12. Barbor TF, Higgins-Biddle JC, Saunders JB, Monteiro MG. Manual for the alcohol use disorders identification test (AUDIT). 2nd ed. Geneva: World Health Organization; 2001. pp. 1–40.

13. Bauchowitz A, Gonder-Frederick L, Olbrisch M, et al. Psychosocial evaluation of bariatric surgery candidates: a survey of present practices. Psychosom Med. 2005;67:825–32.

14. Beck AT, Ward CH, Mendelson M, et al. An inventory of measuring depression. Arch Gen Psychiatry. 1961;4:53–63.

15. Beck AT, Epstein N, Brown G, Steer RA. An inventory for measuring clinical anxiety: psychometric properties. J Consult Clin Psychol. 1988;56:893–7.

16. Becker ES, Margraf J, Türke V, Soeder U, Neumer S. Obesity and mental illness in a representative sample of young women. Int J Obes Relat Metab Disord. 2001;25(Suppl 1):S5–9.

17. Busch AM, Whited MC, Appelhans BM, Schneider KL, Waring ME, DeBiasse MA, Oleski JL, Crawford SL Pagoto SL. Reliable change in depression during behavioral weight loss treatment among women with major depression. Obesity. 2013;21:E211–8.

18. Chaput JP, Drapeau V, Hetherington M, et al. Psychobiological impact of a progressive weight loss program in obese men. Physiol Behav. 2005;86(1–2):224–32.

19. Chen EY. Depressed mood in class III obesity predicted by weight-related stigma. Obes Surg. 2007;17:470–7.

20. Clark MM, Balsinger BM, Sletten CD, et al. Psychosocial factors and 2-year outcome following bariatric surgery for weight loss. Obes Surg. 2003;13:739–45.

21. Colles SL, Dixon JB, O'Brien PE. Grazing and loss of control related to eating: two high-risk factors following bariatric surgery. Obesity. 2008;16(3):615–22.

22. Cunningham JL, Merrell CC, Sarr M, et al. Investigation of antidepressant medication usage after bariatric surgery. Obes Surg. 2012;22(4):530–5.

23. Dallman MF, Pecoraro NC, la Fleur SE. Chronic stress and comfort foods: self-medication and abdominal obesity. Brain Behav Immun. 2005;19(4):275–80.

24. de Zwaan M, Mitchell JE, Seim HC, et al. Eating related and general psychopathology in obese females with binge eating disorder. Int J Eat Disord. 1994;15:43–52.

25. de Zwaan M, Hilbert A, Swan-Kremeier L, et al. Comprehensive interview assessment of eating behavior 18–35 months after gastric bypass surgery for morbid obesity. Surg Obes Relat Dis. 2010;6(1):79–85.

26. de Zwaan M, Enderle J, Wagner S, Mühlhans B, Ditzen B, Gefeller O, Mitchell JE, Müller A. Anxiety and depression in bariatric surgery patients: a prospective, follow-up study using structured clinical interviews. J Affect Disord. 2011;133:61–8.

27. Derogatis LR. Symptom Checklist-90-Revised: Administration, scoring and procedures manual. 3rd ed. Minneapolis:National Computer Systems, Inc.; 1994.
28. Dixon JB, Dixon ME, O'Brien PE. Quality of life after lab-band placement: influence of time, weight loss, and comorbidities. Obes Res. 2001;9:713–21.
29. Dixon JM, Dixon ME, O'Brien PE. Body image: appearance orientation and evaluation in the severely obese: changes with weight loss. Obes Surg. 2002;12:65–71.
30. Dixon JB, Dixon ME, O'Brien PE. Depression in association with severe obesity: changes with weight loss. Arch Intern Med. 2003;163(7):2058–65.
31. Elfhag K, Rossner, S, Barkeling B, Rooth P. Sibutramine treatment in obesity: initial eating behavior in relation to weight loss results and changes in mood. Pharmacol Res. 2005;51:159–63.
32. Ertelt TW, Mitchell JE, Lancaster K, Crosby RD, Steffen KJ, Marino JM. Alcohol abuse and dependence before and after bariatric surgery: a review of the literature and report of a new data set. Surg Obes Rel Dis. 2008;4(5):647–50.
33. Fabricatore AN, Wadden TA. Obesity. Annu Rev Clin Psychol. 2005;2:357–77.
34. Faulconbridge LF, Wadden TA, Berkowitz RI, et al. Changes in symptoms of depression with weight loss: results of a randomized trial. Obesity (Silver Springs). 2009;17(5):1009–16.
35. Fossati M, Amati F, Painot D, et al. Cognitive-behavioral therapy with simultaneous nutritional and physical activity education in obese patients with binge eating disorder. Eat Weight DIsord. 2004;9(2):134–8.
36. Foster GD, Wadden TA, Vogt RA. Body image in obese women before, during, and after weight loss treatment. Health Psychol. 1997;16:226–9.
37. Friedman KE, Reichmann SK, Costanzo PR, et al. Weight stigmatization and ideological beliefs: relation to psychological functioning obese adults. Obes Res. 2005;13:907–16.
38. Friedman KE, Ashmore JA, Applegate KL. Recent experiences of weight-based stigmatization in a weight loss surgery population: psychological and behavioral correlates. Obesity. 2008;2(Suppl. 16):69–74.
39. Gariepy G, Nitka D, Schmitz N. The association between obesity and anxiety disorders in the population: a systematic review and meta-analysis. Int J Obes (Lond). 2010;34(3):407–19.
40. Gorin AA, Raftopoulos I. Effect of mood and eating disorders on the short-term outcome of laparoscopic Roux-en-Y gastric bypass. Obes Surg. 2009;19(12):1685–90.
41. Gormally J, Black S, Daston S, Rardin D. The assessment of binge eating severity among obese persons. Addict Behav. 1982;7:47–55.
42. Greenber I, Sogg S, Perna F. Behavioral and psychological care in weight loss surgery: best practice update. Obesity. 2009;17:880–84.
43. Grilo CM, Masheb RM, Brody M, Burke-Martindale CH, Rothschild BS. Binge eating and self-esteem predict body image dissatisfaction among obese men and women seeking bariatric surgery. Int J Eat Disord. 2005;37:347–51.
44. Grucza RA, Przybeck TR, Cloninger CR. Prevalence and correlates of binge eating disorder in a community sample. Compr Psychiatry. 2007;48:124–31.
45. Hainer V, Kunesova M, Bellisle F, et al. Psychobehavioral and nutritional predictors of weight loss in obese women treated with sibutramine. Int J Obes. 2005;29:208–16.
46. Hasin DS, Stinson FS, Ogburn E, Grant BF. Prevalence, correlates, disability, and comorbidity of DSM-IV alcohol abuse and dependence in the United States: results from the national epidemiologic survey on alcohol and related conditions. Arch Gen Psychiatry. 2007;64(7):830–42.
47. Hayden MJ, Dixon JB, Dixon ME, Shea TL, O'Brien PE. Characterization of the improvement in depressive symptoms following bariatric surgery. Obes Surg. 2011 Mar;21(3):328–35.
48. Heinberg LJ, Ashton K. History of substance abuse relates to improved postbariatric body mass index outcomes. Surg Obes Relat Dis. 2010;6:417–21.
49. Heinberg LJ, Keating K, Simonelli L. Discrepancy between ideal and realistic goal weights in three bariatric procedures: who is likely to be unrealistic? Obes Surg. 2009;20:148–53.

50. Heinberg LJ, Ashton K, Coughlin J. Alcohol and bariatric surgery: review and suggested recommendations for assessment and management. Surg Obes Rel Dis. 2012;8:357–63.
51. Heneghan H, Heinberg LJ, Windover A, Rogula T, Schauer PR. Weighing the evidence for an association between obesity and suicide risk. Surg Obes Relat Dis. 2012;8:98–107.
52. Hotter A, Mangweth B, Kemmler G, et al. Therapeutic outcome of adjustable gastric banding in morbid obese patients. Eat Weight Disord. 2003;8:218–24.
53. Hrabosky JI, Masheb RM, White MA, et al. A prospective study of body dissatisfaction and concerns in extremely obese gastric bypass patients: 6- and 12-month postoperative outcomes. Obes Surg. 2006;16:1615–21.
54. Hudson JI, Hiripi E, Pope HG, Kessler RC. The prevalence and correlates of eating disorders in the national comorbidity survey replication. Biol Psychiatry. 2007;61(3):438–58.
55. Huizinga MM, Cooper LA, Bleich SN, Clark JM, Beach MC. Physician respect for patients with obesity. J Gen Intern Med. 2009;24(11):1236–9.
56. Javaras KN, Pope HG, Lalonde JK, Roberts JL, Nillni YI, Laird NM, Bulik CM, Crow SJ, McElroy SL, Walsh BT, Tsuang MT, Rosenthal NR, Hudson JI. Co-occurrence of binge eating disorder with psychiatric and medical disorders. J Clin Psychiatry. 2008a;69(2):266–73.
57. Jones-Corneille LR, Wadden RA, Sarwer DB, et al. Axis I psychopathology in bariatric surgery candidates with and without binge eating disorder: results of structured clinical interviews. Obes Surg. 2012;22:389–97.
58. Kalarchian M, Wilson G, Brolin R, Bradley L. Effects of bariatric surgery on binge eating and related psychopathology. Eat Weight Disord. 1999;4:1–5.
59. Kalarchian M, Marcus M, Wilson G, Labouvie E, Brolin R, LaMarca L. Binge eating among gastric bypass patients at long-term follow-up. Obes Surg. 2002;12:270–5.
60. Kalarchian MA, Marcus MD, Levine MD, et al. Psychiatric disorders among bariatric surgery candidates: a relationship to obesity and functional health status. Am J Psychiatry. 2007;164:328–34.
61. Kalarchian MA, Marcus, MD, Levine MD, Soulakova JN, Courcoulas AP, Wisinski MSC. Relationship of psychiatric disorders to 6-month outcomes after gastric bypass. Surg Obes Relat Dis. 2008a;4:544–9.
62. Karlsson J. Sjostrom L, Sullivan M. Swedish obese subjects (SOS)-an intervention study of obesity: two-year follow-up of health-related quality of life (HRQL) and eating behavior after gastric surgery for severe obesity. Int J Obes Relat Metab Disord. 1998;22:113–26.
63. Karlsson J, Taft C, Ryden A, Sjostrom L, Sullivan M. Ten-year trends in health-related quality of life after surgical and conventional treatment for severe obesity: the SOS intervention study. Int J Obes (Lond). 2007;31:1248–61.
64. Kessler RC, Wang PS. The descriptive epidemiology of commonly occurring mental disorders in the United States. Annu Rev Public Health. 2008;29:115–29.
65. Kessler RC, Berglund P, Demler O, Jin R, Merikangas KR, Walters EE. Lifetime prevalence and age-of-onset distributions of DSM-IV disorders in the national comorbidity survey replication. Arch Gen Psychiatry. 2005;62(6):593–602.
66. King WC, Chen J-Y, Mitchell JE, et al. Prevalence of alcohol use disorders before and after bariatric surgery. JAMA. 2012;307(23):2516–25.
67. Kiortis DN, Tsouli S, Flippatos TD, Konitsiotis S, Elisaf MS. Effects of sibutramine and orlistat on mood in obese and overweight participants: a randomized study. Nutr Metab Cardiovasc Dis. 2008;18:207–10.
68. Kolotkin RL, Crosby RD, Williams GR. Health-related quality of life varies among obese subgroups. Obes Res. 2002;10:748–56.
69. Kolotkin RL, Crosby RD, Gress RE, Hunt SC, Engel SG, Adams TD. Health and health-related quality of life: differences between men and women who seek gastric bypass surgery. Surg Obes Rel Dis. 2008;4:651–9.
70. Kolotkin RL, Crosby RD, Gress RA, Hunt SC, Adams TD. Two-year changes in health-related quality of life in gastric bypass patients compared with severely obese controls. Surg Obes Rel Dis. 2009;5:250–6.

71. Kolotkin RL, Davidson LE, Crosby RD, Hunt SC, Adams TD. Six-year changes in health-related quality of life in gastric bypass patients versus obese comparison groups. Surg Obes Relat Dis. 2012;8:625–33.

72. Kroenke K, Spitzer RL, Williams JB. The PHQ-9: validity of a brief depression severity measure. J Gen Intern Med. 2001;16(9):606–13.

73. Linde JA, Simon GE, Ludman EJ, Ichikawa LE, Operskalski BH, Arterburn D, et al. A randomized controlled trial of behavioral weight loss treatment versus combined weight loss/depression treatment among women with comorbid obesity and depression. Ann Behav Med. 2011;41:119–30.

74. Livhits M, Mercado C, Yermilov I, et al. Preoperative predictors of weight loss following bariatric surgery: systematic review. Obes Surg. 2012;22(1):70–89.

75. Luppino FS, de Wit LM, Bouvy PF, Stijnen T, Cuijpers P, Penninx BW, Zitman FG. Overweight, obesity, and depression: a systematic review and meta-analysis of longitudinal studies. Arch Gen Psychiatry. 2010;67(3):220–9.

76. Madan AK, Beech BM, Tichansky DS. Body esteem improves after bariatric surgery. Surg Inov. 2008;15:32–7.

77. Masheb RM, Grilo CM, Burke-Martindale CH, et al. Evaluating oneself by shape and weight is not the same as being dissatisfied about shape and weight: a longitudinal examination in severely obese gastric bypass patients. Int J Eat Disord. 2006;39:716–20.

78. Matz PE, Foster GD, Faith MS, Wadden TA. Correlates of body image dissatisfaction among overweight women seeking weight loss. J Consul Clin Psychol. 2002;70:1040–4.

79. Mechanick JI, Youdim A, Jones DB, et al. Clinical practice guidelines for the perioperative nutritional, metabolic, and nonsurgical support of the bariatric surgery patient-2013 update: cosponsored by American association of clinical endocrinologists, the obesity society, and American society for metabolic & bariatric surgery. Obesity. 2013;21:S1–27.

80. Mitchell J, Lancaster K, Burgard M, et al. Long-term follow-up in patients' status after gastric bypass. Obes Surg. 2001;11:464–8.

81. Mitchell JE, Selzer F, Kalarchian MA, et al. Psychopathology before surgery in the Longitudinal Assessment of Bariatric Surgery-3 (LABS-3) psychosocial study. Surg Obes Relat Dis. 2012a;8:533–541.

82. Munoz D, Chen EY, Fischer S, et al. Changes in desired body shape after bariatric surgery. Eat Disord. 2010;18:437–54.

83. National Institute on Alcohol Abuse and Alcoholism (NIAAA). Helping patients who drink too much: a clinician's guide and related professional support resources. http://pubs.niaaa.nih.gov/publications/practitioner/cliniciansguide2005/clinicans_guideHYPERLINK "http://pubs.niaaa.nih.gov/publications/practitioner/cliniciansguide2005/clinicans_guide.htm".htm. Accessed: 1 July 2013.

84. Neven K, Dymek M, le Grange D, Maasdam H, Boogerd AC, Alverdy J. The effects of Roux-en-Y gastric bypass surgery on body image. Obes Surg. 2002;12:265–9.

85. Nickel C, Widermann C, Harms D, et al. Patients with extreme obesity: changes in mental symptoms three years after gastric banding. Int J Psychiatry Med. 2005;35(2):109–22.

86. Nickel MK, Loew TH, Bachler E. Change in mental symptoms in extreme obesity patients after gastric banding, part II: six-year follow up. Int J Psychiatry Med. 2007;37:69–79.

87. O'Reardon JP, Ringel BL, Dinges DF, et al. Circadium eating and sleeping patterns in the night eating syndrome. Obes Res. 2004;12:1789–96.

88. Onyike CU, Crum RM, Lee HB, Lyketsos CG, Eaton WW. Is obesity associated with major depression? Results from the Third National Health and Nutrition Examination Survey. Am J Epidemiol. 2003;158(12):1139–47.

89. Pagoto S, Bodenlos JS, Kantor L, Gitkind M, Curtin C, Ma Y. Association of major depression and binge eating disorder with weight loss in a clinical setting. Obesity (Silver Spring). 2007;15(11):2557–9.

90. Pagoto S, Schneider KL, Whited MC, Oleski JL, Merriam P, Appelhans B, Ma Y, Olendzki B, Waring ME, Busch AM, Lemon S, Ockene I, Crawford S. Randomized controlled trial of behavioral treatment for comorbid obesity and depression in women: the Be Active Trial. Int J Obes. 2013;5:1–8.

91. Puhl RM, Brownell KD. Confronting and coping with weight stigma: an investigation of overweight and obese adults. Obesity. 2006;14(10):1802–15.
92. Puhl RM, Heuer CA. The stigma of obesity: a review and update. Obesity. 2009;17(5):941–64.
93. Puhl RM, Moss-Racusin CA, Schwartz MB. Internalization of weight bias: implication for binge eating and emotional well-being. Obesity. 2007;15:19–23.
94. Puhl RM, Andreyeva T, Brownell KD. Perceptions of weight discrimination: prevalence and comparison to race and gender discrimination in America. Int J Obes. 2008;32:992–1000.
95. Puhl RM, Gold JA, Luedicke J, DePierre JA. The effect of physicians' body weight on patient attitudes: implications for physician selection, trust and adherence to medical advice. Int J Obes. 2013;37:1–7.
96. Radloff LS. The CES-D Scale: A self-report depression scale for research in the general population. Appl Psychological Meas. 1977;1(3):385–401.
97. Rosenberger PH, Henderson KE, Grilo CM. Correlates of body image dissatisfaction in extremely obese female bariatric surgery candidates. Obes Surg. 2006a;16(10):1331–6.
98. Rosenberger PH, Henderson KE, Grilo CM. Psychiatric disorder comorbidity and association with eating disorders in bariatric surgery patients: a cross-sectional study using structured interview-based diagnosis. J Clin Psychiatry. 2006b;67:1090–5.
99. Rosenström T, Jokela M, Hintsanen M, Josefsson K, Juonala M, Kivimäki M, Pulkki-Råback L, Viikari JS, Hutri-Kähönen N, Heinonen E, Raitakari OT, Keltikangas-Järvinen L. Body-image dissatisfaction is strongly associated with chronic dysphoria. J Affect Disord. 2013. Epub ahead of print.
100. Rubio JM, Markowitz JC, Alegría A, Pérez-Fuentes G, Liu SM, Lin KH, Blanco C. Epidemiology of chronic and nonchronic major depressive disorder: results from the national epidemiologic survey on alcohol and related conditions. Depress Anxiety. 2011;28(8):622–31.
101. Rucker D, Padwal R, Li SK, Curioni C, Lau DC. Long term pharmacotherapy for obesity and overweight: updated meta-analysis. BMJ. 2007;335:1194–99.
102. Rutledge T, Braden AL, Woods G, Herbst KL, Groesz LM, Savu M. Five-year changes in psychiatric treatment status and weight-related comorbidities following bariatric surgery in a veteran population. Obes Surg. 2012;22:1734–41.
103. Sarwer DB, Wadden TA, Foster GD. Assessment of body image dissatisfaction in obese women: specificity, severity, and clinical significance. J Consult Clin Psychol. 1998;66:651–4.
104. Sarwer DB, Thompson JK, Cash TF. Body image and obesity in adulthood. Psych Clin North Am. 2005;28:69–78.
105. Sarwer DB, Wadden TA, Moore RH, Eisenberg, MH, Raper SE, Williams NN. Changes in quality of life and body image after gastric bypass surgery. Surg Obes Rel Dis. 2010;6:608–14.
106. Saules KK, Wiedemann A, Ivezaj V, Hopper JA, Foster-Hartsfield J, Schwartz D. Bariatric surgery history among substance abuse treatment patients: prevalence and associated features. Surg Obes Rel Dis. 2010;6:615–21.
107. Saunders R. Binge eating in gastric bypass patients before surgery. Obes Surg. 1999;9:72–6.
108. Schwartz MB, Brownell KD. Obesity and body image. Body Image. 2004;1:43–56.
109. Scott KM, McGee MA, Wells JE, Oakley Browne MA. Obesity and mental disorders in the adult general population. J Psychosom Res. 2008;64(1):97–105.
110. Semanscin-Doerr DA, Windover A, Ashton K, Heinberg LJ. Mood disorders in laparoscopic sleeve gastrectomy patients: does it affect early weight loss? Surg Obes Relat Dis. 2010;6(2):191–6.
111. Sjostrom L, Lindroos AK, Peltonen M, et al. Swedish Obese Subjects Study Scientific Group. Lifestyle, diabetes, and cardiovascular risk factors 10 years after bariatric surgery. N Engl J Med. 2004;12:473–81.

112. Soczynska JK, Kennedy SH, Woldeyohannes HO, Liauw SS, Alsuwaidan M, Yim CY, Mc-Intyre RS. Mood disorders and obesity: understanding inflammation as a pathophysiological nexus. Neuromolecular Med. 2011;13(2):93–116.

113. Song AY, Rubin JP, Thomas V, et al. Body image and quality of life in post massive weight loss body contouring patients. Obesity. 2006;14:1626–36.

114. Specker S, de Zwaan M, Raymond N, et al. Psychopathology in subgroups of obese women with and without binge eating disorder. Compr Psychiatry. 1994;35:185–90.

115. Spitzer RL, Kroenke K, Williams JB. Validation and utility of a self-report version of PRIME-MD: the PHQ primary care study. Primary care evaluation of mental disorders. Patient health questionnaire. JAMA. 1999;282(18):1737–44.

116. Stunkard AJ, Wadden TA. Psychological aspects of severe obesity. Am J Clin Nutr. 1991;55:524S–32S.

117. Stunkard AJ, Faith MS, Allison KC. Depression and obesity. Biol Psychiatry. 2003;54(3):330–7.

118. Suzuki J, Haimovici F, Chang G. Alcohol use disorders after bariatric surgery. Obes Surg. 2012;22(2):201–7.

119. Teufel M, Rieber N, Meile T, et al. Body image after sleeve gastrectomy: reduced dissatisfaction and increased dynamics. Obes Surg. 2012;22:1232–7.

120. Torres SJ, Nowson CA. Relationship between stress, eating behavior and obesity. Nutrition. 2007;23:887–94.

121. van Hout MS, van Oudheusden I, van Heck GL. Psychological profile of the morbidly obese. Obes Surg. 2004;14:579–88.

122. van Hout GC, Fortuin FA, Pelle AJ, et al. Psychosocial functioning, personality, and body image following vertical banded gastroplasty. Obes Surg. 2008;18:115–20.

123. Vanina Y, Podolskaya A, Sedky K, et al. Body weight changes associated with psychopharmacology. Psychiatr Serv. 2002;53:842–47.

124. Vartarian LR, Shaprow JG. Effects of weight stigma on exercise motivation and behavior: a preliminary investigation among college-aged females. J Health Psychol. 2008;13:131–8.

125. Vartanian LR. "Obese people" vs "Fat people": impact of group label on weight bias. Eat Weight Disord. 2010;15(3):e195–8.

126. Wadden TA, Didie E. What's in a name? Patients' preferred terms for describing obesity. Obes Res. 2003;11(9):1140–6.

127. Wadden TA, Sarwer DB. Behavioral assessment of candidates for bariatric surgery: a patient-oriented approach. Surg Obes Rel Dis. 2006;2:171–9.

128. White MA, Kalarchian MA, Masheb RM, Marcus MD, Grilo CM. Loss of control over eating predicts outcomes in bariatric surgery: a prospective 24-month follow-up study. J Clin Psychiatry. 2010;71(2):175–84.

129. Yoon CK. Weight gain and first-generation antipsychotics: experience from a developing country. J Clin Psychopharmacol. 2008;28:574–76.

Chapter 4
Dietary and Lifestyle Strategies for Weight Loss

Jennifer Arussi

The combination of dietary modification, increased physical activity, and behavioral therapy is the most effective nonsurgical obesity treatment available [1]. The US Preventative Services Task Force is recommending that clinicians refer obese individuals to "intensive, multicomponent behavioral interventions" and is consequently a mandate under the Affordable Care Act [2, 3]. Additionally, the Centers for Medicare and Medicaid Services recently added a provision calling for "intensive behavioral counseling" to obese seniors [4]. As a result of these national changes, health-care providers familiarizing themselves with the fundamentals of behavioral therapy is apropos and will be outlined as such in this chapter.

Defining Lifestyle Modification

Lifestyle modification programs are composed of caloric restriction, physical activity expenditure, and behavioral therapy. The overriding feature of behavioral therapy is to help patients develop specific strategies to increase compliance with diet and exercise [5–7]. The short-term treatment traditionally involves attendance of 20–26 weekly group meetings yielding a mean weight loss of 9% (8.5 kg). Losing 5–10% of initial weight is a goal set forth by the Institute of Medicine of the National Academy of Sciences, the World Health Organization, and the National Heart, Lung and Blood Institute to ultimately improve obesity-associated comorbidities [8]. Educating patients regarding these modest weight loss targets *may* help alleviate their dissatisfaction with their weight losses and prevent possible premature forfeiture of their participation.

J. Arussi (✉)
Change My Eating, Inc., 861 North Vista Street, Los Angeles, CA 90046, USA
e-mail arussij@me.com

© Springer Science+Business Media New York 2015
A. Youdim (ed.), *The Clinician's Guide to the Treatment of Obesity,*
Endocrine Updates, DOI 10.1007/978-1-4939-2146-1_4

The traditional characteristics of behavioral treatment are multiple and include food and activity journaling, frequent weigh-ins, caloric restriction through consumption of low-energy-dense foods, high levels of physical activity, improved food environments, problem-solving and cognitive therapy. Skilled providers of behavioral therapy guide patients to identify what behavior needs changing with examination of possible elements that may help or hinder goal attainment. This process-oriented, patient-centered approach is collaborative and a defining feature of motivational interviewing, a form of therapy used in the behavioral treatment of obesity [9].

Well-known investigators, such as the Diabetes Prevention Program research group (DPP), afforded evidence that behavioral treatment is valid and reliable [10]. The DPP's purpose was to evaluate the effectiveness of lifestyle interventions in reducing the incidence of prediabetic individuals from progressing to type II diabetes mellitus. This randomized, controlled intervention involved over 3000 obese individuals in 27 centers across the country. The lifestyle intervention group was able to reduce the incidence of diabetes by 58%, outperforming the metformin and placebo counterparts. As a result of these impressive results, YMCAs across the country offer DPP programs for prediabetic individuals.

The Look AHEAD (action for health in diabetes) study similarly depicts the effectiveness of lifestyle interventions [11]. This study is considered the largest prospective, ethnically diverse lifestyle intervention to date. The study authors recruited over 5000 men and women at 16 different centers with type II diabetes mellitus and randomly assigned them to one of the two groups: the intensive lifestyle intervention group or the control group. The lifestyle intervention group participated in 42 group and/or counseling sessions over a year's time, while the control group met only three times for educational sessions. The intensive lifestyle group was able to achieve the gold standard with weight loss—just over 8%, while the control group was unable to achieve significant weight losses.

Treatment Delivery

Lifestyle modification programs can be delivered in groups, one-on-one sessions, or a combination of both. Sessions typically meet weekly in 60–90-minute intervals and are facilitated by registered dietitians (RDs), behavioral psychologists, and/or exercise specialists. The group may begin with a didactic component, with presentation of a nutrition/behavioral topic, followed by planning for the upcoming week [12]. The meeting's focus is program adherence, problem-solving specific steps to accomplish desired behaviors, relapse prevention, and recovery in addition, to review of alternative coping strategies exclusive of food.

Groups

Facilitating patients to support each other in a group process can be effective in getting patients to change their behavior, as well as taking some of the burden off the provider. Other benefits to the group process include helping patients not feel alone with their weight struggle, reducing the cost of individual appointments typically not covered by insurance, and increasing patients' motivation to comply as their weight change is made public during meetings [12]. This accountability and support is what attracts patients to these groups. Perri and colleagues demonstrated significantly greater weight reductions in subjects when behavioral therapy was conducted in groups versus individually [13].

Additionally, group commercial weight loss programs enhanced induction of clinically significant weight losses in the Lighten Up Study. This randomized controlled trial compared one-on-one counseling sessions conducted in primary care offices to group commercial weight loss programs in over 700 subjects. The study authors suspect the primary care providers' less than superior results may have been due in part to the missing group dynamic. [14].

Group attendance is often predictive of weight loss [15, 16]. While the data supporting group behavioral therapy may be more apparent, groups are not ideal for every patient. It is anecdotally true that patients can and do *hide out* in groups.

Remote Support

Appel et al. recently found remote support equally effective at producing clinically significant weight losses in obese subjects when compared with *in-person* behavioral treatment [17]. Both the in-person and remote support patients attended follow-up visits at 6, 12, and 24 months with the primary care physician (PCP) where they were weighed and provided guidance on their computer-generated report accessed from the website. Trained weight loss coaches worked in collaboration with the PCP in delivering group or individual sessions to the *in-person* intervention, while those in the *remote support* intervention were counseled via telephone. The delivery of the behavioral counseling, not the frequency, was the defining characteristic between the two interventions.

At the conclusion of 2 years, the weight change from baseline was 1.1% in the control group, 5% receiving remote support, and 5.2% in the group receiving in-person treatment. These results demonstrate that the remote behavioral counseling can be just as effective as face-to-face counseling in achieving clinically significant weight losses.

Internet behavioral counseling was also compared to standard Internet treatment. All participants were asked to submit their weight and food records via a web-based diary. Email reminders were submitted weekly for the entire 12 months of the study. The behavioral counseling group received feedback on their food records, reinforcement for identified behaviors, and recommendations for change. At 12 months, the addition of e-counseling doubled the percentage of initial weight loss from 2.2 to 4.8 % [18] compared to the standard treatment group.

The paradigm of remote counseling with reinforcement has far-reaching implications. Consider the patient's reduced burden from missing time from work, finding and paying for a parking space, and cost of commuting. While more studies are needed to confirm its effectiveness, this and other recent studies are promising.

Weight Loss Surgery Candidates

Although surgical weight losses produce the maximum results, not every patient is a candidate for weight loss surgery or open to this type of intervention. Furthermore, the realities of weight regain after bariatric surgery have been demonstrated [19]. Encouraging surgical patients both pre- and postoperatively to practice specific lifestyle interventions may help bode for a more successful outcome and dismiss patient's false belief that surgery will "cure their obesity" and reduce postsurgical complications [20].

A randomized controlled trial found Hispanic subjects who received "comprehensive nutrition and lifestyle education" sessions experienced significantly greater excess weight losses at 1 year following, gastric bypass than their control counterparts [21]. Additionally, postoperative gastric bypass subjects who engaged in dietary self-monitoring were less likely to suffer from weight regain [22, 23]. Further studies are needed that examine the impact of lifestyle modification on pre- and postsurgery subjects since there are a limited number of well-designed randomized controlled trials [24].

Choose Your Words Wisely

It is important to put yourself in the shoes of the patient, especially since negative biases from health-care providers towards their obese patients have been demonstrated [7]. Barbara Rolls [25] and her colleagues from the Department of Nutritional Science at Pennsylvania State University found that subjects are more apt to change their behavior after hearing *what to do* in lieu of *what not to do*. Two types of messages were delivered to two randomly assigned groups of obese women. The first group of women was counseled to reduce their fat intake, while the second group was advised to increase the energy density of their diet. Energy density is the amount of total calories of a food, related to its weight. Influencers of food's energy density include water, fiber, and fat. Fruits and vegetables are a mainstay of low-energy-dense or low-calorie diets.

Throughout the year, both groups received individualized counseling with weigh-ins and participated in group lessons consisting of holiday eating, label reading, dining out, grocery shopping, and recipe modification. Both groups were asked to keep food records and these records were reviewed individually with the dietitian.

Significant weight losses were achieved in both groups. However, the group that was advised to add more water-rich foods, was able to lose 33 % more weight at 6 months compared to the group coached in the more traditional restrictive messages to eat less. Additionally, records kept by the participants indicated that those who ate more water-rich foods consumed 25 % greater food by weight and experienced less hunger than those on the reduced fat approach. The authors speculate that the increased compliance was also attributable to the increased satiety from the high volume of food consumed.

This study coincides with American beliefs reported in the International Food Information Council Foundation in which 78 % of Americans identified themselves as preferring to hear what they should eat rather than what they *should not eat* [26].

A smaller-scale study done by Epstein [27] and colleagues found encouraging consumption of fruit and vegetables to families with children at high risk of obesity experienced better outcomes, compared to the group who received messages to *decrease* their fat and sugar intake. Interestingly, the parents of the high-risk children, not the children, experienced significant weight losses and increased their fruit and vegetable intake by approximately three servings per day; in contrast to their low-fat, low-sugar group counterparts.

Self-monitoring With Food Journaling

Self-monitoring is the cornerstone of many weight loss interventions. Albert Bandera, the father of social cognitive theory (SCT), asserts that self-monitoring is a process which forces us to pay attention to our own behavior. SCT assumes that without this focus, undesired actions, such as eating foods that we otherwise would not eat or know we should not eat, cannot be modified. Ultimately, self-monitoring promotes self-regulation [28]. A meta-analysis published in the *Journal of the American Dietetic Association* reviewed the effectiveness of dietary self-monitoring and its effects on weight loss in 15 studies. Associations between self-monitoring and weight loss were consistently found. As one might estimate, weight losses are highly correlated with frequent and more thorough food records [29, 30].

Dietary Self-monitoring Using Technology

While self-monitoring is effective, providers need strategies to increase compliance with this essential behavior. Self-monitoring using technology is one recently identified strategy. As of now, greater weight losses occur when remote technology is added to in-person patient provider contact [31–33].

Lora Burke and her colleagues discovered increased compliance with food re-cording using personal digital assistants (PDAs). This advantage was noted to be most beneficial in the first 6 months of the study, where PDA users self-monitored 80–90 % of the time, compared to their paper recording counterparts who only self-monitored 55 % of the time [16].

The greatest adherence and weight losses were witnessed in the group that re-ceived personalized feedback messages through the PDA platform. PDA messages were tailored to the individual and included such reminders as "taking a few min-utes to record will help you meet your goals" *or* "watch portion sizes to control calories." All study groups (paper method, PDA, and PDA with feedback) experi-enced some weight regain in the 2nd year of the study, with the *least* amount in the PDA with feedback. The authors concluded that the additive *coaching* may have been responsible for the superior results.

Similar results were published in the *Journal of Internal Medicine* where pre-dominantly male subjects were randomized into a technology or *standard* interven-tion group [34]. The technology group received coaching calls, was advised to re-cord food intake throughout the day via their PDA, and attended behavioral classes led by a psychologist, dietitian, or physician. The standard group did not receive coaching calls but tracked their food via paper method and attended group meet-ings. The technology group achieved and *sustained* significantly greater weight losses contrasted with the standard group. This benefit occurred for the remainder of the study (7–12 months), even after cessation of the coaching calls. The enhanced weight losses may have been due to the combination of individualized coaching calls and tracking technology.

Using technology to increase compliance of self-monitoring shows promise and is aligned with our technology-centered world. Once patients learn how to self-monitor using specific *apps* and software, most of them are relieved at the ease of entering their food. They have access to a large database of foods; foods are subto-taled as they are entered and the ability to reach calorie and protein goals are con-cretely assessed on a day-to-day basis. Additional benefits include easy retraction of frequently eaten meals and portability of the "paperless notebook" in the event a smart phone or tablet is used.

According to SCT, not all patients possess the "behavioral capability" to perform self-monitoring effectively. This process of skills training may need to be part of in-clinic consultations or group meetings.

Another strategy to increase compliance with self-monitoring and behavior change, in general, may be reminding patients they do not have to be perfect. Patients hold themselves to very high standards and this "perfectionist" mentality may often be a barrier to change or managing unexpected setbacks. In Lora Burke's study [16], subjects who adhered to food recording 30–59 % of the time were nonetheless able to lose significant weight. Consistency with self-monitoring should ultimately be the focus, as this will have the greatest impact with weight loss. However, benefits are achieved even when our patients have not been compliant all the time. Studies have shown that early compliance (with self-monitoring and attendance) predicts long-term weight losses in the POUNDS LOST study (prevention of obesity using novel dietary strategies) [35].

Improving Underreporting of Food Intake

It is estimated that underreporting is more common in the obese population, which have been known to underestimate their caloric intake by as much as 20–40 % [7]. These uncounted calories could prevent patients from losing weight. While meal replacements may help alleviate some of these errors, it is desirable for patients to improve upon their ability to estimate portion sizes. Several researchers have invariably found improvements in reporting errors with specialized self-monitoring training [36]. The various teaching media include food models, food photographs, illustrations or graphs. A focus group acknowledged that this type of food estimation training improved their comfort in reporting less socially desirable food choices. The goal of this specialized training is to mitigate underreporting errors, not necessarily ameliorate this phenomenon. A registered or licensed dietitian professional is highly skilled at this type of instruction.

Self-monitoring With Weighing

Similar to self-monitoring of food consumed, regular weighing can both slow weight regain and facilitate weight losses. While the necessary frequency is debated, individuals who weigh at least once weekly can more quickly identify a lapse or obtain reinforcement for a behavioral accomplishment. The Institute of Medicine of the National Academy of Sciences, the World Health Organization, and the National Heart, Lung and Blood Institute all recommend regular weighing to help ensure long-term weight maintenance [1].

A review article by VanWormer and colleagues examined the evidence of 12 studies that included frequent self-weighing. They concluded from 11 out of the 12 studies that frequent self-weighing is a good predictor of moderate weight loss and weight maintenance. This is true for both for individuals who have lost weight and are attempting to keep it off, and for individuals who are attempting to avoid weight gain in the first place [37, 38].

The Health Works trial examined the efficacy of preventing weight gain via frequent weighing. Six worksites with more these 250 employees in the Minneapolis area were recruited. Three of the worksites received a weight gain prevention intervention and the other three worksites received no treatment. Weights were measured at baseline and 24-month follow-up. The intervention group had access to stations with scales where they recorded and submitted their weight into a locked box. At 2-year follow-up, monthly self-weighers ended up gaining weight, while daily self-weighers experienced the greatest weight losses [39].

The study to prevent regain (STOP) tested the efficacy of weekly weighing as a self-regulation strategy to prevent weight regain after significant weight loss. Over 300 subjects who had lost at least 10% of their initial body weight within 2 years prior were recruited to either a face-to-face intervention, Internet intervention, or control group. Both intervention groups were given a scale, weighed and submitted their weekly weight through the telephone or Internet. They were taught to compare their maintenance start weight with their current weight. If they had gained more than 3 pounds, they were instructed to use the weight loss approach that afforded them the initial weight loss or a standard behavioral approach.

Both groups attended weekly meetings in the first month and then monthly thereafter throughout the 18-month study. The Internet group participated in their meetings via a chat room led by the same nutritionist, exercise physiologist, and clinical psychologist who led the face-to-face group. Clinic assessments occurred for all groups at 6, 12, and 18 months. During the 18-month period, 72% of the control group regained greater than 5 pounds, compared with only 54.8% in the Internet group and 45.7% in the face-to-face group. While the face-to-face group produced the most superior results, the Internet intervention should be considered a viable option to help patients prevent weight regain [40].

The evidence supports encouraging patients to weigh often. Reminding resistant patients of the benefits of weighing and that their weight is unrelated to their worth is appropriate.

Macronutrients and Dietary Interventions

Only one in three Americans realizes that *all* calorie sources influence weight gain. Equally troubling, only 38% of Americans give serious thought about the number of calories they consume [26].

Providers and patients inquire what specific macronutrient or macronutrient combination will afford the greatest weight loss. Sacks and colleagues set out to investigate this pressing question and recruited over 800 subjects and randomly assigned them to one of four diet groups, including: low fat, average protein; low fat, high protein; high fat, average protein; or high fat, high protein. Meal plans, group and individual sessions were provided over 2 year's time. Each diet, irrespective of macronutrient intake, was *equally* successful at achieving clinically significant weight loss and maintenance [15]. Similarly, Dansinger and colleagues found that diet compliance, irrespective of dietary intervention type (Atkins, Ornish, Weight Watchers, and the Zone), was the greatest determinant in predicting weight losses [41].

Superior initial weight losses have been demonstrated in the low-carbohydrate diet approach when contrasted with the conventional low-fat diet. However, these weight loss differences become statistically insignificant at 1 year [42–44].

One identified limitation of these specific low-carbohydrate dietary interventions is the lack of behavioral counseling. Subsequently, Foster and colleagues sought out to investigate the effects of a low-carbohydrate approach compared with a low-fat diet; this time, with the incorporation of intensive lifestyle counseling. Interestingly, the results of this 2-year trial echo Sacks' conclusions; that lifestyle modification programs help facilitate greater adherence to *any* dietary approach [45].

While Mediterranean diets have the potential to be calorically dense, they are showing promise with weight loss. Common foods consumed with this approach are nuts at 175 kcal/ounce, olive oil at 120 kcal/tablespoon and avocado, one-half of whole equal to 150 kcal. The dietary intervention randomized controlled trial (DIRECT) study evaluated a calorie-restricted Mediterranean diet, different from the traditional Mediterranean diet. They randomly assigned over 300 moderately obese adults to one of the three diet interventions. The dietary interventions included a calorie-restricted low-fat diet, a Mediterranean calorie-restricted diet, or a low-carbohydrate noncalorie restricted diet over 2 year's time. The subjects in the Mediterranean arm were advised to not exceed 35% of the calories coming from fat. They consumed 2–3 tablespoons of olive oil and 5–7 nuts per day, fish and . chicken, and high quantities of vegetables. The intervention model used dietary group sessions by an RD, spousal support, food labels in the cafeteria, and monthly weighing—all conducted in the subject's workplace. At the conclusion of 2 years, both the Mediterranean and low-carbohydrate groups' weight losses were greatest when compared to the calorie-controlled low-fat diet [46].

Similarly, a low-carbohydrate Mediterranean (LCM) diet was compared to a standard Mediterranean and American Diabetes Association (ADA) diet in a community-based intervention [47]. The subjects were overweight individuals with type II DM and randomly assigned to one of the dietary interventions. All of the subjects met individually with the dietitian every 2 weeks for 1 year. While the weight loss in the LCM group was greatest, this difference was not considered significant. It is notable that the LCM group achieved the greatest metabolic benefit. High-density lipoprotein (HDL) levels in the LCM group increased by 12% and low-density lipoprotein (LDL) levels were reduced by an additional 8% when compared to the other diet intervention. This type of dietary intervention should be considered for patients with diabetes who are at high risk of cardiovascular events [47, 48].

Meal Replacements Accelerate Weight Loss

Meal replacements are premeasured portioned food products that are used to replace conventional meals or snacks. Protein shakes, preportioned entrees, and protein-rich bars are available both over-the-counter or at medically supervised weight loss clinics. Meal replacement usage is a common dietary intervention of lifestyle programs and should be considered as a viable weight loss approach.

Besides replacing higher calorie conventional food choices, meal replacements are thought to enhance compliance through simplifying food choices, controlling portions, and providing easy-to-prepare meals and snacks. When a two preportioned entree-per day-regimen was compared to a self-select diet group, the subjects consuming preportioned entrees were able to lose 56% more weight [49]. Meal replacements exceed patients' ability to choose, prepare, measure, and consume foods in the recommended portions.

A study by Ashley and colleagues analyzed the effectiveness of using meal replacements in premenopausal overweight women. Over 100 subjects were randomized into one of the three groups: RD visits without meal replacements (MRs), RD group visits with MRs *or* 10-min nurse/MD visits with MRs. In the second year, all of the groups attended monthly seminars with quick visits with the RD. The group with the RD group visits and MR showed the greatest differences in weight loss with increased ability to maintain their weight losses [50].

Very low calorie diets (VLCDs) are dietary interventions comprising complete meal replacement usage totaling as low as < 500 kcal per day. The long-term efficacy of the VLCD approach is and has been questioned. In 1994, Wadden and Foster were able to show the superior weight loss effect of VLCDs at 6 months; however, this group regained approximately 50 % of the weight they initially lost at 1 year when compared to their balanced deficit diet (BDD) counterparts who successfully maintained all of their initial losses [51]. This study supports proponents of "slow and steady" weight loss.

Anderson and colleagues sought out to examine long-term weight loss maintenance of individuals completing a structured weight loss program. This meta-analysis examined four very low energy diets (VLEDs) with eight hypo-energetic balanced diets (HBDs). Both groups had follow-up weights at 4.5 years. The comparison found that subjects who had greater initial weight losses were able to maintain three times more weight loss at 4.5 years than their HBD counterparts. Thus, while both subsets ended up with some weight regain, the VLED subjects fared better both with initial weight losses and sustaining their weight losses. In fact, the VLED individuals were successfully maintaining 23.4 % of their initial weight loss at 5 years [52]. These results support the hypothesis that momentous weight losses keep patients more engaged and motivated, hence, ultimately more successful.

The benefit of using meal replacements has also been demonstrated in maintenance. Anderson and colleagues prospectively identified patients who lost at least 100 pounds. The subjects participated in an intensive, medically-supervised, behavioral weight management intervention using meal replacements. These subjects attended weekly behavioral education classes for 18 months and then returned to the program for re-treatment during the 5 years they were followed. During maintenance, they were counseled to consume a minimum of 2 MRs per day, greater than 2000 kcal/week of physical activity expenditure, and ≥35 servings of fruits and vegetables per week. At 5 years, 58 % of the subjects were keeping off on average 66 pounds or 49 % of their initial weight losses [53].

Partial meal replacement (PMR) usage is a compromised approach between a strict VLCD and a balanced deficit diet (BDD). It is composed of one to two portion-controlled MRs along with conventional meals and snacks. Heymsfield and colleagues reviewed six randomized controlled trials using PMRs in a meta-analysis. Weight losses after 1 year in the PMR-treated subjects exceeded the BDD -treated group by 5.3–7.5 pounds. Moreover, the PMR group witnessed a reduced attrition rate [54].

The intervention arm of the Look AHEAD trial additionally used PMRs. Subjects were advised to replace breakfast and lunch with an over-the-counter or physician-prescribed protein-rich shake and one snack with a protein-rich bar. Dinner provided the option of prepared entrees or conventional foods. Two-meal replacement per day were additionally recommended 7–12 months into the study intervention to help maintain the initial weight that was lost. When stratifying meal replacement usage into quartiles, subjects who consumed a greater number of meal replacements lost significantly more weight. Participants with the highest quartile of meal replacement usage had four times greater odds of reaching the 7 % weight loss goal than subjects in the lowest quartile [55].

Despite research available outlining the benefits of VLCDs or PMR programs, consideration of a patient's food preferences in tailoring a particular food plan should be first and foremost. Providing patients with defined food plans outlining specific food types and amounts has also been shown to be effective and should be considered as an alternative to patients who are adverse to meal replacements [56].

Environment Influences Food Choices

According to the 2013 Food & Health Survey, 64 % of Americans identified their lack of taking greater control of their weight, attributable to their "lack of willpower [26]." In truth, environmental cues or triggers such as the oversized dinner plate, family-sized box of breakfast cereal, or option to super-size a meal, may be a greater contributor to overeating. These types of environmental triggers should be assessed when counseling patients desiring to lose weight.

In 2004, both a *Washington Post* article titled, "Whose Fault is Fat?" and Yale Center for Eating and Weight Disorders, director Kelly Brownell's book *Food Fight,* make the argument that "genes load the gun and the environment pulls the trigger [57, 58]." Furthermore, the estimated increase in energy intake of more than 500 calories per day from 1970 to 2000 supports the notion that our environment is the likely culprit of increasing weights in both children and adults from the National Health and Nutrition Examination Survey [59–61].

Examples of environmental strategies that mitigate eating include eating off a small dinner plate, having fruits and vegetables in obvious locations, avoiding purchasing trigger types of foods (i.e., large bag of chips), purchasing preportioned foods, bringing healthier options of foods to events where tempting foods will be present, and sharing restaurant entrees. For a detailed publication to provide to patients, see America on the Move's 100 Ways to Create an Environment for Success [62].

Implementation Intentions (Otherwise Known as Planning)

Eighty-one percent of Americans feel they have direct control over their weight with 88% believing they have control over the healthfulness of their diet [26]. While that belief may exist, there is clearly a gap between good intentions to eat healthfully and actual behavior. A recent meta-analysis sought to investigate if "implementation intentions"—which specify the where, when, and how of goal attainment—improved fruit and vegetable consumption and reduced consumption of unhealthy snacks.

"If I am in the grocery store and tempted to eat a chocolate bar, I will consume the protein bar in my purse instead" is an example of an implementation intention. Implementation intentions which promoted healthy eating behaviors found positive effects in 12 out of 15 studies. Reviewing how patients will achieve specific desired behaviors in classes or appointments is both a relevant and beneficial behavioral tool [63].

Conclusion

Treating obesity as a chronic disease, as recently defined by the American Medical Association, is crucial [64]. With an estimated 80% of people not following the advice of their health-care providers to change health behaviors [65], it should be no surprise that this line of work needs ample follow-up, patience, and fine tuning. Avoidance of losing patients to follow-up should be of primary concern. Recognize that patients feel shame and may avoid confronting their suboptimal performance. Empathize with them and remind them you are there to help problem-solve adherence and not to judge.

The aforementioned strategies of self-monitoring, meal replacement usage, and environmental control into a comprehensive weight loss program or individual patient appointment are viable and vetted components to be considered while treating obese and/or overweight patients. The goal is to find which specific techniques work for your patients while helping them avoid feeling too overwhelmed.

References

1. National Heart, Lung, and Blood Institute and the North American Association for the Study of Obesity. The Practical Guide: Identification, Evaluation, and Treatment of Overweight and Obesity in Adults. National Institutes of Health. MD: Bethesda; 2000.
2. Morton JM. The affordable care act: key elements and what it means for bariatric surgery. 2013;10(1):8.
3. Moyer VA. On behalf of the U.S. preventative services task force. Screening for and management of obesity in adults. U.S. Preventative Services Task Force recommendation statement. Ann Intern Med. 2012;157:373–8.

4. Centers for Medicaid and Medicare Services. Decision memo for behavioral therapy for obesity (CAG-00423N). http://www.cms.gov/medicare-coveragedbase/details/ncadecision-memo.aspx?&NcaName=Intensive%20Behavioral%20Therapy%20for%20Obesity&bc=A CAAAAAAIAAA&NCAId=253. Accessed 29 Nov 2011.
5. Wadden TA, Webb VL, Moran CH, Bailer BA. Lifestyle modification for obesity: new developments in diet, physical activity, and behavior therapy. Circulation. 2012;125:1157–70.
6. Wadden TA, Butryn ML, Byrne KJ. Efficacy of lifestyle modification for long-term weight control. Obes Res. 2004;12:151S–62S.
7. Foster G, Makris A, Bailer B. Behavioral treatment of obesity. Am J Clin Nutr. 2005;82(suppl):230S–5S.
8. Foster GD, Nonas CA. Managing obesity: a clinical guide. American Dietetic Association; 2004. (Insert author query- Author: Please provide publishers' main location for the following references "Foster and Nonas 2004" and "Constance and Sauter 2011".)
9. VanBuskirk KA, Wetherell JL. Motivational interviewing with primary care populations: a systematic review and meta-analysis. J Behav Med. 2013;37:768–80.
10. Diabetes prevention program research group. N Engl J Med. 2002;346(6):393–403.
11. Wadden TA, West DS, et al. One year weight losses in the Look AHEAD study: factors associated with success. Obesity (Silver Spring). 2009;17(4):713–22.
12. Wadden TA, Butryn M, Wilson C. Lifestyle modification for the management of obesity. Gastroenterology. 2007;132:2226–38.
13. Rejilian DA, Perri MG, et al. Individual vs group therapy for obesity: effects of matching participants to their treatment preference. J Consult Clin Psychol. 2001;69:717–21.
14. Jolly K, Lewis A, et al. Comparison of range of commercial or primary care led weight reduction programs with minimal intervention control for weight loss in obesity: lighten Up randomized controlled trial. BMJ. 2011;343:d6500
15. Sacks FM, Bray GA, et al. Comparison of weight-loss diets with different compositions of fat, protein and carbohydrate. N Engl J Med. 2009;360:859–73.
16. Burke LE, Styn MA, et al. Using mHealth technology to enhance self monitoring for weight loss: a randomized trial. Am J Prev Med. 2012;43(1):20–6.
17. Appel, LJ, Clark, JM, et al. Comparative effectiveness of weight loss interventions in clinical practice. N Eng J Med. 2011;365:1959–68.
18. Tate DF, Jackvony EH, Wing RR. Effects of internet behavioral counseling on weight loss in adults at risk for type 2 diabetes: a randomized trial. JAMA. 2003;289(14):1833–6.
19. Sjostrom, L, Narbro, K, et al. Effects of bariatric surgery on mortality in Swedish obese subjects. N Engl J Med. 2007;357:741–52.
20. Benotti P, Still C, et al. Preoperative Weight loss before bariatric surgery. Arch Surg. 2009;144:1150–5.
21. Nijamkin M, Campa A, et al. Comprehensive nutrition and lifestyle education improves weight loss and physical activity in Hispanic Americans following gastric bypass surgery: a randomized controlled trial. J Acad of Nutr and Diet. 2012;112:382–90.
22. Odom J, Zalesin K, et al. Behavioral predictors of weight regain after bariatric surgery. Obes Surg. 2009;20:349–56.
23. Lynch A, Bisogni C. Understanding dietary self-monitoring and self-weighing by gastric bypass patients: a pilot study of self monitoring behaviors and long-term weight outcomes. Obes Surg. 2012;22:1818–26.
24. Cassie S, Menezes, et al. Effect of preoperative weight loss in bariatric surgical patients: a systematic review. Sug Obes Rel Dis. 2011;7:760–8.
25. Rolls BJ, Ello-Martin JA, et al. Dietary energy density in the treatment of obesity: a yearlong trial comparing two weight loss diets. Am J Clin Nutri. 2007;85:1465–77.
26. Food & Health Survey. Consumer Attitudes toward Food Safety, Nutrition & Health. International Food Information Council Foundation; 2013.
27. Epstein LH, Gordy CC, et al. Increasing fruit and vegetable intake and decreasing fat and sugar intake in families at risk for childhood obesity. Obes Res. 2001;3:171–8.

28. Bandura A. Social cognitive theory of self-regulation. Org Behav Hum Decis Process. 1991;50:248–187.
29. Burke LE, Wang J. Self-monitoring in weight loss: a systematic review of the literature. J Am Diet Assoc. 2011;111:92–102.
30. Streit KJ, Steven NH. Food records: a predictor and modifier of weight change in a long-term weight loss program. J Am Diet Assoc. 1991;1991(2):213–16.
31. Pellegrini CA, Verba SD, et al. The comparison of a technology-based system and an in-person behavioral weight loss intervention. Obesity (Silver Spring). 2012;20(2):356–63.
32. Shuger SL, Barry VW, et al. Electronic feedback in a diet- and physical activity based life-style intervention for weight loss: a randomized controlled trial. Int J Behav Nutr Phys Act. 2011;8:41.
33. Harvey-Berino J, West D, et al. Internet delivered behavioral obesity treatment. Prev Med. 2010;51(2):123–8.
34. Spring B, Duncan JM, et al. Integrating technology into a standard weight loss treatment. JAMA Intern Med. 2013;173(2):105–11.
35. Williamson DA, Anton SD, Han H, Champagne, C, Allen R, LeBlanc E, Ryan D, Rood J, McManus K, Laranjo N, Carey VJ, Loria CM, Bray GA, Sacks FM. Early behavioral adherence predicts short and long-term weight loss in the POUNDS LOST study. J Behav Med. 2010;33(4):305–14.
36. Scagliusi FB, Polacow VO, Guilherme AG, Benatti FB, Lancha AH. Selective underreporting of energy intake in women: magnitude, determinants and effect of training. J Am Diet Assoc. 2003;103:1306–13. (36–40).
37. Van Wormer JJ, French SA, Pereira MA, Welsh EM. The impact of regular self-weighing on weight management: a systematic review. Intl J of Behav Nutr and Phys Activity. 2008;5(54).
38. Van Wormer JJ Martinez AM Martinson BC Crain AL Benson G Cosentino DL Pronk NP. Self weighing promotes weight loss for obese adults. Am J Prev Med. 2009;36(1):70–3.
39. Van Wormer JJ, Linde JA, Harnack LJ, Stovitz SD, Jeffery RW. Self-weighing frequency is associated with weight gain prevention over 2 years among working adults. Int J Behav Med. 2012;19:351–8.
40. Wing, RR, Tate DF, Gorin AA, Raynor HA, Fava JL. A self-regulation program for maintenance of weight loss. N Engl J Med. 2006;355(15):1563–71.
41. Dansiger ML, et al. Comparison of the Atkins, Ornish, Weight Watchers, and Zone diets for weight loss and heart disease risk factors: a randomized trial. JAMA. 2005;293:43–53.
42. Foster GD, Wyatt HR, et al. A randomized trial of a low-carbohydrate diet for obesity. New Eng J Med. 2003;348:2082–90.
43. Stern L, Iqbal N, et al. The effects of a low-carbohydrate versus conventional weight loss diet in severely obese adults: one-year follow-up of a randomized trial. Ann Intern Med. 2004;140:778–85.
44. Nordmann AJ, et al. Effects of low-carbohydrate vs low-fat diets on weight loss and cardiovascular risk factors: a meta-analysis of randomized controlled trials. Arch Intern Med. 2006;166:285–93.
45. Foster GD, Wyatt HR, et al. Weight and metabolic outcomes after 2 years on a low-carbohydrate versus low-fat diet: a randomized trial. Ann Intern Med. 2010;153:147–57.
46. Shai I, Schwarzfuchs D, et al. Weight loss with a low-carbohydrate, Mediterranean, or low-fat diet. N Engl J Med. 2008;359:229–41.
47. Elhayany A, Lustman A, et al. A low carbohydrate Mediterranean diet improves cardiovascular risk factors and diabetes control among overweight patients with type 2 diabetes mellitus: a 1 year prospective randomized intervention study. Diabetes Obes Metab. 2010;12:204–9.
48. Ajala O, English P, et al. Systematic review and meta-analysis of different dietary approaches to the management of type 2 diabetes. Am J Clin Nutr. 2013;97:505–16.
49. Hannum SM, et al. Use of portion-controlled entrees enhances weight loss in women. Obes Res. 2004;12(3):538–46.
50. Ashley, JM, St. Jeor ST, Perumean-Chaney S, Schrage, J, Bovee V. Meal replacements in weight intervention. Obes Res. 2001;9(suppl 4):312S–20S.

51. Wadden TA, Foster GD, Letizia KA. One-year behavioral treatment of obesity: comparison of moderate and severe caloric restriction and the effects of weight maintenance therapy. Consult Clin Psychol. 1994;62:165–71.
52. Anderson JW, Konz EC, Frederich RC, Wood CL. Long term weight loss maintenance: a meta-analysis of US studies. Am J Clin Nutr. 2001:74:579–84.
53. Anderson JW, Conley SB, Nicholas AS. One hundred pound weight losses with an intensive behavioral program: changes in risk factors in 118 patients with long-term follow up. Am J Clin Nutr. 2007;86:301–7.
54. Heymsfield SB, et al. Weight management using a meal replacement strategy: Meta and pooling analysis from six studies. Int J of Obes. 2003;27:537–49.
55. Wadden TA, West DS., et al. One year weight losses in the Look AHEAD study: factors associated with success. Obesity (Silver Spring). 2009;17(4):713–22.
56. Wing, RR, Jeffery RW. Food provision as a strategy to promote weight loss. Obes Res. 2001;9(Suppl 4):271S–5S.
57. Tallmadge K. Whose fault is fat? Washington Post. http://www.washingtonpost.com/wp-dyn/articles/A46127-2004Jul13.html. Accessed 14 July 2004.
58. Brownell K, Horgen KB. Food fight: the inside story of the food industry, America's obesity crisis, and what we can do about it. NY: McGraw-Hill; 2004.
59. Wansink B, Ittersum KV, Painter, J. Ice cream illusions; bowls, spoons, and self-served portion sizes. Am J Prev Med. 2006;31(3):240–3.
60. Swinburn B, Sacks G, Ravussin E. Increased food energy supply is more than sufficient to explain the US epidemic of obesity. Am J Clin Nutr. 2009;90:1453–6.
61. Wansink B, Painter JE, Lee Y-K. The office candy dish: proximity's influence on estimated and actual consumption. Intl J of Obes. 2006;30:871–5.
62. America on the Move Steps to a Healthier Life. 100 ways to surround your family with success. https://aom3.americaonthemove.org/~/media/91787CD757B64955A5D04FFC9D3EA4F5.ashx (2007).
63. Adriaanse MA, Vinkers CDW, et al. Do implementation intentions help to eat a healthy diet? A systematic review and meta-analysis of the empirical evidence. Appetite. 2011;56:183–93.
64. American Medical Association House of Delegates (Internet). (cited 2013 May 16). http://www.npr.org/documents/2013/jun/ama-resolution-obesity.pdf (2013).
65. Constance A, Sauter, C. Inspiring and supporting behavior change: a food and nutrition professional's counseling guide. American Dietetic Association; 2011. (Publisher Location is missing, author query required)

Chapter 5
Physical Activity and Writing an Exercise Prescription

Alexis Peraino

Physical Activity trends

Obesity trends have demonstrated a steady rise over the past several decades (www.cdc.gov/obesity/data/trends) [1]. Obesity has increased as a major public health concern over the last several decades, and so has the focus on identifying the risk factors and lifestyle habits that contribute to this epidemic. Physical activity and exercise are seen as markers of health and fitness; however, as a whole the American population repeatedly falls short on meeting minimum activity recommendations. Optimal physical activity levels help to combat and prevent obesity and many of its comorbidities. The benefits of exercise not only include weight loss and weight maintenance but also go well beyond just weight management. Physicians are fundamental to addressing obesity in the office as well as encouraging patients to alter unhealthy lifestyle habits. Just as physicians provide prescriptions to aid with smoking cessation or hypertension, physicians also need to play a role in addressing and encouraging Americans of all ages to participate in regular physical activity. Unfortunately, many physicians lack the time or expertise to counsel patients regarding the benefits of activity as well as the steps needed to begin an exercise program.

Multiple measures of activity levels in Americans show consistent and underwhelming trends—essentially most Americans do not exercise routinely or enough to receive many of the benefits for optimal health and wellness. Leisure-time physical activity measures from 1988 to 2008 demonstrate consistent rates of inactivity ranging from 31% in 1988 to about 25% of the population in 2008 [2]. Essentially, one person in four did not participate in any consistent or regular leisure-time activity in 2010 according to the Centers for Disease Control and Prevention's (CDC)

A. Peraino (✉)
Internal Medicine, California Health and Longevity Institute,
2 Dole Drive, Westlake Village, CA 91362, USA
e-mail: aperaino@CHLI.com

© Springer Science+Business Media New York 2015
A. Youdim (ed.), *The Clinician's Guide to the Treatment of Obesity*,
Endocrine Updates, DOI 10.1007/978-1-4939-2146-1_5

Table 5.1 General physical activities defined by level of intensity. The following is in accordance with CDC and ACSM guidelines. (http://www.cdc.gov/physicalactivity/everyone/measuring/index.html, http://www.cdc.gov/nccdphp/dnpa/physical/pdf/PA_Intensity_table_2_1.pdf)

Moderate intensity 3.0–6.0 METs (3.5–7 kcal/min)	Vigorous intensity Greater than 6.0 METs (than 7 kcal/min)
Walking briskly (3–4.5 mph, but not race walking)	Race walking, jogging, or running
	Swimming laps
Water aerobics	Tennis (singles)
Bicycling slower than 10 miles per hour	Aerobic dancing
Tennis (doubles)	Bicycling 10 miles per hour or faster
Ballroom dancing	Jumping rope
Golf—wheeling or carrying clubs	Heavy gardening (continuous digging or hoeing)
	Hiking uphill or with a heavy backpack

CDC Centers for Disease Control and Prevention, *ACSM* American College of Sports Medicine, *METs* metabolic equivalents

Behavioral Risk Factor Surveillance System (BRFSS) [3]. In 2003, less than half of the US states polled had at least 50 % of the population who achieved recommended levels of physical activity [2]. The recommended levels of activity were defined as 30 min of moderate intensity activity at least 5 days per week or a total of 150 min of activity per week (Table 5.1). Again in 2007, the prevalence of the US adult population to meet recommended physical activity levels was measured between 45 and 50 % in most states [2]. Additionally, in 2005 the BRFSS found that 14 % of Americans were inactive—doing less than 10 min of activity per week [2]. Additionally, 38 % of the population is insufficiently active—they may be doing some activity but not quite enough to gain the health benefits of regular exercise. Between 1997 and 2012, even though there was a trend upward in the number of adults meeting federal recommended activity guidelines, the data still remains unimpressive, see Fig. 5.1. In total, less than 50 % of Americans are achieving the minimum recommended amount of aerobic physical activity on a regular basis, and this number drops to approximately 20 % when you assess the number of Americans achieving the minimum recommended amount of aerobic and resistance activity on a regular basis. This lack of regular activity contributes to an increased risk of obesity as well as an increased risk of mortality from both cardiovascular and noncardiovascular diseases [3–6] (Fig. 5.2).

For decades the CDC and medical societies such as the American College of Sports Medicine (ACSM) and American Heart Association (AHA) have worked to promote physical activity in the American population, however, the results have been disappointing at best. In part, the American population has been inundated with various recommendations from different medical societies as well as the lay press, which has lead to confusion about how much and what type of exercise is really needed on a regular basis for optimal health and fitness. When medical societies

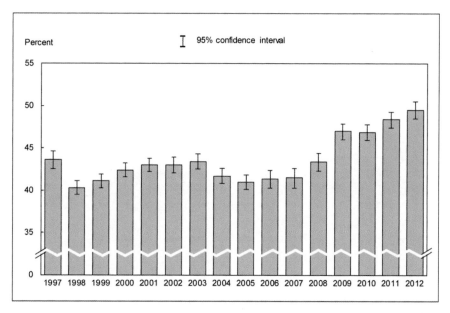

Fig. 5.1 Percentage of adults aged 18 and over who met the 2008 federal physical guidelines for aerobic activity through leisure-time aerobic activity: United States 1997–2012. (Data from the CDC/National Center for Health Statistics (NCHS), National Health Interview Survey, 1997–2002, Sample Adult Core Component)

have quite differing opinions regarding the amount and intensity of activity it leads many to become frustrated. Fortunately, the AHA and the ACSM have helped to clarify the public health recommendations for physical activity. Recommendations are moderate to ensure that they are realistic and achievable, with some of the most recent recommendations in 2008. Additionally, in 2009, the ACSM also published guidelines regarding the amount of physical activity for children, adults and the elderly for weight loss and maintenance. In 1990, 2000 and 2010, physical activity recommendations have been included as a part of the public health goals within the CDC's Healthy People Initiatives. Sadly, as the obesity epidemic continues in the USA, the public health initiatives have not made great strides in significantly impacting physical activity levels.

Definitions

Exercise and physical activity are typically used interchangeably; however, their exact definitions are distinct. Exercise is structured and repetitive physical activity designed to maintain or improve specific components of physical fitness [7, 8]. The components of physical activity include cardiorespiratory endurance, muscular strength, flexibility, and body composition. When individuals train for any activity

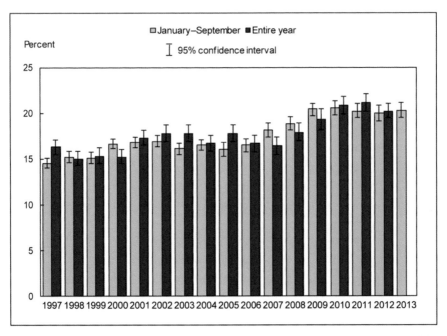

Fig. 5.2 Percentage of adults aged 18 and over who met the 2008 federal physical activity guidelines for both aerobic and muscle-strengthening activities through leisure-time aerobic and muscle-strengthening activities: United States, 1997 to September 2013. (Data from CDC/NCHS, National Health Interview Survey, 1997 to September 2013, Sample Adult Core Component)

or sport, they are performing exercise, examples include running on a treadmill, cycling or taking an aerobics class. While in comparison, the term physical activity includes all leisure and nonleisure body movements resulting in increased energy output from the resting condition [8]. Physical activity includes activities of daily living, occupational activity, transportation, and leisure [7]. Walking your dog, biking to work, vacuuming your home, and gardening are all types of physical activity. All exercise is a type of physical activity; however, all physical activity is not exercise. In short, exercise is intentional physical activity for improving health and fitness [7]. Active daily living, the goal of most health recommendations, is the implementation of physical activity as an integral and meaningful part of daily life. Not only should individuals aim to have structured physical activity daily, they should also focus on being active in nonstructured ways, such as walking to lunch or taking the stairs.

Physical fitness is also used within the literature, and is defined by measured health and skill-related assessments for cardiorespiratory fitness, muscular strength and endurance, body composition, flexibility, balance, agility, reaction time, and power [8]. Different types of exercise and physical activity will help to improve different aspects of physical fitness. For example, running or walking will improve cardiorespiratory fitness while pilates will improve flexibility, balance, and muscular strength. To improve different aspects of one's fitness, it is important to combine a variety of activities.

Exercise can then further be split into aerobic and nonaerobic exercise. Aerobic exercise includes activities that are rhythmic in nature, using large muscle groups at moderate intensities for prolonged periods of time with the goal of keeping the heart rate elevated. The elevation in the heart rate as well as the amount of work performed during the activity determines the intensity of the exercise. The more intense the activity the more energy or calories expended per minute. Typically, intensity is evaluated in terms of metabolic equivalents (METs). METs is the unit used to estimate the amount of oxygen used by the body during physical activity [7, 8].

Moderate intensity physical activity refers to the level of effort in which a person should experience while exercising. There are a variety of definitions of moderate intensity activity and include: some increase in breathing or heart rate, a "perceived exertion" of 11–14 on the Borg scale of 6–20, 3–6 METs, and any activity that burns 3.5–7 calories per minute [7, 8]. While participating in moderate intensity activity patients should be able to hold a conversation with someone; this can be an easy guideline to help patients monitor intensity levels. Examples of moderate intensity activity include walking briskly, dancing, swimming, or bicycling. Vigorous activity levels are typically intense enough to represent a substantial challenge to an individual. With vigorous activity there will be a large increase in heart rate and breathing rate, a perceived exertion score of 15 or greater on the Borg scale of 6–20, a METs of 6 or greater and includes any activity that burns more than 7 calories per minute [7, 8]. Patients will no longer be able to hold a conversation with someone while exercising. Examples of vigorous activity include jogging, high-impact aerobic dancing, swimming continuous laps, or bicycling uphill.

Resistance activity or weight training is nonaerobic activity, which includes movements that use repeated and progressive contractions of specific muscle groups to increase muscle strength, endurance, and power. Traditional resistance training consists of lifting heavier weights with long rest periods in between. In comparison, circuit training includes lifting lighter weights with shorter rest periods in between, which allows for an aerobic component to the workout [9].

Benefits of Exercise

Physical activity and exercise are recommended as fundamental components of weight management programs by most public health agencies and scientific organizations. However, for many patients exercise is seen as a means to an end: you exercise to lose weight. When activity is not combined with other lifestyle interventions, such as dietary change, the results can be disappointing at best [10]. The real benefit of exercise and activity during weight loss is the increased caloric expenditure, which can induce greater weight loss compared with diet alone, even in patients with severe obesity [5]. Physical activity will help to prevent loss of lean body mass during weight loss and will assist with greater reductions in abdominal visceral fat [5, 9]. In addition to the role regular activity plays in active weight loss, studies demonstrate even greater benefit of regular activity in long term weight maintenance and prevention of weight regain [11]. Preventing weight regain can be more difficult than the initial weight loss process itself and physical activity is seen as a must for optimal long-term management [12, 13]. Studies of the National Weight Control Registry point to the inclusion of regular physical activity as one of the cornerstone themes for successful long-term weight management—suggesting the need for higher levels of activity than previously recommended [11]. Weight loss, weight maintenance, and prevention of weight gain are fundamental benefits of regular activity; However, they must be used in combination with diet and life-style change for optimal results.

The benefits of regular physical activity go well beyond weight loss and management. Studies have showed that the relative risk of death from any cause as well as from cardiovascular causes is elevated in patients who are unfit [14]. Furthermore, Myers group has shown that relative risk of death in patients with cardiovascular risk factors was reduced among men who reached an exercise capacity of at least 5 METs. A 1-MET improvement on an exercise test was associated with a 12 % improvement in survival in men [14]. Studies in women have demonstrated similar, if not more impressive, survival benefits as well [15]. Kokkinos et al. demonstrated survival benefits in older men aged 65–92 who were able to achieve an exercise capacity of >5 METs [16]. The Aerobics Center Longitudinal Study of Healthy Women compared death rates of overweight and obese women and found that unfit women had a death rate more than double those of fit women [17]. Additionally, patients do not need to become athletes to reach these benefits. Small improvements in fitness, such as moving from a sedentary to an unsedentary lifestyle can reap the largest health benefits [16, 18, 19]. Blair et al., demonstrated the survival curves for change and lack of change in physical fitness in a study of healthy and unhealthy men, suggesting improved survival benefit for all men moving from unfit to fit quintiles by the end of the trial [20]. Collectively these studies and others suggest that fitness lowers cardiovascular death by a graded and inverse association with cardiovascular and all-cause mortality [14, 15, 17, 21, 22].

The well defined benefits of regular activity include: a reduction in all-cause mortality, heart disease, stroke, type II diabetes, hypertension, hyperlipidemia, metabolic syndrome, colon cancer, and breast cancer [23–25]. Improvements in cholesterol include reductions in total cholesterol, triglyceride and low-density lipoprotein (LDL) levels as well as increases in high-density lipoprotein (HDL) levels [24, 25]. Other important benefits continue to emerge in the literature and include reduced depression, reduced falls, and improved cognitive functioning [25]. And most importantly, lack of weight loss does not diminish these benefits, but lack of consistency with activity does [25]. Some exercise and activity benefits can dissipate after as little as 3 weeks of cessation of activity, so consistent activity is key for persistent long-term benefits [25].

The use of exercise and activity to target a specific disease—for either prevention or treatment—has long been recommended. Chronic diseases including cardiovascular disease, hypertension, hyperlipidemia, hepatic steatosis, diabetes, and arthritis have been shown to improve with regular and consistent physical activity. In severely obese adults, exercise is important for reduction in hepatic steatosis as well abdominal fat [5]. The benefits of physical activity and regular exercise on blood sugar control have long been documented in diabetics as well. Boule et al. demonstrated a reduction in HbA1c of 0.66 % after 8 weeks of exercise intervention despite stable weights following the intervention, suggesting that the impact on HbA1c reduction is independent of weight loss [26]. Exercise increases glycogen synthesis as well as improves free fatty acid delivery and uptake in the muscle, stabilizes key proteins in insulin signaling, improves mitochondrial function, improves capillary blood flow into the muscle, and reduces inflammation via tumor necrosis factor (TNF) alpha [27]. When evaluating the impact of fitness on mortality in diabetics, Church et al. demonstrated that obese men in the lowest fitness group had a 5.6 times higher risk of death compared with normal-weight men in the highest fitness group [28]. Studies have shown that the duration of activity is the primary factor in response to insulin action, with a minimum of 170 min of activity needed per week, regardless of intensity, suggesting that the current guidelines regarding physical activity would prove adequate for diabetics [23, 29]. Not only does physical activity reduce mortality and improve blood sugar in diabetics but also it helps with the prevention of diabetes. The Diabetes Prevention Program Research Group demonstrated a reduction in the risk of developing diabetes early on as well as at the 10-year follow-up in the lifestyle intervention group [30, 31]. These studies demonstrated that lifestyle modification can delay and prevent the development of diabetes and in some cases more effectively than the use of pharmacologic agents. For years, lifestyle changes, i.e., diet and exercise, have been on the forefront of diabetes care, but patients rarely dedicate themselves to making consistent change and physicians do not always have the time to stress its importance. However, the continued support, education, and accountability for each patient are crucial for lifestyle changes to be consistent and successful.

The benefits of resistance activity or strength training have become clearer in the last decade. Classically, resistance training improves muscular strength, muscular endurance, and muscle mass but will not lead to significant weight loss [11]. Strength training does contribute to an increase in basal energy expenditure as well as help to reduce visceral adipose tissue, which is associated with metabolic syndrome [6, 9, 25]. Weight bearing activity on the skeletal system can also stimulate bone formation in young adults and slow bone loss in the middle aged, all of which has helped to lower the risk of osteoporosis, osteopenia, and bone fractures [6, 7, 9, 18, 25]. Resistance activity can also improve glucose metabolism, with improvements in HbA1c of 1.1–1.2 % following consistent strength training activity [26, 32]. Frequently, aerobic activity is thought of as the primary activity to improve cardio-metabolic risk factors, but resistance training can also impact cardio-metabolic risk factors, including improving lipid profiles and aiding with glucose metabolism in diabetics as well as prediabetics [9, 11, 25].

The importance of strength training is frequently overlooked in older patients. However, the benefits of strength training in the elderly are quite impressive and include an improvement in balance and a reduction in falls, as well as improved quality of life, physical independence, and improved skeletal muscle neuromuscular function and structure [9]. There are no age limits to these benefits. Studies have documented improved strength and daily functioning in elderly men and women even after as little as 10 weeks of activity [10]. Benefits seen in seniors included quicker walking speed, ability to climb more stairs, and increased muscle size in the thighs as well as decreased falls [10]. Encouraging elderly patients to incorporate resistance activity into exercise routines can reap large benefits for daily functioning and prolonged independence.

Physical Activity Guidelines

The current guidelines from the US Department of Health and Human Services for adults aged 18–64 years of age are 150 min of moderate intensity cardiovascular activity per week or 75 min of vigorous activity per week, plus 2 or more nonconsecutive days of muscle strengthening activity per week [23]. For adults over 65 years of age the recommendations are the same. However, if adults suffer from a chronic illness, the recommendations stress that older adults should be as active as the disability allows. The guidelines emphasize that inactivity should be avoided and that the more activity individuals participate in, the greater the health benefits. Keep in mind that these guidelines are for attaining health benefits, and not for optimizing weight loss or weight maintenance. Regardless of the initial goal of activity, this is a good starting place for most patients, especially if they are currently sedentary.

The recommendations for weight loss and weight maintenance start at the same point—150 min of cardiovascular activity per week. But according to the ACSM, overweight and obese patients will see greater weight loss and enhanced prevention of weight gain with doses of activity at 250–300 min per week plus two nonconsecutive days of resistance activity per week [11]. It is at this point that the recommendations and guidelines become blurred for patients and truly require individualization. Many others argue that for weight loss and for prevention of weight regain, patients will require much higher levels of physical activity and the more activity the greater reduction in weight [32]. The National Weight Control Registry has demonstrated consistently that high levels of activity, upwards of 60 min per day, are critical for long-term weight loss success [33]. Additionally, research done on groups of identical twin pairs has demonstrated significant individual variability in response to identical exercise interventions, again suggesting that the amount of activity required for weight loss and maintenance will vary from person to person and require personalization [10, 11, 25].

So how much activity is really enough? It really depends on each patient's goals. Is the ultimate goal weight loss, blood pressure reduction, improved functional status, or weight maintenance? For many patients who are losing weight or maintaining weight loss the amount of activity they need to reach the goal varies—for some 45 min per day is sufficient, while others may need more. For those aiming for fitness goals or preserving lean body mass during active weight loss, recommendations become specifically focused for each patient in regards to the combination of resistance and cardiovascular activity. So the basic exercise and activity recommendations are an ideal starting place for each patient, however, over time and as the patient focuses on their desired goals, the recommendations need to be individualized for optimal results.

The bottom line regarding exercise recommendations—some activity is better than none and starting patients slowly helps to limit injury and fatigue. Patients just need to become active whether it is walking regularly or going to the gym for a structured exercise class. Finding activities patients will continue long term is most important. In fact, studies suggest patients lose similar amounts of weight regardless of whether they participate in structured exercise or increased daily activity [34]. Yet, in the long term, patients who increase their daily activity are more likely to remain active longer and maintain their weight loss [34]. Additionally, exercise and activity sessions can be split up over the course of the day into smaller 10-min sessions if needed. Jakicic et al. demonstrated that dividing one long exercise bout into several smaller bouts over the day might help to improve patients' adherence to regular and consistent activity [35]. Finally, pedometers can serve as an inexpensive tool to aid in motivation and tracking of activity levels and studies demonstrate that pedometers are associated with significant increases in physical activity as well as weight loss [36, 37]. Finding ways for patients to remain compliant with activity for the long term is key to making successful progress with lifestyle changes for weight loss, weight maintenance, and disease prevention.

Activity recommendations for the diabetic patient should start with the same goal of at least 150 min of moderate intensity physical activity per week in combination with 2 days of resistance activity, as this is a good starting place for most patients. However, for optimal blood sugar control requesting that patients aim for 150 min per week to be split up into at least 3 days per week, with no more than 2 consecutive days without activity [38]. Patients need to be encouraged to participate in both aerobic and anaerobic activity on a regular basis [38]. The improvements to blood sugar are transient, and if patients discontinue regular aerobic physical activity the benefits are lost as well; however, resistance training benefits from increased muscle mass may persist longer despite cessation of activity [38].

Physical activity recommendations specifically for the bariatric patients have not yet been defined and only a handful of studies have looked at the impact of activity on weight loss post surgery. However, there are data to suggest that patients will experience improved weight loss and decreased loss of lean body mass with regular and consistent physical activity post surgery [39–41]. Additionally, individuals who were active after surgery had greater improvements on the quality of life scores related to mental health, general health, and vitality [39]. Initially after surgery, high intensity exercise is not advised during the initial catabolic phase following surgery [42]. Walking can be the primary activity in the first 3–6 months following surgery [42]. To prevent loss of lean mass during rapid weight loss, encourage patients to participate in strength training regularly. Several studies confirm an association between regular physical activity and increased weight loss, decreased body mass index (BMI) and improved postsurgical outcomes, so advising patients to start slow and providing them the tools and regular follow-up for success will be key to ensuring long-term weight loss maintenance [41, 42].

According to the CDC, patients without a diagnosed chronic condition (diabetes, coronary artery disease (CAD), arthritis) and who do not have symptoms of cardiovascular disease do not need to consult a physician prior to initiating physical activity [23]. In any patient, regardless of age, who has signs or symptoms of CAD or with a history of CAD, exercise testing should be performed prior to starting an exercise program [43]. In asymptomatic healthy patients, who are not planning vigorous activity there is no indication to undergo cardiac stress testing prior to activity, regardless of age [43]. However, exercise stress testing is appropriate in asymptomatic women ≥50 and men ≥40 who plan to engage in vigorous intensity activity. Finally, consider testing asymptomatic patients with two or more risk factors for CAD, a 10-year cardiovascular disease (CVD) risk of >10% or in patients with diabetes who plan to start a vigorous intensity program. Risk factors include hyperlipidemia, smoking, myocardial infraction (MI) in a relative <60 years of age, and diabetes [43].

The Exercise Prescription

Most physicians encourage physical activity and regular exercise, but many unfortunately, do not know how to write an exercise prescription or are not aware of the current guidelines and recommendations for physical activity. As office appointments become shorter and physician time is limited, there is simply less time to counsel patients. The healthcare community needs to refocus our patients to look at the importance of prevention and healthy habits. Physical inactivity is a modifiable risk factor that can help improve health, lower disease burden, and reduce mortality. Physicians need to provide solid, evidence-based activity recommendations and remind patients that there is no "silver bullet" or "quick fix" to getting fit; instead, fitness requires dedicated lifestyle changes, including regular and consistent exercise.

Most patients want to lose weight, get healthy, and be fit. Unfortunately, all too often patients state that they know what to do to be healthy, but they just cannot seem to stick to it for the long term. This problem sadly occurs too frequently, and particularly in patients who have battled their weight most of their lives. Giving patients concrete directions and guidance regarding their diet and exercise regimens, in as little as 3–8 min of interaction [44], has been shown to positively impact activity levels. This is the theory behind the US Surgeon General and the Institute of Medicine's (IOM) 2010 Campaign: Exercise Is Medicine [45]. This slogan encourages physicians and other healthcare professionals to take a more active role in motivating patients to meet exercise and physical activity recommendations for prevention and treatment of disease. Some studies have suggested that <35% of adult patients receive activity counseling during their clinic visits [46, 47]. This low rate of physician counseling is a missed opportunity for prevention of obesity especially in the setting of increasing obesity prevalence as well as stable trends towards inactive lifestyles [47]. Patients need to think of exercise as medicine, just as they would take a prescription medication daily, they too need to exercise daily with the same diligence. Studies demonstrate that exercise counseling is most effective when a prescription is provided and is accompanied with regular follow-up [44]. Follow-up at subsequent visits is important; studies suggest that overweight patients are 5.5 times more likely to continue the activity when doctors follow-up on the exercise recommendations compared with patients who received less counseling [44].

So where should physicians and health care providers start? First, identify realistic goals for each patient. Evaluate and consider each patient's individual needs. For example, when patients are unstable on their feet, consider physical therapy to optimize balance. Patients with no physical activity experience may benefit from group classes or one-on-one instruction with a trainer for guidance and safety. Identify activities they enjoy and think of activities outside of the gym—do they like to swim, dance (such as ballroom or ballet), or perform martial arts? Make a plan; set a goal with a follow-up appointment to discuss results.

Writing a prescription provides structure to the recommendations and gives patients a concrete goal. The FITT principle—prescribing frequency, intensity, time, and type of activity can provide the basic outline for a safe program in overweight and obese patients. [46]. Write out for patients how frequently they need to participate in the activity—daily or a few times per week. Start patients slowly with achievable goals to motivate them and not overwhelm them. Recommend the intensity you would like them to exercise at—a healthy young female who has been exercising for several months may be able to reach a vigorous intensity, where most older patients are likely going to do best at a low to moderate intensity level. Teach patients to check their heart rate or give them an objective measure to ensure they stay at the right intensity. Consider the Borg scale or articulate clearly that they should be able to hold a conversation while walking on the treadmill at moderate intensity. Start patients on a gradual progression of time using 10–20-min increments, keeping in mind that several short bouts can be just as effective as one long bout of activity daily [28]. Finally, focus on types of activity that will be convenient, accessible, and enjoyable for the patient as this will help to encourage compliance [46].

Identifying and addressing barriers to activity can help to prevent poor compliance in advance. Barriers include advancing age and disabilities, low income, low motivation, unrealistic expectations of benefits, poor self perception to participate in activity, lack of support or limited facilities, and unsafe neighborhoods [23]. Assessing the barriers at the initial visit can help patients to find ways around them so that activity is more likely. If patients lack time related to employment or family obligations, the use of a pedometer can allow then to track their daily activity to better assess the need for additional activity. A reasonable goal when using a pedometer is to increase the number of steps walked daily by 1,000 each month until you walk at least 5,000 steps per day at baseline. Patients can continue to increase to an optimal goal of 10,000 steps per day [36].

The importance of regular physical activity and exercise cannot be undervalued. As the rates of diabetes and obesity remain elevated, the steps for prevention and treatment must include lifestyle changes, and specifically include increased physical activity. Health-care professionals need to stress this with their patients at every visit. The health benefits of activity occur regardless of age and weight loss, and no patient is exempt from the need for activity. The CDC emphasizes the importance of getting Americans moving, with fairly modest recommendations that are designed to be reasonable and obtainable by the majority of patients. These guidelines are a great starting place and patients need to be pushed beyond them on an individual basis regardless of whether they are losing weight after bariatric surgery, maintaining a recent weight loss, or optimizing blood glucose levels. With every refill for a medication or prescription for a lab test physicians need to include a prescription for exercise. All health-care partners must remind patients of the benefits of an active lifestyle because the long-term risks of inactivity are far too great—for everyone.

References

1. Flegal KM, Margaret CD, Ogden CL, Curtin LR. Prevalence and trends in obesity among US Adults, 1999–2008. JAMA. 2010;303(3)235–41.
2. Behavioral Risk Factor Surveillance System. 2003, 2005, 2007. www.CDC.gov/datastatistics/archive/physical-activity.html.
3. Moore LV, Harris CD, Carlson SA, Kruger J, Fulton JE. Trends in no leisure-time physical activity—United States, 1988–2010. Res Q Exerc Sport. 2012;83(4):587–91.
4. CDC National Health Interview Survey. http://www.cdc.gov/nchs/data/nhis/earlyrelease/earlyrelease201306_07.pdf (2012).
5. Goodpasture BH, Delany JP, Otto AD, Kuller L, Vockley J, South-Paul JE, Thomas SB, Brown J, McTigue K, Hames KC, Lang W, Jakicic JM. Effects of diet and physical activity interventions on weight loss and cardiometabolic risk factors in severely obese adults. JAMA. 2010;304(16):1795–02.
6. Warburton D, Nicol CW, Bredin S. Health benefits of physical activity: the evidence. Can Med Assoc J. 2006;174(6):801–9.
7. ACSM/AHA. Physical activity and public health updated recommendations for adults. Circulation. 2007;116:1081–93.
8. CDC Physical Activity Terms. WWW.cdc.gov/nccdphp/dnpa/physical/terms/index.htm.
9. Williams MA, Haskell WL, Ades PA, Amsterdam EA, Bittner V, Franklin BA, et al. american heart association council on clinical cardiology; American heart association council on nutrition, physical activity, and metabolism. Resistance exercise in individuals with and without cardiovascular disease: 2007 update: a scientific statement from the American Heart Association Council on Clinical Cardiology and Council on Nutrition, Physical Activity, and Metabolism. Circulation. 2007;116:572–84.
10. Wilmore JH. Increasing physical activity: alterations in body mass and composition. Am J Clin Nutr. 1996;63(Suppl):456S–60S.
11. Donnelly J, Blair S, Jakicic J, Manore MM, Rankin JW, Smith BK. American college of sports medicine. American college of sports medicine position stand: appropriate physical activity intervention strategies for weight loss and prevention of weight regain for adults. Med Sci Sports Exerc. 2009;41(2):459–71.
12. Tate DF, Jeffery RW, Sherwood NE, Wing RR. Long-term weight losses associated with prescription of higher physical activity goals. Are higher levels of physical activity protective against weight regain? Am J Clin Nutr. 2007;85:954–9.
13. Blair SN, LaMOnte MJ, Nichaman MZ. The evolution of physical activity recommendations: how much is enough? Am J Clin Nutr. 2004;79(Suppl):913S–20S.
14. Myers J, Prakash M, Froelicher, V, Do D, Partington S, Atwood JE. Exercise capacity and mortality among men referred for exercise testing. N Engl J Med. 2002;346:793–801.

15. Gulati M, Pandey DK, Arnsdorf MF, Lauderdale DS, Thisted RA, Wicklund RH, Al-Hani AJ, Black HR. Exercise capacity and the risk of death in women: the St James women take heart project. Circulation. 2003;108(13):1554–9.

16. Kokkinos P, Myers J, Faselis C, Panagiotakos DB, Doumas M, Pittaras A, Manolis A, Kokkinos JP, Karasik P, Greenberg M, Papademetriou V, Fletcher R. Exercise capacity and mortality in older men A 20-year follow-up study. Circulation. 2010;122:790–7.

17. Lyerly GW, Sui X, Lavie CJ, Church TS, Hand GA, Blair SN. The association between cardiorespiratory fitness and risk of all-cause mortality among women with impaired fasting glucose and undiagnosed diabetes mellitus. Mayo Clin Proc. 2009;84(9):780–6.

18. Wadden. Nutrition and Health Management, Obesity: management; chapter 64, pp. 1029–42.

19. Blair SN, Kampert JB, Kohl HW, Barlow CE, Macera CA, Paffenbarger RS Jr, Gibbons LW. Influences of cardiorespiratory fitness and other precursors on cardiovascular disease and all-cause mortality in men and women. JAMA. 1996;276(3):205–10.

20. Blair SN, Kohl HW, Barlow CE, Paffenbarger RS Jr, Gibbons LW, Macera CA. Changes in physical activity and all-cause mortality. A prospective study of healthy and unhealthy men. JAMA. 1995;273(14):1093–8.

21. Franklin BA. Cardiorespiratory fitness: an independent and additive marker of risk stratification and health outcomes. Mayo Clin Proc. 2009;84(9):776–9.

22. Lee D, Artero E, Sui X, Blair SN. Mortality trends in the general population: the importance of cardiorespiratory fitness. J Psychopharmacol. 2010;24(11,Suppl 4):27–35.

23. Physical Activity Guidelines Advisory Committee. Physical activity guidelines advisory committee report. Washington DC: U.S. Department of Health and Human Services. www.health.gov/PAGuidelines (2008).

24. Cannon CP, Kumar A. Treatment of overweight and obesity: lifestyle, pharmacologic, and surgical options. Clin Cornerstone. 2009;9(4):55–71.

25. Garber CE, Blissmer B, Deschenes MR, Franklin BA, Lamonte MJ, Lee I, Nieman DC, Swain DP. ACSM position stand: quantity and quality of exercise for developing and maintaining cardiorespiratory, musculoskeletal, and neuromotor fitness in apparently healthy adults: guidance for prescribing exercise. Med Sci Sports Exerc. 2011;43:1334–59.

26. Boule NG, Kenny GP, Haddad E, Wells GA, Sigal RJ. Effects of exercise on glycemic control and body mass in type 2 diabetes mellitus: a meta-analysis of controlled clinical trials. JAMA. 2001;286:1228–7.

27. Corcoran MP, Lamon-Fava S, Fielding RA. Skeletal muscle lipid deposition and insulin resistance: effect of dietary fatty acids and exercise. Am J Clin Nutr. 2007;85:662–77.

28. Church TS, Cheng YJ, Earnest CP, Barlow CE, Gibbons LW, Priest EL, Blair SN. Exercise capactiy and body composition as predictors of mortality among men with diabetes. Diabetes Care. 2004;27:83–8.

29. Houmard J, Tanner CJ, Slentz CA, Duscha BD, McCartney JS, Kraus WE. Effect of volume and intensity of exercise training on insulin sensitivity. J Appl Physiol. 2004;96:101–6.

30. Diabetes Prevention Program Research Group. Reduction in the incidence of type 2 diabetes with lifestyle intervention or metformin. N Engl J Med. 2002;346(6):393–403.

31. Diabetes Prevention Program Research Group. 10-year follow up of diabetes incidence and weight loss in the diabetes prevention program outcomes study. Lancet. 2009;374(9702):1677–86.

32. Look AHEAD Research Group. Look AHEAD (Action for Health in Diabetes). One-year weight losses in the look AHEAD study: factors associated with success. Obesity (Silver Sping). 2009;17(4):713–22.

33. Catenacci VA, Wyatt HR. The role of physical activity in producing and maintaining weight loss. Nat Clin Pract Endocrinol Metab. 2007;3(7):518–529.

34. Anderson RE, Wadden TA, Bartlett SJ, Zemel B, Verde T, Franckowiak S. Effects of lifestyle activity vs structured aerobic exercise in obese women: a randomized trial. JAMA. 1999;281:335–40.

35. Jakicic JM, Wing RR, Butler BA, Robertson RJ. Prescribing exercise in multiple short bouts versus one continuous bout: effects on adherence, cardiorespiratory fitness, and weight loss in overweight women. Int J Obesity. 1995;19:893–01.

36. Bravata, D, Smith-Spangler C, Sundaram V, Gienger AL, Lin N, Lewis R, Stave CD, Olkin I, Sirard JR. Using pedometers to increase physical activity and improve health. JAMA. 2007;298(19):2296–04.

37. Richardson CR, Newton TL, Abraham JJ, Sen A, Jimbo M, Swartz AM. A meta-analysis of pedometer-based walking interventions and weight loss. Ann Fam Med. 2008;6(1) 69–77.

38. Sigal, RJ, Kenny GP, Wasserman DH, Castaneda-Sceppa C, White RD. Physical activity/exercise and type 2 diabetes: a consensus statement from the American Diabetes Association. Diabetes Care. 2006;29(6):1433–8.

39. Bond DS, Phelan S, Wolfe LG, Evans RK, Meador JG, Kellum JM, Maher JW, Wing RR. Becoming physically activity after bariatric surgery is associated with improved weight loss and health related quality of life. Obesity (Silver Spring). 2009;17(1):78–83.

40. Evans RK, Bond DS, Wolfe LG, Meador JG, Herrick JE, Kellum JM, Maher JW. Participation in 150 min/wk of moderate or higher intensity physical activity yields greater weight loss after gastric bypass surgery. Surg Obes Relat Dis. 2007;3:526–30.

41. Silver H, Torquati A, Jensen GL, Richards WO. Weight, dietary and physical activity behaviors two years after gastric bypass. Obes Surg. 2006;16:859–64.

42. Petering R, Webb CW. Exercise, fluid, nutrition recommendations for the post gastric bypass exerciser. Curr Sports Med Rep. 2009;8(2):92–7.

43. ACC/AHA. Guideline update for exercise testing: summary article: a report of the American college of cardiology/American Heart Association task force on practice guidelines (committee to update the 1997 exercise testing guidelines). J Am Coll Cardiol. 2002;40(8):1531–40.

44. Weidinger KA, Lovegreen SL, Elliott MB, Hagood L, Haire-Joshu D, McGill JB, Brownson RC. How to make exercise counseling more effective: lessons from rural America. J Fam Pract. 2008;57(6):394–402.

45. Exercise is Medicine. http://exerciseismedicine.org/physicians.htm.

46. Mcinnis KJ, Franklin BA, Rippe JM. Counseling for physical activity in overweight and obese patients. Am Fam Physician. 2003;67:1249–56, 1266–8.

47. Wee CC, McCarthy EP, Davis RB, Phillips RS. Physician counseling about exercise. JAMA. 1999;282:1583–8.

Chapter 6
The Doctor's Tool Kit: Pharmacotherapy for the Patient with Obesity

George A. Bray and Donna H. Ryan

Introduction

The prevalence of obesity now exceeds 34 % for US adults [1], and the prevalence of more severe obesity (body mass index (BMI)/40 kg/m^2) continues to rise [2]. Excessive weight is a health risk for children and adolescents too [3]. The fundamental problem producing obesity is a small, but prolonged, positive energy balance, where energy derived from food exceeds energy expended for everyday living [4, 5]. Obesity is associated with many illnesses that are related to and may be caused by excess fat [6].

In response to the impact of obesity on morbidity and health-care costs, and the health and potential cost benefits of modest weight loss, the Center for Medicare Services (CMS) announced in 2012 that reimbursement would be provided for up to 14 sessions of intensive behavioral therapy for obesity, when delivered by primary care providers [7]. Primary care physicians are at the forefront of attempts to manage the chronic conditions (type 2 diabetes, hypertension, dyslipidemia, sleep apnea, nonalcoholic fatty liver disease) that result from obesity as a root cause. This practice group is compelled to help their patients in achieving and sustaining weight loss, so as to prevent and improve these chronic diseases.

In this chapter, we will discuss the pharmacological treatment of the patient with obesity from two perspectives—use of medications approved for obesity per se and the selection of medications that affect body weight for obese patients who already have complications from their obesity and who are receiving these

G. A. Bray (✉)
Pennington Biomedical Research Center, 6400 Perkins Road, Baton Rouge, LA 70808, USA
e-mail: George.Bray@pbrc.edu

D. H. Ryan
Pennington Biomedical Research Center, Louisiana State University System,
6400 Perkins Road, Baton Rouge, LA 70808, USA
e-mail: ryandh@pbrc.edu

© Springer Science+Business Media New York 2015   91
A. Youdim (ed.), *The Clinician's Guide to the Treatment of Obesity,*
Endocrine Updates, DOI 10.1007/978-1-4939-2146-1_6

medications for chronic disease management. Although some medications are appropriate for both groups, others are only approved for the obese patient who has already developed comorbidity, but if they also produce weight loss so much the better for the patient.

Medications Approved by the US Food and Drug Administration (FDA) for the Treatment of the Patient with Obesity

Two groups of medications are described below. The first are the agents approved for long-term treatment of obesity which include, orlistat, lorcaserin, the combination of phentermine and topiramate as an extended release (PHEN/TPM ER) formulation, and the combination of bupropion and naltrexone in a sustained release form. Liraglutide, which is anticipated to become available in later 2015, has also been approved by the FDA for long term use. The second are the medications approved by the US Food and Drug Administration (FDA) for short-term use. Interestingly, the FDA has given the last three drugs approved for treatment of weight an indication for "chronic weight management" indicating that management of obesity is like other chronic diseases in that it requires long-term, chronic care. The drugs approved for obesity are shown in Table 6.1.

Orlistat (Marketed as Xenical in the USA)

Orlistat (tetrahydrolipstatin) is approved by the US FDA for long-term management of obesity. Orlistat is a potent and selective inhibitor of pancreatic lipase that reduces intestinal digestion of fat. It is available as a prescription drug (120 mg tid (three times a day) before meals). A number of long-term clinical trials with orlistat have been published using patients with uncomplicated obesity and patients with obesity and diabetes [8]. A 4-year double-blind, randomized, placebo-controlled trial with orlistat in 3304 overweight patients, 21 % of whom had impaired glucose tolerance [9], achieved a weight loss during the first year of more than 11 % below baseline in the orlistat-treated group compared to 6 % below baseline in the placebo-treated group. Over the remaining 3 years of the trial, there was a small regain in weight, with the orlistat-treated patients remaining 6.9 % below baseline, compared with 4.1 % for those receiving placebo. There was a reduction of 37 % in the conversion of patients from impaired glucose tolerance to diabetes.

Use of orlistat has also been studied in children; 539 adolescents received 120 mg three times per day compared to placebo [10]. BMI decreased by 0.55 kg/m^2 in the drug-treated group compared to an increase of +0.31 kg/m^2 in the placebo group [10]. In a meta-analysis of trials with orlistat, the weighted mean weight loss in the placebo group was -2.40 ± 6.99 kg and the weight loss in those treated with orlistat was -5.70 ± 7.28 kg for a net effect of -2.87 (95 % CI -3.21 to -2.53) [11].

Table 6.1 Drugs approved by the US Food and Drug Administration that produce weight loss. (Adapted from Bray Obesity 2013)

Generic name	Trade name(s)	Dosage	DEA schedule
Pancreatic lipase inhibitor approved by FDA for long-term use			
Orlistat	Xenical	120 mg three times daily before meals	Not scheduled
Serotinin-2C receptor agonist approved by FDA for long-term use			
Lorcaserin	Belviq	10 mg twice daily	IV
Combination of phentermine–topiramate approved by FDA for long-term use			
Phentermine–topiramate ER	Qsymia	3.75/23 mg 7.5/46 mg 11.25/69 mg 15/92 mg	IV, because of phentermine component
Combination naltrexone–bupropion approved by FDA for long-term use			
Naltrexone–bupropion SR	Contrave	8/90 mg tablets: 2 in morning and 2 in evening with carbo-hydrate meal	Not scheduled
Noradrenergic drugs approved for short-term use			
Diethylpropion	Tenuate Tenuate dospan	25 mg three times daily 75 mg every morning	IV
Phentermine	Adipex and many others	15–30 mg/day	IV
Benzphetamine	Didrex	25–50 mg three times daily	III
Phendimetrazine	Bontril Prelu-2	17.5–70 mg three times daily 105 mg daily	III
Liraglutide 3 mg, approved by the FDA for long-term use			
Liraglutide 3 mg	Saxenda	3.0 mg by injection	Not Scheduled

FDA Food and Drug Administration, *DEA* Drug Enforcement Agency, *ER* extended release
[a] Drug Enforcement Agency Schedule IV
[b] Drug Enforcement Agency Schedule III

Safety Profile of Orlistat

Orlistat is not absorbed to any significant degree, and its side effects are thus related to the blockade of triglyceride digestion in the intestine [12]. Fecal fat loss and related gastrointestinal (GI) symptoms are common initially, but they subside as patients learn to use the drug. Orlistat can cause small but significant decrease in fat-soluble vitamins. Levels usually remain within the normal range, but a few patients may need vitamin supplementation. Because it is clinically challenging to tell which patients need vitamins, it is thus wise to provide a multivitamin routinely with instructions to take it before bedtime. Orlistat does not seem to affect the absorption of other drugs, except acyclovir. Rare cases of severe liver injury have been reported with the use of orlistat; at a time when an estimated 40 million people took orlistat, only one case of severe liver injury occurred in the USA, and 13 elsewhere. A causal relationship has not been established, but patients who take orlistat should contact their health-care provider if itching, jaundice, pale color stools, or anorexia develop [5].

Lorcaserin, (Marketed as BELVIQ® in the USA)

Lorcaserin Belviq®, Arena Pharmaceuticals and Esai Pharmaceuticals) is approved by the US FDA for a long-term weight management. Serotonergic drugs have been used in the past to treat obesity (fenfluramine and dexfenfluramine), but were removed from the market because of damage to the heart valves [13]. Lorcaserin selectively targets the serotonin 2c receptor, which when activated in the hypothalamus reduces food intake, [14]and avoids the serotonin 2b heart valve target. Lorcaserin is prescribed at 10 mg twice daily (Belviq prescribing information).

Efficacy of Lorcaserin

Three clinical studies provided evidence [15] for approval of lorcaserin. Two of these studies called Behavioral Modification and Lorcaserin for Overweight and Obesity Management (BLOOM) [16] and Behavioral Modification and Lorcaserin Second Study for Obesity (BLOSSOM) [17] enrolled volunteers who were obese or had BMI >27 kg/m^2 with one comorbidity. The third study called BLOOM diabetes mellitus (DM) [18] enrolled diabetic patients with hemoglobin A1C of 7–10 % and a BMI of 27–45 kg/m^2. In this study, all patients (including the placebo group) received counseling in diet and physical activity. There was modest weight loss (5 %) with lorcaserin at 1 year. There were improvements in cardiovascular risk factors particularly when the patient population had abnormal risk factors at baseline. In the BLOOM-DM study, HbA1c decreased 0.9 ± 0.06 with lorcaserin BID, compared to 0.4 ± 0.06 with placebo ($P<0.001$) and fasting glucose decreased 27.4 ± 2.5 mg/dL compared to a decrease of 11.9 ± 2.5 mg/dL for placebo ($P<0.001$) [18]. Weight maintenance was demonstrated in the BLOOM-DM study with a small amount of regain in the second year.

Safety Profile of Lorcaserin

Lorcaserin was scrutinized for potential effects on heart valves during phase III studies where echocardiograms were done on more than 5200 subjects. There was no statistically significant increase in FDA-defined valvulopathy with drug treatment as compared to placebo. In the FDA briefing report [15], using combined data on all patients who were exposed to lorcaserin or to placebo in the three studies, the relative risk of FDA-defined valvulopathy in lorcaserin-treated participants, as compared with those who received placebo, was reported as 1.16 (95% CI, 0.81–1.67) which is not statistically significant. However, since lorcaserin has much greater selectivity for the 5-HT2c receptor than the 5-HT2b receptor, it is very unlikely that lorcaserin will increase the risk of valvulopathy in humans and the FDA has not recommended routine echocardiography for prescription of lorcaserin

Another issue with lorcaserin was found in preclinical toxicology studies, where an increased numbers of brain and mammary tumors were reported in rats. These were reanalyzed and there were fewer malignant tumors than first thought [15]. Additionally, the drug does not have high levels in the central nervous system of humans, whereas it does in rats [15].

Lorcaserin is well tolerated. The most common adverse events in clinical trials were headache, nausea, dizziness, fatigue, dry mouth, and constipation (Belviq prescribing information). These were mild and resolved quickly. However, a primary concern is that the drug should not be used with selective serotonin reuptake inhibitors (SSRIs) or with monoamine oxidase inhibitors (MAOIs), because of the risk of serotonin syndrome.

In summary, the remarkable aspect of lorcaserin seems to be in its safety and tolerability not in the magnitude of its weight loss [34]. The only issue is the risk of serotonin syndrome and because the background use of SSRI antidepressants in overweight and obese patients is so high, physicians should be watchful and not prescribe lorcaserin in patients taking SSRIs.

Phentermine/Topiramate ER (Marketed as QSYMIA™ in the USA)

The combination PHEN/TPM ER is marketed as Qsymia™ by Vivus Inc. and is the first new drug combination approved for chronic weight management in overweight and obese persons in more than a decade. The combination uses lower doses of phentermine (3.75 mg in the starting dose, 7.5 mg in the recommended dose, and 15 mg in the top dose) than are usually prescribed when phentermine is used as a single agent. The topiramate is an extended release (ER) formulation, not available other than in this combination and the dose of topiramate in the combination is 23 mg in the starting dose, 46 mg in the recommended dose, and 92 mg in the top dose and is also lower than when topiramate is used for migraine prophylaxis or to control seizures. In terms of mechanism of action, phentermine acts to reduce appetite through increasing norepinephrine in the hypothalamus and topiramate's appetite-reducing mechanism is not thoroughly understood, although it may be through its effect on γ-aminobutyric acid (GABA) receptors.

Efficacy of PHEN/TPM ER Two clinical studies [19, 20] provided efficacy and safety data that formed the basis [21] for approval of the medication. The first called EQUIP [19] enrolled subjects <70 years of age with BMI >35kg/m² who had one of the following: blood pressure to be controlled (<140/90 mmHg using

0–2 antihypertensive medications), fasting blood glucose <110 mg/dL, and triglyc-erides <200 mg/dL using 0 or 1 lipid-lowering medication. The other study called CONQUER [20]enrolled adults <70 years of age with BMI >27 and <45 kg/m², but for patients with type 2 diabetes, no lower BMI limit was required. The CON-QUER study also required patients to have two or more of the following comorbidi-ties: hypertension, hypertriglyceridemia, dysglycemia (impaired fasting glucose, impaired glucose tolerance or type 2 diabetes), or an elevated waist circumference (>40 inches for men or >35 inches for women). Thus, the patient population in these two studies represents those with higher risk profiles from the consequences of excess weight. A titration period of 2 weeks is recommended for PHEN/TPM ER, starting at 3.75/23 mg dosage, although in these studies it was shorter. All subjects in these studies received a lifestyle modification program based on the LEARN manual [22, 23]. This combination medication has produced the largest weight losses observed in clinical trials of obesity medications approaching 10% on average.

The CONQUER study was extended for a second year of observation with pa-tients keeping their treatment assignment; this was called the SEQUEL study [2] At the end of the second year of treatment, patients completing the trial taking the recommended dose (7.5/46 mg) maintained a weight loss of 9.3% below baseline and those on the top dose maintained a 10.7% weight loss from baseline.

The weight loss with PHEN/TPM ER is accompanied by improvements in most risk factors. In the CONQUER study [20], there were clinically and statistically significant improvements in blood pressure, glycemic measures, high-density lipo-protein (HDL) cholesterol, and triglycerides with both the recommended and the top doses of the medication. In the EQUIP, CONQUER, and SEQUEL studies, im-provements in risk factors were related to the amount of weight loss, with greater benefit being observed with greater weight loss. Further, a population with abnor-mal risk factors is more likely to demonstrate improvement in those risk factors. PHEN/TPM ER has also been studied in patients with sleep apnea and has shown to reduce the severity of symptoms from sleep apnea [24].

Safety Profile of PHEN/TPM ER

The most commonly observed side effects in the clinical trials were paresthesia, diz-ziness, dysgeusia (altered taste particularly with carbonated beverages), insomnia, constipation, and dry mouth (Qsymia prescribing information). These side effects are related to the constituents of PHEN/TPM ER or, in the case of constipation, to weight loss per se. Phentermine, as a sympathomimetic agent, causes insomnia and dry mouth, usually early in treatment, which then resolve. Topiramate is a carbonic anhydrase inhibitor that is associated with altered taste for carbonated beverages and tingling in fingers, toes, and perioral areas and may lead to mild metabolic acidosis.

Safety concerns(Qsymia™ prescribing information) with PHEN/TPM ER are also associated with the two components. Weight loss is contraindicated in preg-nancy, as are all weight loss medications. Topiramate is associated with oral clefts if used during pregnancy and PHEN/TPM ER is pregnancy category X. A rare side effect of topiramate is acute glaucoma and the drug is contraindicated in glaucoma. PHEN/TPM ER is also contraindicated in hyperthyroidism and within 14 days of treatment with MAOIs and in patients with hypersensitivity to any of the ingredients in the medication. Because of the risk of oral clefts, a negative pregnancy test before treatment and monthly thereafter and use of effective contraception are required. If a patient becomes pregnant while taking PHEN/TPM ER, treatment should be immediately terminated. Other potential issues, though rare, includes risk of kidney stones (associated with topiramate) mild metabolic acidosis (associated with topiramate) and increased heart rate in patients susceptible to sympathomimetic drugs (associated with phentermine).

Naltrexone/Bupropion (NB) Combination in Sustained Release Formulation (Marketed as Contrave in the USA)

Bupropion (± 1-(3-chlorophenyl)-2-[(1,1-dimethylethyl)amino)-1-propanone) reduces food intake by acting on adrenergic and dopaminergic receptors in the hypothalamus. Naltrexone (17-(cyclopropylmethyl)-4,5-alpha-epoxy-3,14-dihydroxy-morphinan-6-1) is an opioid receptor antagonist with minimal effect on weight loss on its own. The rationale for combining bupropion with naltrexone is that naltrexone might block inhibitory influences of opioid receptors activated by the β-endorphin which is released in the hypothalamus and stimulates feeding, while allowing α-melanocyte stimulating hormone (α-MSH) which reduces food intake to inhibit food intake [25]. The combination was favorably reviewed by an FDA advisory panel in 2012 [26]. However, because bupropion increases pulse and both bupropion and naltrexone increase blood pressure and in the phase III studies, the FDA has required a premarketing study of the combination drug with assessment of cardiovascular outcomes. An interim analysis of the trial was favorable and the drug is now marketed.

Efficacy of NB SR

Weight loss with the NB combination at 1 year was intermediate to that of PHEN/TPM ER and lorcaserin. This produced improvement in risk factors. However, the effect on blood pressure is not as great as one would expect with this degree of weight loss in the two studies that comprised the phase III trials of NB, called the Contrave Obesity Research (COR) [27] and COR and Behaviour Modification (COR BMOD) trials [28].

What is of concern is the outlier effect of NB, not the mean blood pressure effect, which is reduced, albeit not as much as expected. This has implications for patients with hypertension, as we discuss later. In the COR BMOD trial (http://www.accessdata.fda.gov/scripts/cder/drugsatfda/ http://www.accessdata.fda.gov/scripts/

cder/drugsatfda/), the authors describe a post hoc subgroup analysis of 50 individuals who had systolic blood pressure > 130 mmHg at baseline. For individuals who received NB 32/360+ BMOD, mean systolic blood pressure declined at all visits with mean reductions 3.4–11.4 mm Hg. In this same set of subjects, mean diastolic blood pressure also declined by 1.0–6.5 mm Hg. This would seem to indicate that there was no increased risk for those with higher blood pressure who take the drug. However, in the COR I trial [27], there were transient increases in mean blood pressure of 1.5 mm Hg systolic, while the placebo-treated group had transient decreases of 1.5 mm Hg. The amount of weight loss may modify the blood pressure response. In the COR BMOD trial [28], the authors report that changes in blood pressure in the NB 32/360+ BMOD group were correlated with weight loss.

Safety Profile of NB SR

The label (http://www.accessdata.fda.gov/scripts/cder/drugsatfda/ http://www.accessdata.fda.gov/scripts/cder/drugsatfda/) for this medication recommends following blood pressure in the first few weeks of prescribing. Of course, over time, weight loss will have a beneficial effect on blood pressure. Other safety issues relate to the individual components. Like all medications for depression in the USA, a black box warning cautions about increased risk of suicidal thinking, especially in young individuals. This has carried over to the indication for weight loss, although there was no signal of suicidality in the clinical trials with the combination. Bupropion lowers the seizure threshold and the combination is contraindicated in those with history of seizures. Naltrexone is an opioid antagonist and should not be given with opiates or opiate inducers because it will negate their effects. There are some tolerability issues, chiefly nausea on initiating the drug [27],and potential issues with SSRIs or MAOIs [27]. However, a dose escalation over 3 weeks is recommended to minimize nausea and vomiting. But the medication could offer another option for physicians prescribing to aid patients in behavioral attempts at weight loss.

Liraglutide 3 mg (Marketed as Saxenda in the USA) Under Consideration for FDA Approval, Tentatively Named Saxenda

Liraglutide is a glucagon-like peptide (GLP)-1 agonist that has a 97% homology to GLP-1. This molecular change extends the circulating half-life from 1–2 min to 13 h. Liraglutide is approved in doses up to 1.8 mg for the treatment of type 2 diabetes. This molecule, like other GLP-1 agonists has a multiplicity of actions besides effects on the pancreas to promote glycemic control [29]. One such effect is reduction in food intake [30].

Efficacy of Liraglutide 3 mg

In a 20-week multicenter European clinical trial, Astrup et al. [31] reported that daily injections of liraglutide at 1.2, 1.8, 2.4, or 3.0 mg produced weight losses of 4.8, 5.5, 6.3, and 7.2 kg, respectively, compared to a loss of 2.8 kg in the placebo-treated group and 4.1 kg in the orlistat-treated comparator group. In the group treated with 3.0 mg/day, 76% achieved a >5% weight loss compared to 30% in the placebo group. Blood pressure was significantly reduced, but there were no changes in lipids. The prevalence of prediabetes was reduced by liraglutide.

Liraglutide 3 mg was studied following a highly structured diet where patients who achieved 5% or more weight loss over 4–12 weeks (77% of enrollees achieved this benchmark) were randomized to liraglutide 3.0 mg or placebo. Mean percentage weight loss (± standard deviation) in the run-in was −6.0% (±0.9). At 56 weeks, subjects in the liraglutide group lost an additional −6.2% (±7.3) compared with −0.2% (±7.0) in the placebo group. This reflects a mean −12.2% reduction from initial baseline body weight for those in the liraglutide treatment [32].

Safety Profile of Liraglutide 3 mg

Liraglutide will carry many of the safety and tolerability warnings that are known from the 1.8 mg dose, including increased risk for pancreatitis and a warning about potential for thyroid C cell tumors. The tolerability issues are the same as with the drug when used at a lower dose for type 2 diabetes. Nausea and vomiting mandate a dose escalation over 5 weeks. Of course, liraglutide must be given by injection and it is unknown how this will affect the use in obese patients. Liraglutide is an important addition to the obesity therapeutic toolbox, when made available. It marks the first time our understanding of the biology of food intake regulation has yielded a biological therapy.

Drugs Approved by the US FDA for Short-Term Use in Treating the Patient with Obesity

The sympathomimetic drugs, benzphetamine, diethylpropion, phendimetrazine, and phentermine are grouped together because they act like norepinephrine and were tested before 1975. Phentermine and diethylpropion are classified by the US Drug Enforcement Agency as schedule intravenous (IV) drugs; benzphetamine and phendimetrazine are schedule III drugs. This regulatory classification indicates the government's belief that these drugs have the potential for abuse, although this potential appears to be very low [12]. Phentermine and diethylpropion are approved for only a "few weeks," which usually is interpreted as up to 12 weeks.

Most of the data on these drugs come from short-term trials.

Phentermine

Phentermine, as a single agent, remains the most often prescribed drug for weight loss in the USA. Because phentermine was approved in 1959 for short-term use for weight loss, there are little current data to evaluate its long-term efficacy. In 2011, the FDA approved a new formulation of the drug (http://www.accessdata.fda.gov. drugsatfda_docs/nda/2011/201088_suprenza_toc.cfm) called Suprenza, and marketed by Akrimax Pharmaceuticals, LLC. Since the FDA only approved the new orally disintegrating formulation, there was no clinical weight loss data submitted with the NDA application. However, several studies are worthy of note because they provide recent data on safety and efficacy of phentermine as a single agent.

A study of 6 months duration that was presented to the FDA in the briefing document [33] for topiramate/phentermine combination had four treatment arms and 200 subjects with 158 subjects completing 6 months. For the phentermine 15 mg daily treatment group, weight loss at 6 months was 4.6%, compared to a loss of 2.1% for placebo. Another phentermine study that is relatively current was presented as a poster at the European Congress of Obesity in 2009 [35]. This study also explored phentermine topiramate combination and overall had seven treatment arms among 756 subjects; it is thus one of the largest studies of phentermine alone at two doses (>100 subjects per dose) with over 6 months of observation. In that study, at 28 weeks, completion rates were 65%. Weight loss at 28 weeks for the placebo group was 1.7% from baseline; for phentermine 7.5 mg/day it was 5.5%; and for phentermine 15 mg/day it was 6.1%. Finally, a report from Korea [31]evaluated a diffuse, controlled release form of phentermine at 30 mg ($n=37$) versus placebo ($n=37$). At 12 weeks, mean weight loss was 8.1 ± 3.9 kg for drug-treated patients versus 1.7 ± 2.9 kg for placebo patients. These trials suggest that the effect on weight loss with phentermine is dose related.

Safety Profile of Phentermine

The sympathomimetic drugs produce central excitation, manifested clinically as insomnia and in some individuals as nervousness. This effect is most obvious shortly after the drug is started and wanes substantially with continued use. Dry mouth is among the most common side effects. To a variable extent, these drugs may also increase heart rate and blood pressure. The prescribing information usually recommends that the drugs not be given to individuals with a history of cardiovascular disease. There is little evidence of quantitative effects on blood pressure and pulse, especially after 6 months or more of treatment. A short-term study evaluating phentermine and taranabant [36] administered singly or together for up to 28 days, showed that there were no significant differences in blood pressure and heart rate versus placebo in that study. In a 12-week study [37] from Korea, 68 obese individuals were randomized to either phentermine HCl 37.5 mg per day or placebo. There were no significant differences in mean blood pressure changes between groups at 12 weeks although the phentermine group lost significantly more weight on average (7.2 ± 2.7 kg vs. 1.9 ± 2.7 kg, $P<0.001$). In the Korean study [36] of a new formulation of phentermine (diffuse controlled release; not marketed in the USA), at 12 weeks, mean weight loss was significantly greater in the phentermine group $(8.1 \pm 3.9$ vs. 1.7 ± 2.9 kg, $P < 0.001$). However, there were no significant differences in systolic and diastolic blood pressure. Despite clinically significant weight loss, one does not observe the expected decreases in blood pressure. Furthermore, the phentermine group had a mean increase in blood pressure of 2.7 ± 11.4 beats/min, compared to a decrease of 4.3 ± 12.5 in the placebo-treated subjects [36].

Lacking good quantitative measures of the effects of phentermine on heart rate and pulse, we recommend caution in prescribing drugs in this group. They should not be prescribed to persons with a history of cardiovascular disease. The blood pressure and pulse should be monitored while taking sympathomimetics. Even though there is no convincing evidence of mean blood pressure increases, the lack of the expected reductions in blood pressure with weight loss is an indication that the drugs do have some stimulatory effect on blood pressure.

In one survey of bariatric physicians, use of sympathomimetic amines was more frequent than orlistat and they were often used for longer than approved by the FDA [38]. However, prescribers should be aware of the local and federal regulations governing prescribing limits and the lack of long-term clinical trial data for phentermine.

Treatment of the Overweight or Obese Patient Who has Diabetes, Depression, Migraine Prophylaxis, or Epilepsy

Weight gain or weight loss is the side effect of many drugs used by physicians to treat their patient's diseases. If there is a reasonable choice when selecting medications for chronic disease management that will produce weight loss for the patient with obesity, good clinical practice would seem to recommend the choice of the drug that produces weight loss and avoidance of drugs that produce gain.

Treatment of the Obese Patient with Diabetes

The epidemic of diabetes is following closely on the heels of the obesity epidemic. The rate of developing diabetes can clearly be slowed by weight loss [39–42], which is the first line of treatment. There is growing interest in the ability of weight loss to "reverse" diabetes, and this has been demonstrated in association with various surgical procedures [42] and even with a lifestyle intervention [43]. Table 6.2 lists the drugs that are available to treat diabetes. Insulin produces a weight gain that ranges from 1.8 to 6.6 kg [44]. Two widely used sulfonylurea drugs (glipizide and glibenclamide) also produce weight gain in most studies which ranges from −0.3 to 4.0 kg [44], and this is also true for the thiazolidinediones (rosiglitazone and pioglitazone) which lead to weight gains of 0.18–1.5 kg or more [44]. Other drugs are weight neutral or can cause weight loss [45].

Table 6.2 Categorization of antidiabetic drugs by their effects on body weight

Produce weight loss	Are weight neutral	Produce weight gain
Metformin	Dipeptidyl peptidase-4 inhibitors (DPP-4)	Insulin
Pramlintide	Acarbose	Sulfonylureas[a]
Exenatide	Miglitol	Glitinides
Liraglutide	Bromocriptine	Thiazolidinediones[b]
SGLT2 inhibitors—dapagliflozin and canagliflozin		

SGLT2 sodium-glucose cotransporter 2

[a] Glipizide, glimepride, glibenclamide, chlorpropamide

[b] Pioglitazone, rosiglitazone

Metformin

Metformin is a biguanide that is approved by the US FDA for the treatment of DM, and has a good safety profile. This drug reduces hepatic glucose production, decreases intestinal glucose absorption from the GI tract and enhances insulin sensitivity. One mechanism for the reduction in hepatic glucose production by metformin may depend on the phosphorylation of a nuclear binding protein (cyclic adenosine monophosphate (cAMP) response element binding (CREB) binding protein (CBP) at (Ser436) AMP-activated protein kinase (AMPK)). This disrupts a number of other signals, including a master transcription factor, peroxisome proliferator-activated receptor-γ coactivator 1A (PPARGC1A), which in turn leads to the suppression of hepatic glucose output [46].

The longest and best study of metformin on body weight comes from the Diabetes Prevention Program [47]. During the first 2.8 years of the double-blind, placebo-controlled trial, the metformin-treated group lost 2.9 kg (2.5 %) of their body weight versus a loss of only 0.42 kg in the placebo group ($P<0.001$). The degree of weight loss was related to the adherence to metformin. Those who were the most adherent lost 3.5 kg at 2 years, compared with a small weight gain of 0.5 kg in those who were assigned to, but never took metformin. This differential weight loss persisted throughout the 8 years of follow-up with highly adherent patients remaining 3–4 kg below baseline and those who were not adherent being no different from placebo [47].

Metformin has been used to reduce weight gain in people treated with antipsychotic drugs. In a systematic review, Bushe et al. [48] found that metformin may have some value in reducing or preventing weight gain and change in metabolic parameters during treatment with antipsychotic medications.

Pramlintide

Pramlintide is a modified form of amylin, a peptide secreted from the beta cell of the pancreas along with insulin. Pramlintide has been approved by the FDA for treatment of diabetes and in clinical trials produced weight loss. The combination of phentermine with pramlintide produced additive weight loss in a 6-month clinical trial that may offer weight loss in the patient with diabetes [49].

Glucagon-Like Peptide-1 (GLP-1)

This naturally occurring peptide released by the GI track in response to food. It is a known suppressor of food intake. Two GLP-1 agonists may be of value in treating the patient.

Exenatide

Exenatide (exendin-4) is a 39-amino acid peptide that is produced in the salivary gland of the Gila monster lizard. It has 53 % homology with GLP-1, but it has a much longer half-life. Exenatide has been approved by the FDA for treatment of type 2 diabetics who are inadequately controlled while being treated with either metformin or sulfonylureas. In human beings, exenatide reduces fasting and postprandial glucose levels, slows gastric emptying, and decreases food intake by 19 % [50]. A systematic review of incretin therapy in type 2 diabetes [51] showed a weight loss of 2.37 kg for all GLP-1 analogues versus control, 1.44 for exenatide versus placebo injection, and a loss of 4.76 for exenatide versus insulin (which often leads to weight gain). The side effects of exenatide in humans are headache, nausea, and vomiting that are lessened by gradual dose escalation [52]. The interesting feature of this weight loss is that it occurred without prescribing lifestyle modification, diet, or exercise. A 26-week randomized control trial of exenatide produced a weight loss of 2.3 kg compared to a gain of 1.8 kg in the group receiving the glargine form of insulin [53].

Liraglutide 3 mg

Liraglutide has been approved by the European Medicines Agency and the FDA for the treatment of diabetes at a dose up to 1.8 mg/day. This chapter discusses the weight loss efficacy of liraglutide in obesity treatment in a preceding section and we refer our readers to that. It would be a good choice for the diabetic patient with obesity.

SGLT2 Inhibitors

Sodium-glucose cotransporter (SGLT2) inhibitors (dapagliflozin and canagliflozin) are a new class of antidiabetic drugs. They reduce renal glucose reabsorption in the proximal convoluted tubule, leading to increased urinary glucose excretion [54].

These agents not only have effects on glycemic control but also produce weight loss. In a systematic review and meta-analysis [55], the SGLT2 inhibitors produced placebo-subtracted weight loss of -2.37% (95% CI: -2.73 to -2.02) in eight studies of 12 or more weeks duration. There was slightly more weight loss on average with canagliflozin. In three studies with dapagliflozin versus placebo, there was mean loss of -2.06% (95% CI: -2.38 to -1.74) and in five studies of canagliflozin versus placebo there was -2.61% loss (95% CI: -3.09 to -2.13). Since studies of 12 weeks were included, this is probably an underestimation of weight loss response to the SGLT2 inhibitors.

Treatment of the Patient with Obesity and Neurobehavioral Disorders such as Depression, Epilepsy, and Migraine

This category includes patients with obesity who are depressed, those with migraine symptoms and those needing antipsychotic drugs. Some of the approved drugs in this class produce weight gain, and others are associated with weight loss (Table 6.3). One option for the health provider is to change to an effective medication that produces weight loss from one that produces weight gain. The magnitude of weight gain ranges from 1.2 to 5.8 kg for valproate, 4.0 kg for lithium, 2.1–2.3 for resperidone, 2.8–7.1 kg for olanzapine, and 4.2–9.9 kg for clozapine for the drugs in the weight gain column [44]. This degree of weight gain can make continuation of treatment more difficult, and using weight neutral or the alternatives produce weight loss, particularly for the obese and overweight individual is good clinical practice.

Table 6.3 Categorization of neurobehavioral drugs by their effects on body weight

Produce weight loss	Are weight neutral	Produce weight gain
Bupropion	Haloperidol	Tricyclic antidepressants[a]
Venlafaxine	Aripiprazole	Monoaine oxidase inhibitors
Desvenlafaxine		Paroxetine
Topiramate		Escitalopram
Zonisamide		Lithium
Lamotrigine		Olanzapine
Ziprasidone		Clozapine
Topiramate		Resperidone
		Carbamazepine
		Valproate
		Divalproex
		Mirtazapine

[a] Nortriptyline, amitriptyline, doxepin

Bupropion

Bupropion is an approved drug for treatment of depression and as an aid in helping patients stop smoking. It reduces food intake by acting on adrenergic and dopaminergic receptors in the hypothalamus. These neurotransmitters are involved in the regulation of food intake.

In a study with uncomplicated and nondepressed people with obesity, 327 subjects were randomized to bupropion 300 mg/day, bupropion 400 mg/day, or placebo in equal proportions [56]. All patients were prescribed a hypocaloric diet that included the use of liquid meal replacements. At 24 weeks, 69 % of those randomized remained in the study and body weight was reduced by 5.0, 7.2, and 10.1 % for the placebo, bupropion 300 mg, and bupropion 400 mg groups, respectively ($P < 0.0001$). The placebo group was randomized to the 300- or 400-mg group at 24 weeks and the trial was extended to week 48. By the end of the trial, the dropout rate was 41 %, and the weight losses in the bupropion 300 mg and bupropion 400 mg groups were 6.2 and 7.2 % of initial body weight, respectively [56].

Topiramate

Topiramate is an anticonvulsant drug that is approved for the use in certain types of epilepsy and for the prophylaxis of migraine headache. It was shown to reduce food intake, but was not developed clinically because of the side effects at the doses selected for trial. Topiramate was found to induce weight loss in clinical trials for epilepsy treatment. Weight losses of 3.9 % of initial weight at 3 months and 7.3 % of initial weight at 1 year were seen. In a 6-month, placebo-controlled, dose-ranging study [57], 385 subjects were randomized to five groups: topiramate at 64, 96, 192, or 384 mg/day or placebo. These doses were gradually increased over 12 weeks and were tapered off in a similar manner at the end of the trial. Weight loss from baseline to 24 weeks was 5.0, 4.8, 6.3, 6.3, and 2.6 %, in the five groups, respectively. The most frequent adverse events were paresthesias (tingling or prickly feelings in skin), somnolence, and difficulty with concentration, memory, and attention.

Conclusion

Medications are useful in treatment of the patient with obesity because they can reinforce behavioral intentions that lead to lifestyle change. The current approach to managing most obese patients is often to wait until comorbidity has developed and to then use a medication approved for that comorbidity. There are now four medications approved by the FDA for long-term weight loss and a fifth may be available soon. This makes treating the root cause (obesity) of many chronic diseases increasingly feasible. Still, adopting a weight-centric prescribing approach to chronic disease management is also important. In the management of obesity-associated chronic diseases, physicians should adopt an attitude in their prescribing of, first, doing no harm, i.e., avoiding medications that promote weight gain. Second, whenever possible patients should be counseled to lose weight as a pathway to health improvement. When they struggle, medications approved for long-term weight management are appropriate. Last, when necessary for chronic disease management, medications that promote weight loss should be prescribed. While the future points to use of combinations of medications for weight management and evaluation of anti-diabetic drugs for weight loss indication, it is time for physicians to incorporate weight loss counseling in their practices and to engage weight-centric management in their prescribing.

The lessons of the past in prescribing for obese patients and their medical problems are several. First, we learned that prescribing for weight loss in obesity, like prescribing for hypertension, is a chronic disease management paradigm. Drugs must be prescribed over the long term for chronic weight management; they do not produce permanent weight loss. Second, we learned the importance of understanding the mechanism by which drugs produce weight loss, so that the medication can be prescribed along with appropriate instruction in diet and physical activity. Third, safety and tolerability are key factors. By increasing doses of a single agent to maximize weight loss, adverse consequences arise. Thus, combination therapy using lower drug doses are carrying the day. Last, we have learned the hard lessons of unexpected consequences. Because one can never predict these, the current trend is to prescribe for patients with health consequences of their weight status, who will benefit from weight loss. Prescribing for cosmetic weight loss is unacceptable, given the wide margin of safety required for cosmetic intervention. The new medications for obesity take advantage of old targets, old compounds, and old principles learned from chronic disease management. Surely, we are finally entering an age where primary care physicians will feel responsible for helping patients manage their weight and for managing their chronic diseases in a weight-centric manner.

References

1. Flegal KM, Carroll MD, Ogden CL, Curtin LR. Prevalence and trends in obesity among US adults, 1999–2008. JAMA. 2010;303:235–41.
2. Prevalence of Overweight, Obesity and Extreme Obesity among adults: United States, Trends 1976–1980 through 2007–2008. www.cdc.gov/nch/data/hestat/obesity-adult_07_08. Posted 6/4/10.
3. Ogden CL, Carroll MD, Curtin LR, Lamb MM, Flegal KM. Prevalence of high body mass index in US children and adolescents, 2007–2008. JAMA. 2010;303:242–9.
4. Bray GA. The low-fructose approach to weight control. Pittsburgh: Dorrance Publishing; 2009.
5. Bray GA. A guide to obesity and the metabolic syndrome. Boca Raton: CRC Press; 2011.
6. Klein S, Burke LE, Bray GA, Blair S, Allison DB, Pi-Sunyer X, Hong Y, Eckel RH. Clinical implications of obesity with specific focus on cardiovascular disease: a statement for professionals from the American Heart Association Council on Nutrition, Physical Activity, and Metabolism: endorsed by the American College of Cardiology Foundation. Circulation. 2004;110:2952–67.

7. Decision Memo for Intensive Behavioral Therapy for Obesity (CAG-00423N). www.hhs. gov/medicare-coverage-database/details/nca-decision-memo.
8. LeBlanc ES, O'Connor E, Whitlock EP, Patnode CD, Kapka T. Effectiveness of primary care—relevant treatments for obesity in adults. A systematic evidence of review for the U.S. preventive task force. Ann Int Med. 2011;155:434–47.
9. Torgerson JS, Hauptman J, Boldrin MN, Sjöström L. XENical in the prevention of diabetes in obese subjects (XENDOS) study: a randomized study of orlistat as an adjunct to lifestyle changes for the prevention of type 2 diabetes in obese patients. Diabetes Care. 2004;27:155–61.
10. Chanoine JP, Hampl S, Jensen C, Boldrin M, Hauptman J. Effect of orlistat on weight and body composition in obese adolescents: a randomized controlled trial. JAMA. 2005;293:2873–83.
11. Rucker D, Padwal R, Li SK, Curioni C, Lau DC. Long term pharmacotherapy for obesity and overweight: updated meta-analysis. BMJ. 2007;335:1194–9.
12. Bray GA, Greenway FL. Pharmacological treatment of the overweight patient. Pharmacol Rev. 2007;59:151–84.
13. Rothman RB, Baumann MH. Serotonergic drugs and valvular heart disease. Expert Opin Drug Saf. 2009;8:317–29.
14. Halford JC, Harrold JA, Boyland EJ, Lawton CL, Blundell JE. Serotonergic drugs: effects on appetite expression and use for the treatment of obesity. Drugs. 2007;67:27–55.
15. FDA briefing information: meeting of the Endocrinologic and Metabolic Drugs Advisory Committee. http://www.fda.gov/downloads/AdvisoryCommittees/CommitteesMeetingMaterials/Drugs/EndocrinologicandMetabolicDrugsAdvisoryCommittee/UCM303198.pdf. Accessed 10 May 2012.
16. Smith SR, Weissman NJ, Anderson CMS, M, Chuang E, Stubbe S, Bays H, Shanahan WR, the Behavioral Modification and Lorcaserin for Overweight and Obesity Management (BLOOM) Study Group. Multicenter, placebo-controlled trial of lorcaserin for weight management. N Engl J Med. 2010;363:245–56.
17. Fidler MC, Sanchez M, Raether B, Weissman NJ, Smith SR, Shanahan WR, Anderson CM, for the BLOSSOM Clinical Trial Group. A one-year randomized trial of lorcaserin for weight loss in obese and overweight adults: the blossom trial was significantly greater than with placebo. J Clin Endocrinol Metab. 2011;96:3067–77.
18. O'Neil PM, Smith SR, Weissman NJ, Fidler MC, Sanchez M, Zhang J, Raether B, Anderson CM, Shanahan WR. Randomized placebo-controlled clinical trial of lorcaserin for weight loss in type 2 diabetes mellitus: the BLOOM-DM study. Obesity (Silver Spring). 2012;20(7):1426–36. doi:10.1038/oby.2012.66. (Epub 2012 Mar 16).
19. Allison DB, Gadde KM, Garvey WT, Peterson CA, Schwiers ML, Najarian T, Tam PY, Troupin B, Day WW. Controlled-release phentermine/topiramate in severely obese adults: a randomized controlled trial (EQUIP). Obesity. 2012;20(2):330–42.
20. Gadde KM, Allison DB, Ryan DH, Peterson CA, Troupin B, Schwiers ML, Day WW. Effects of low-dose, controlled-release, phentermine plus topiramate combination on weight and associated comorbidities in overweight and obese adults (CONQUER): a randomised, placebo-controlled, phase 3 trial.Lancet. 2011;377(9774):1341–52.
21. FDA briefing information : meeting of the Endocrinologic and Metabolic Drugs Advisory Committee. http://www.fda.gov/downloads/AdvisoryCommittees/CommitteesMeetingMaterials/Drugs/EndocrinologicandMetabolicDrugsAdvisoryCommittee/UCM292315.pdf. Accessed 22 Feb 2012.
22. Colman E, Golden J, Roberts M, Egan A, Weaver J, Rosebraugh C. The FDA's assessment of two drugs for chronic weight management. N Engl J Med. 25;367(17):1577–9. doi:10.1056/NEJMp1211277. Epub 2012 Oct 10.
23. Brownell KD. The learn manual for weight management. Dallas; Tex: American Health Publishing Co; 2000.
24. Garvey WT, Ryan DH, Look M, Gadde KM, Allison DB, Peterson CA, Schwiers M, Day WW, Bowden CH. Two-year sustained weight loss and metabolic benefits with controlled-release phentermine/topiramate in obese and overweight adults (SEQUEL): a randomized, placebo-controlled, phase 3 extension study. Am J Clin Nutr. 2012;95:297–308.

25. Greenway FL, Whitehouse MJ, Guttadauria M, Anderson JW, Atkinson RL, Fujioka K, Gadde KM, Gupta AK, O'Neil P, Schumacher D, Smith D, Dunayevich E, Tollefson GD, Weber E, Cowley MA. Rational design of a combination medication for the treatment of obesity. Obesity (Silver Spring). 2009;17:30–9.

26. CONTRAVE (NALTREXONE SR/BUPROPION SR COMBINATION) ADVISORY COMMITTEE BRIEFING DOCUMENT. NDA 200063. Endocrinologic and Metabolic Drugs Advisory Committee Meeting, December 7, 2010.

27. Greenway FL, Fujioka K, Plodkowski RA, Mudaliar S, Guttadauria M, Erickson J, Kim DD, Dunayevich E, for the COR-I Study Group. Effect of naltrexone plus bupropion on weight loss in overweight and obese adults (COR-I): a multicenter, randomised, double = blind, placebo-controlled, phase 3 trial. Lancet. 2010;376:595–605.

28. Wadden TA, Foreyt JP, Foster GD, Hill JO, Klein S, O'Neil PM, Perri MG, Pi-Sunyer FX, Rock CL, Erikson JS, Maier HN, Kim DD, Dunayeich E. Weight loss with naltrexoneSR/ bupropion SR combination therapy as an adjunct to behavior modification: the COR-BMOD trial. Obesity. 2011;19:110–20.

29. Seufert J, Gallwitz B. The extra-pancreatic effects of GLP-1 receptor agonists:a focus on the cardiovascular, gastrointestinal and central nervous systems. Diabetes Obes Metab. 2014;16:673–88.

30. van Can J, Sloth B, Jensen CB, Flint A, Blaak EE, Saris WH. Effects of the once-daily GLP-1 analog liraglutide on gastric emptying, glycemic parameters, appetite and energy metabolism in obese, non-diabetic adults. Int J Obes (Lond). 2014;38(6):784–93. doi:10.1038/ijo.2013.162. Epub 2013 Sept 3.

31. Astrup A, Rössner S, Van Gaal L, Rissanen A, Niskanen L, Al Hakim M, Madsen J, Rasmussen MF, Lean ME. NN8022-1807 Study Group. Effects of liraglutide in the treatment of obesity: a randomised, double-blind, placebo-controlled study. Lancet. 2009;374:1606–16.

32. Wadden TA, et al. Weight maintenance and additional weight loss with liraglutide after low-calorie-diet-induced weight loss: the SCALE Maintenance randomized study. Int J Obes (Lond). 2013;37(11):1443–51.

33. VI-0521 (QNEXA®) ADVISORY COMMITTEE BRIEFING DOCUMENT. NDA 022580. Endocrinologic and Metabolic Drugs Advisory Committee Meeting. July 15, 2010 www.fda. gov/.../AdvisoryCommittees/CommitteesMeetingMaterials/. Accessed 15 March 2012.

34. Ryan D, Peterson C, Troupin B, Najarian T, Tam P, Day W. Weight loss at 6 months with VI-0521 (PHEN/TPM combination) treatment. Obes Facts. 2010;3:139–46.

35. Kang JG, Park C-Y, Kang JH, Park Y-W, Park SW. Randomized controlled trial to investigate the effects of a newly developed formulation of phentermine diffuse-controlled release for obesity. Diabetes Obes Metab. 2010;12:876–82.

36. Addy C, Rosko JP, Li S, Li H, Maes A, Johnson-Levonas, AO, Chodakewitz J, Stoch SA, Wagner JA. Pharmacokinetics, safety, and tolerability of phentermine in healthy participants receiving taranabant, a novel cannabinoid-1 receptor (CB1R) inverse agonist. J Clin Pharmacol. 2009;49(10):1228–38.

37. Kim KK, Cho H-J, Kang J-C, Youn B-B, Lee K-R. Effects on weight reduction and safety of short-term phentermine administration in Korean obese people. Yonsei Med J. 2006;47(5):614–25.

38. Hendricks EJ, Rothman RB, Greenway FL. How physician obesity specialists use drugs to treat obesity. Obesity (Silver Spring). 2009;17:1730–5.

39. Knowler WC, Barrett-Connor E, Fowler SE, Hamman RF, Lachin JM, Walker EA, Nathan DM. Reduction in the incidence of type 2 diabetes with lifestyle intervention or metformin. NEJM. 2002;346:393–403.

40. Knowler WC, Fowler SE, Hamman RF, Christophi CA, Hoffman HJ, Brenneman AT, Brown-Friday JO, Goldberg R, Venditti E, Nathan DM. 10-year followup of diabetes incidence and weight loss in the diabetes prevention program outcomes study. Lancet. 2009;374:1677–86.

41. Tuomilehto J, Lindström J, Eriksson JG, Valle TT, Hämäläinen H, Ilanne-Parikka P, Keinänen-Kiukaanniemi S, Laakso M, Louheranta A, Rastas M, Salminen V, Uusitupa M. Finnish

diabetes prevention study group. Prevention of type 2 diabetes mellitus by changes in lifestyle among subjects with impaired glucose tolerance. N Engl J Med. 2001;344:1343–50.

42. Buchwald H, Avidor Y, Braunwald E, Jensen MD, Pories W, Fahrbach K, Schoelles K. Bariatric surgery: a systematic review and meta-analysis. JAMA. 2004;292:1724–37.

43. Gregg EW, Chen H, Wagenknecht LE, Clark JM, Delahanty LM, Bantle J, Pownall HJ, Johnson KC, Safford MM, Kitabchi AE, Pi-Sunyer FX, Wing RR, Bertoni AG, Look AHEAD Research Group. Association of an intensive lifestyle intervention with remission of type 2 diabetes. JAMA. 2012;308(23):2489–96.

44. Leslie W, Hankey CR, Lean MEJ. Weight gain as an adverse effect of some commonly prescribed drugs: a systematic review. Quart J Med. 2007;100:395–404.

45. Bray GA, Ryan DH. Medical therapy for the patient with obesity. Circulation. 2012;125:1695–1703.

46. He L, Sabet A, Djedjos S, Miller R, Sun X, Hussain MA, Radovick S, Wondisford FE. Metformin and insulin suppress hepatic gluconeogenesis through phosphorylation of CREB binding protein. Cell. 2009;137:635–46.

47. Diabetes Prevention Program Research Group, DPP, Bray G, Edelstein S, Crandall J, Aroda V, Franks P, Fujimoto W, Horton E, Jeffries S, Montez M, Mudaliar S, Pi-Sunyer X, White N, Knowler W. Long term safety, tolerability and weight loss associated with metformin in the diabetes prevention program outcomes study. Diab Care. 2012;35:731–7.

48. Bushe CJ, Bradley AJ, Doshi S, Karagianis J. Changes in weight and metabolicparameters during treatment with antipsychotics and metformin: do the data inform as to potential guideline development? A systematic review of clinical studies. Int J Clin Pract. 2009;63:1743–61.

49. Aronne LJ, Halseth AE, Burns CM, Miller S, Shen LZ. Enhanced weight loss following co-administration of pramlintide with sibutramine or phentermine in a multicenter trial. Obesity (Silver Spring). 2010;18(9):1739–46. Epub 2010 Jan 21.

50. Edwards CM, Stanley SA, Davis R, Brynes AE, Frost GS, Seal LJ, Ghatei MA, Bloom SR. Exendin-4 reduces fasting and postprandial glucose and decreases energy intake in healthy volunteers. Am J Physiol Endocrinol Metab. 2001;281:E155–61.

51. Amori RE, Lau J, Pittas AG. Efficacy and safety of incretintherapy in type 2 diabetes: systematic review and meta-analysis. JAMA. 2007;298:194–206.

52. Apovian CM, Bergenstal RM, Cuddihy RM, Qu Y, Lenox S, Lewis MS, Glass LC. Effects of exenatide combined with lifestyle modification in patients with type 2 diabetes. Am J Med. 2010;123:e9–e17.

53. Fineman MS, Shen LZ, Taylor K, Kim DD, Baron AD. Effectiveness of progressive dose-escalation of exenatide (exendin-4) in reducing dose-limiting side effects in subjects with type 2 diabetes. Diabetes Metab Res Rev. 2004;20:411–7.

54. Ferrannini E, Solini A. SGLT2 inhibition in diabetes mellitus: rationale and clinical prospects. Nat Rev Endocrinol. 2012;8:495–502.

55. Vasilakou D, Karaglannis T, Athanasladou E, Mainou M, Liakos A, Bekiari E, Sarigianni M, Matthews DR. Tsapas A 2013 Sodium-glucose cotransporter 2 inhibitors for type 2 diabetes: a systematic review and meta-analysis. Ann Intern Med 159:262–274.

56. Anderson JW, Greenway FL, Fujioka K, Gadde KM, McKenney J, O'Neil PM. Bupropion SR enhances weight loss: a 48-week double-blind, placebo- controlled trial. Obes Res. 2002;10:633–41.

57. Bray GA, Hollander P, Klein S, Kushner R, Levy B, Fitchet M, Perry BH. A 6-month randomized, placebo-controlled, dose-ranging trial of topiramate for weight loss in obesity. Obes Res. 2003;11:722–33.

Chapter 7
Roux-en-Y Gastric Bypass: Procedure and Outcomes

Seth Felder and Scott Cunneen

Introduction

Roux-en-Y gastric bypass (RNYGB), the most commonly performed bariatric (weight loss) operation in the USA, involves two surgical alterations: restriction of gastric volume and diversion of ingested nutrients away from the proximal small intestine [1, 2] (Fig. 7.1). The strength of the RNYGB lies in the hybridization of restriction and bypass into one procedure. The reduction of food intake mediated by restriction is accompanied by dynamic changes in nutrient transport along the gastrointestinal tract. Thus, resultant changes in hormonal profiles constitute one of the first and most important roles of RNYGB [3]. Although the physiological changes contributing to loss of body weight and improvements in obesity-related comorbidities are incompletely understood, the complexities of neurohormonal changes and precise mechanisms resulting in durable weight loss and reduction in associated comorbidities continue to be elucidated. Even though we continue to learn and progress in understanding the intricate interplay between the alimentary tract and neurohormonal axis, the benefits of gastric bypass are clear and well-documented with long-term follow-up results of surgery demonstrating obesity-related mortality and morbidity significantly reduced [4–6].

S. Felder (✉)
Surgery, Cedars-Sinai Medical Center, Los Angeles, CA, USA
e-mail: seth.felder@cshs.org

S. Cunneen
Department of Surgery, Cedars-Sinai Medical Center, Los Angeles, CA, USA
e-mail: Scott.Cunneen@cshs.org

© Springer Science+Business Media New York 2015   111
A. Youdim (ed.), *The Clinician's Guide to the Treatment of Obesity,*
Endocrine Updates, DOI 10.1007/978-1-4939-2146-1_7

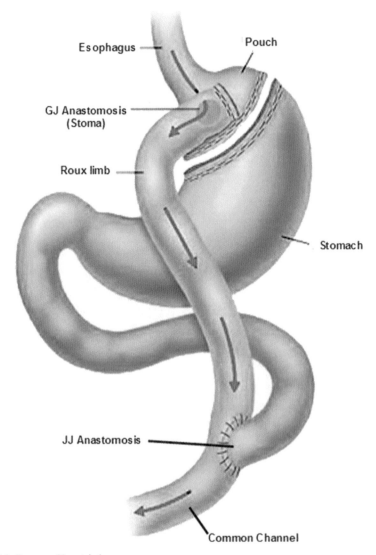

Fig. 7.1 Roux-en-Y gastric bypass

History of Gastric Bypass

The origins of the gastric bypass operation date back to the 1960s and the contributions of Dr. Mason. While searching for a weight loss operation without the detrimental side effects often seen with the jejuno-ileal bypass, he noted that patients with peptic ulcer disease who had undergone a partial gastrectomy with Billroth II gastrojejunostomy subsequently experienced weight loss and had difficulty regaining that lost weight. Based on these findings, Mason described the original gastric bypass in 1967 using a technique that divided the stomach and anastomosed a jejunal loop to the proximal gastric pouch [7, 8]. His original description emphasized a small pouch as well as a small diameter anastomosis to delay gastric emptying and enhance satiety [8]. Over the ensuing several decades, there have been a variety of technical modifications, including attempted calibration and standardization of gastric pouch size [9] and the replacement of the loop gastrojejunostomy with a Roux-en-Y configuration [10]. In 1995, Wittgrove reported the first laparoscopic RNYGB [11]. Since this time, data from the Nationwide Inpatient Sample from 2003 through 2008 have documented an increase of laparoscopic bariatric operations from 20% in 2003 to 90% in 2008 [12]. Minimally invasive techniques now account for the vast majority of bariatric procedures performed today and should be considered the standard of care in primary procedures.

Operative and Technical Details

Despite the evolution and almost universal adoption to a laparoscopic technique, there still remain significant technical variations in the way a RNYGBP can be performed. Owing to its complexity and the need for a high degree of laparoscopic technical skills, the relative risk of complications has been reported to diminish following a 500-procedure learning curve [13]. The number of surgeries performed, or experience of the operating surgeon, and the standardization of the laparoscopic technique have been cited as main factors contributing to improved rates of postoperative complications, mortality, and decrease in conversion to open rates [13]. The currently adopted surgical principles, as described by Pories et al. include the exclusion of a majority of the stomach ($\sim 90\%$) except for a 15–30-ml pouch created around the gastroesophageal junction, and transection of the jejunum 30–60 cm from the ligament of Treitz [14]. The distal jejunal segment (Roux limb) is then anastomosed to the gastric pouch and the proximal jejunal segment (biliopancreatic limb) connected distally as a jejunojejunostomy approximately 75–150 cm from the ligament of Treitz, providing secretory drainage of the bypassed stomach, duodenum, and proximal jejunum (common channel limb). The Roux limb, or alimentary limb, carries ingested food and is delineated between the gastrojejunostomy and the jejunojejunostomy. The Roux limb, the excluded or remnant stomach, duodenum, and proximal jejunum represent the bypassed section of the RNYGB [3, 14]. Variations in operative techniques other than gastric pouch size and Roux limb length have included various positionings of the Roux limb and gastrojejunal anastomosis in relation to other body structures. Combinations have included antecolic (above colon) versus retrocolic (behind colon) placement of the Roux limb and antegastric (above stomach) versus retrogastric (behind stomach) creation of the gastrojejunostomy. Techniques for construction of the gastrojejunostomy have included: one layer versus two-layered anastomosis, stapled versus hand-sewn anastomosis or combinations of techniques. Other major variations include routine versus selective closure of mesenteric defects [15, 16].

Outcomes

Multiple studies have demonstrated that among morbidly obese patients, compared with nonsurgical control patients, the use of RNYGB has been associated with higher rates of diabetes remission and lower risk of cardiovascular and other negative health outcomes over long-term follow up [17–20]. In contrast, the cardiovascular and metabolic status of obese control participants generally worsens over time, despite aggressive medical management. When comparing RNYGB with lifestyle and intensive medical management, achievement of primary end points including hemoglobin A1C level, low-density lipoprotein cholesterol levels, systolic blood pressure, and the number of medications needed to manage these co-morbidities, the literature has consistently supported gastric bypass, although at the potential expense of increased nutritional deficiencies and potential surgical complications [21].

Weight Loss

Several studies have evaluated the degree of weight loss following gastric bypass, and the durability of the lost weight. A meta-analytic review of the recent published surgical experience found an excess weight loss of 68.2% (61.5–74.8%) for RNYGB [22]. A randomized series reported by Nguyen et al. examined 111 laparoscopic RNYGB during a 4-year follow-up period. The authors reported 68.4% excess weight loss (EWL) for RNYGB with a mean body mass index (BMI) decrease of 15 kg/m^2 [23]. In a smaller series, Spivak et. al. reported an EWL of 58.6% at 7 years follow-up [24]. However, after an initial 4 years of progressive weight loss,the authors reported that most patients experience a certain weight regain during a long-term follow-up period [24]. The prospective, controlled Swedish Obese Subjects study reported a 7% mean weight regain among patients after gastric bypass surgery from 2 years to 10 years [20]. A more recent study described similar results, with a weight regain of approximately 7% at 2 years following gastric bypass surgery [17]. Overall, it has been found that for the majority the weight loss is durable and weight regain is modest. It is unclear, at present, if the weight regain represents the normal weight trajectory of the patient's weight over time or a consequence of physiological or behavioral adaptations to the surgical changes performed.

Diabetes Mellitus

Insulin resistance constitutes a central pathophysiology of type II diabetes mellitus (DM) in the obese. Long-standing remission of DM has been reported to occur in up to 83% of individuals undergoing RNYGB [3, 18, 25, 26]. In the Surgical Treatment and Medications Potentially Eradicate Diabetes Efficiently (STAMPEDE) trial, intensive medical therapy was compared to surgical treatment (gastric bypass or sleeve gastrectomy) as a means of improving glycemic control. The proportion of patients with the primary end point was 12 % in the medical-therapy group versus 42 % in the gastric bypass group ($P=0.002$) [27]. The mechanisms by which gastric bypass results in prolonged improvement in glycemic control have been the subject of a great deal of scientific study. Weight loss, reduced oral intake, altered enteric hormonal secretion (glucagon-like peptide-1, glucose-dependent insulinotropic peptide, ghrelin), and changes to the gastrointestinal tract microflora, all having been proposed as playing a part in this phenomenon [28–34]. Caloric restriction in obese patients without surgery improves insulin sensitivity and glucose homeostasis significantly before any evidence of weight loss is seen [35]. Similarly, all types of bariatric surgery include an element of caloric restriction, which may be the common cause for the associated improvements in insulin sensitivity independent of anatomic changes [3, 36]. However, the immediate effects in glycemic control often precede substantial weight loss typically associated with insulin sensitivity [3]. These observations are consistent with findings by Schauer et al. where reductions in the use of diabetes medications occurred before the achievement of maximal weight loss, suggesting that caloric restriction alone is unable to explain the complex effects RNYGB has on DM [21, 27, 37–39].

Despite the expectation that DM may undergo remission, or at least improve following RNYGB, there is a relative paucity of data attempting to identify patient-specific predictive factors. Hayes et al. used 13 preoperative parameters and a variety of statistical techniques to create mathematical models able to correctly identify which patients would experience remission of DM at 12 months follow-up in 82.7–87.4 % of cases[40]. The two strongest predictors of DM resolution were low HbA1c and the nature and level of preoperative DM control [25, 40, 41]. Other predictive factors that have been proposed for long-term DM remission have included gender (males more likely than women), younger age, and percentage of postoperative EWL [42, 43].

Dyslipidemia

Hyperlipidemia plays a major role in the excess morbidity and premature mortality of the morbidly obese. Improvements in coronary risk factors, including hyperlipidemia, after gastric bypass have been predicted to lower the 10-year risk of ischemic heart disease events by approximately 50 % [44]. Nguyen et al. showed a significant positive effect on atherogenic lipids with improvement of favorable lipoprotein levels after RNYGB that were sustained for the duration of the study [45]. Improvement in lipid profiles was observed as early as 3 months postoperatively and sustained at 2 years follow-up. One year after gastric bypass, mean total cholesterol levels decreased by 16 %; triglyceride levels decreased by 63 %; low-density lipoprotein cholesterol levels decreased by 31 %; very-low-density lipoprotein cholesterol decreased by 74%; total cholesterol/high-density lipoprotein cholesterol risk ratio decreased by 60%, and high-density lipoprotein cholesterol levels increased by 39%. Also, within 1 year, 82% of patients requiring lipid-lowering medications preoperatively were able to discontinue their medications [45].

Operative Risk Stratification

A large meta-analysis of over 29,000 patients reported mortality of gastric bypass to be 0.5%.(4) The obesity surgery mortality risk score (OS-MRS) developed by a single institution experience of 2075 patients and subsequently validated used a 90-day all-cause death rate, not just hospitalization, and confirmed a high-risk predictive score [46, 47]. The OS-MRS assigns 1 point to each of 5 preoperative variables, including body mass index >=50 kg/m2, male gender, hypertension, known risk factors for pulmonary embolism (previous thromboembolism, preoperative vena cava filter, hypoventilation, pulmonary hypertension), and age >=45 years [48, 49]. Overall mortality for the validation cohort was 0.7%, consistent with published standards, and represents an average mortality risk among all patient subgroups. Although the highest-risk group class based on the OS-MRS score experienced a 12-fold increase in mortality compared with the lowest-risk group patients, the authors emphasized that the increased risk should not preclude consideration for surgical treatment, as these high-risk patients represent those with a high-risk of early death from their associated comorbidities of obesity.

Postoperative Adverse Outcomes

Anastomotic Leak

Unexplained tachycardia, dyspnea, oliguria, and hypoxia may be warning signs of a leak; however, initial signs and symptoms may be minimal in the morbidly obese. An expected leak rate has been reported to be 0.5% for laparoscopic RNYGB and remains the most common cause of death after bariatric surgery, followed by pulmonary embolism [50]. A high index of suspicion is warranted and emergent re-exploration may be indicated in patients with unexplained septic physiology.

The primary goal is to obtain adequate drainage of the leak (thereby creating a controlled fistula), bowel rest, broad-spectrum antibiotics, and nutritional support either parenterally or by distal enteral feeding through a gastrostomy tube placed in the excluded stomach to promote healing of the leak. Imaging studies that may assist in diagnosing a leak include an upper gastrointestinal (UGI) study or computerized tomography (CT) scan with oral contrast.

Internal Hernia/Small Bowel Obstruction

Defects in the mesentery are created when transecting the small intestine and reconstructing continuity in a Roux-en-Y configuration. Several potential spaces allow for small bowel herniation with the possibility for strangulation and necrosis of a large intestinal segment. Despite this, routine closure of mesentery is controversial. According to the literature, nonclosure of the defects with the laparoscopic RNYGB technique (antegastric, antecolic), results in an internal hernia rate of 6.9% [51]. Higa recently demonstrated that after systematic closure of both the mesenteric defect and the Petersen defect with nonresorbable material, the occurrence of internal hernia after transmesocolic, antegastric laparoscopic RNYGB decreased from 16% to <1% [52]. Conversely, Rosenthal's group reported that the chances of developing an internal hernia are low and do not justify the additional time and possible complications associated with closure of defects [53].

Any patient having undergone RNYGB presenting with abdominal pain and signs or symptoms consistent with bowel obstruction must be considered to have an internal hernia until proven otherwise. The consequence of a delayed diagnosis of an internal hernia is infarction of an extensive portion of small bowel. Persistent abdominal pain in the setting of a negative radiologic study does not rule out the possibility of internal herniation. Diagnostic laparoscopy may serve as the most expeditious diagnostic and potentially therapeutic modality for post-gastric bypass patients with abdominal pain, either definitively "ruling-out" or "ruling-in" an internal hernia while allowing for immediate repair.

In the immediate postoperative period, obstruction distal to the jejunojejunostomy can cause acute distention of the gastric remnant, which is a surgical emergency. Patients may present with severe bloating and persistent hiccups with a plain abdominal X-ray demonstrating dilatation of the remnant stomach.

Marginal Ulceration

The incidence of marginal ulceration at the gastrojejunal anastomosis ranges from 0.6 to 16% [54–57]. This number increases to 53.3% when the complication of gastrogastric fistula is also present [58]. Several factors, including gastric acid, foreign body reaction, exogenous substances such as alcohol, nicotine, and nonsteroidal anti-inflammatory drugs, and *Helicobacter pylori* infection, have been implicated as potential etiologies causing mucosal ischemia and subsequent marginal ulcer formation [57, 59]. The majority (>90%) of patients diagnosed with a marginal ulcer will experience complete resolution of symptoms with proton pump inhibitors and sucralfate.

Anastomotic Stricture

Factors associated with the formation of strictures include operative technique, tension and ischemia at the anastomosis, and ulcer formation [60]. Gradual onset of intolerance to solids or liquids, epigastric pain, and vomiting may signify the development of a stricture. Stricturing at the gastrojejunostomy presents differently than a stricture distally at the jejunojenostomy, as the biliopancreatic limb would contribute bile reflux. A UGI study may assist in diagnosis, however, endoscopic evaluation may be both diagnostic and therapeutic. Dilatation is generally recommended if the gastrojejunostomy anastomosis stoma diameter is less than 15 mm, with serial dilations sometimes required. After 3 balloon treatments, however, surgical revision is generally recommended. Jejunojejunostomy anastomotic narrowing more often requires operative revision, as they are less amenable to endoscopic intervention. The efficacy of newer endoscopic techniques, such as stenting, is yet to be validated.

Gastrogastric Fistula

An abnormal reconnection between the gastric pouch and remnant stomach occurs in approximately 1.2% of patients following RNYGB [58]. Risk factors for developing a gastrogastric fistula include marginal ulceration and postoperative leak. Symptoms are vague but include nausea, vomiting, and epigastric pain in the majority of patients, as well as insufficient weight loss or weight regain in a minority of patients. The most sensitive test for diagnosing a gastrogastric fistula is an UGI study. Medical treatment may be attempted initially, consisting of acid suppression therapy, particularly if associated with a concomitant marginal ulcer. However, persistent pain, weight regain, and ulceration refractory to optimal medical treatment requires revisional surgery with ligation of the fistula [58].

Weight Regain

Failure to sustain weight loss is often cited as the most common indication for revisional gastric bypass surgery [8, 10]. Loss of restriction in patients with prior RNYGB can occur in three ways: dilation of the gastric pouch, dilation of the gastrojejunostomy anastomosis, or a combination of both. Enlargement over time of the restrictive component can occur secondary to strictures at the gastrojejunostomy anastomosis and maladaptive eating habits which can stress and dilate the gastric pouch over time [61]. Revisional surgery after RNYGB performed for weight regain provides good additional weight loss but carries significant morbidity [62]. Complication rates as high as 33–62% have been reported in the literature, most commonly due to the significant increase in anastomotic leaks [60].

Dumping Syndrome

Typically occurring in patients noncompliant with the recommended bariatric diet, dumping is believed to occur due to exposure of the proximal small bowel to hyperosmolar refined sugars and fats. The small gastric reservoir and the increased gastric emptying lead to rapid filling of the small bowel with hyperosmolar chyme, causing an osmotic overload and shift of extracellular fluid into the bowel to restore isotonicity. This increase of fluid in the small bowel causes intestinal distention, cramping, vomiting, and diarrhea. The late dumping syndrome occurs 1–4 h after eating and is characterized by reactive hypoglycemia with diaphoresis, dizziness, and fatigue. The dumping response may serve as a negative conditioning response against consumption of a high-sugar diet postoperatively [63].

Vitamin Deficiencies

Low levels of iron, vitamin B_{12}, vitamin D, and calcium are predominant after RNYGB [64]. Routine testing for micronutrient deficiency may be required indefinitely following gastric bypass.

Iron-deficiency anemia is estimated to occur in 14–16 % of patients by the American Society of Bariatric and Metabolic Surgery after RNYGB [65]. The etiology is multifactorial, including reduced absorption of dietary iron in association with achlorhydria caused by gastric partitioning. The decreased production of hydrochloric acid in the gastric pouch diminishes the conversion of ferrous iron to the more absorbable ferric iron. Iron absorption occurs predominantly in the duodenum, which is bypassed. Most multivitamin and mineral supplements do not contain sufficient amounts of iron to prevent deficiency. Iron deficiency and anemia sometimes persist despite oral supplementation. Recommended amount of supplemental iron in the RNYGB patient is 45–60 g daily. In refractory cases, intravenous iron may be necessary [64].

Although the body storage of vitamin B_{12} is substantial (about 2000 µg) compared to the small daily needs (2 µg/day), the deficiency is relatively common. The estimated prevalence of vitamin B12 deficiency after RNYGB range from 12 to 33 % [66]. Since there is a risk of irreversible neurological damage if B_{12} deficiency is maintained for an extended period, B12 should be monitored postoperatively. B12 deficiency is due to achlorhydria, suboptimal vitamin consumption, and a reduced production of intrinsic factor, which is required for normal absorption to occur in distal ileum. The absence of hydrochloric acid and pepsin restricts the cleavage of food-bound vitamin B12 from its protein carrier. The use of 350 µg/day generally corrects a low level of this vitamin. Only a small percentage of individuals will require parenteral administration of B_{12} (2000 µg/month) [67].

Folate deficiency after RNYGB range from 0 to 28 % and usually occurs secondary to decreased dietary intake. Additionally, Vitamin B12 is needed for the conversion of inactive folate to the active form of folate. Folate deficiency is preventable and promptly corrected with multivitamin supplementation (400 mcg/day) [64].

Thiamine is absorbed in the proximal small intestine, and may become deficient after a combination of reduced intake, frequent vomiting, and malabsorption. The incidence of thiamine deficiency after bariatric surgery has been reportedly low. Chang et al. found only 29 cases (0.0002%) of thiamine deficiency in a total of 168,010 bariatric cases reported in a survey by members of the American Society for Metabolic and Bariatric Surgery [68]. To prevent potentially catastrophic neurologic consequences (Wernicke-Korsakoff) of Thiamine deficiency, oral supplementation is mandatory because humans cannot synthesize it [69].

Malabsorption of calcium and vitamin D occurs from bypassing the duodenum and proximal jejunum after RYGB. The malabsorption of vitamin D contributes further to calcium malabsorption. With a relative lack of calcium, the production of parathyroid hormone (PTH) is increased, which leads to the release of calcium from bone, potentially causing bone loss and long-term risk of osteoporosis.

The delayed breakdown of dietary fats and delayed formation of micelles limits the fat available for absorption resulting in undigested fat and can cause malabsorption of the fat-soluble vitamins (A, D, E, K) and steatorrhea.

Conclusion

In summary, RNYGB remains a procedure of choice for most metabolic and weight loss surgeons in the USA today. It is a safe, durable procedure which should be offered early and liberally to those who qualify. Its favorable risk to benefit balance has endured decades despite the appearance of popular choices that have gained short-term favor and have subsequently demonstrated inferior durability in fighting the chronic diseases of obesity and the common metabolic derangements that often accompany it.

References

1. Santry HP, Gillen DL, Lauderdale DS. Trends in bariatric surgical procedures. JAMA J Am Med Assoc. 2005;294(15):1909–17.
2. Rubino F, Gagner M, Gentileschi P, Kini S, Fukuyama S, Feng J, et al. The early effect of the Roux-en-Y gastric bypass on hormones involved in body weight regulation and glucose metabolism. Ann Surg. 2004;240(2):236–42.
3. Saliba J, Wattacheril J, Abumrad NN. Endocrine and metabolic response to gastric bypass. Curr Opin Clin Nutr Metab Care. 2009;12(5):515–21.
4. Buchwald H, Avidor Y, Braunwald E, Jensen MD, Pories W, Fahrbach K, et al. Bariatric surgery: a systematic review and meta-analysis. JAMA J Am Med Assoc. 2004;292(14):1724–37.
5. Maggard MA, Shugarman LR, Suttorp M, Maglione M, Sugerman HJ, Sugarman HJ, et al. Meta-analysis: surgical treatment of obesity. Ann Intern Med. 2005;142(7):547–59.
6. Perry CD, Hutter MM, Smith DB, Newhouse JP, McNeil BJ. Survival and changes in comorbidities after bariatric surgery. Ann Surg. 2008;247(1):21–7.
7. Baker MT. The history and evolution of bariatric surgical procedures. Surg Clin North Am. 2011;91(6):1181–201, viii.

8. Mason EE, Ito C. Gastric bypass in obesity. Surg Clin North Am. 1967;47(6):1345–51.
9. Alder RL, Terry BE. Measurement and standardization of the gastric pouch in gastric bypass. Surg Gynecol Obstet. 1977;144(5):762–3.
10. Griffen WO Jr, Young VL, Stevenson CC. A prospective comparison of gastric and jejunoileal bypass procedures for morbid obesity. Ann Surg. 1977;186(4):500–9.
11. Wittgrove AC, Clark GW Tremblay LJ. Laparoscopic gastric bypass Roux-en-Y: preliminary report of five cases. Obes Surg. 1994;4(4):353–7.
12. Nguyen NT, Masoomi H, Magno CP, Nguyen X-MT, Laugenour K, Lane J. Trends in use of bariatric surgery, 2003–2008. J Am Coll Surg. 2011;213(2):261–6.
13. El-Kadre L, Tinoco AC, Tinoco RC, Aguiar L, Santos T. Overcoming the learning curve of laparoscopic Roux-en-Y gastric bypass: a 12-year experience. Surg Obes Relat Dis Off J Am Soc Bariatr Surg. 2013;9(6):867–72
14. Pories WJ, Swanson MS, MacDonald KG, Long SB, Morris PG, Brown BM, et al. Who would have thought it? An operation proves to be the most effective therapy for adult-onset diabetes mellitus. Ann Surg. 1995;222(3):339–50; (discussion 350–352).
15. Bendewald FP, Choi JN, Blythe LS, Selzer DJ, Ditslear JH, Mattar SG. Comparison of hand-sewn, linear-stapled, and circular-stapled gastrojejunostomy in laparoscopic Roux-en-Y gastric bypass. Obes Surg. 2011;21(11):1671–5.
16. Kravetz AJ, Reddy S, Murtaza G, Yenumula P. A comparative study of handsewn versus stapled gastrojejunal anastomosis in laparoscopic Roux-en-Y gastric bypass. Surg Endosc. 2011;25(4):1287–92.
17. Adams TD, Gress RE, Smith SC, Halverson RC, Simper SC, Rosamond WD, et al. Long-term mortality after gastric bypass surgery. N Engl J Med. 2007;357(8):753–61.
18. Adams TD, Davidson LE, Litwin SE, Kolotkin RL, LaMonte MJ, Pendleton RC, et al. Health benefits of gastric bypass surgery after 6 years. JAMA J Am Med Assoc. 2012;308(11):1122–31.
19. Sjöström L, Lindroos A-K, Peltonen M, Torgerson J, Bouchard C, Carlsson B, et al. Lifestyle, diabetes, and cardiovascular risk factors 10 years after bariatric surgery. N Engl J Med. 2004;351(26):2683–93.
20. Sjöström L, Narbro K, Sjöström CD, Karason K, Larsson B, Wedel H, et al. Effects of bariatric surgery on mortality in Swedish obese subjects. N Engl J Med. 2007;357(8):741–52.
21. Ikramuddin S, Korner J, Lee W-J, Connett JE, Inabnet WB, Billington CJ, et al. Roux-en-Y gastric bypass vs intensive medical management for the control of type 2 diabetes, hypertension, and hyperlipidemia: the Diabetes Surgery Study randomized clinical trial. JAMA J Am Med Assoc. 2013;309(21):2240–9.
22. Buchwald H, Estok R, Fahrbach K, Banel D, Jensen MD, Pories WJ, et al. Weight and type 2 diabetes after bariatric surgery: systematic review and meta-analysis. Am J Med. 2009;122(3):248–56.e5.
23. Nguyen NT, Slone JA, Nguyen X-MT, Hartman JS, Hoyt DB. A prospective randomized trial of laparoscopic gastric bypass versus laparoscopic adjustable gastric banding for the treatment of morbid obesity: outcomes, quality of life, and costs. Ann Surg. 2009;250(4):631–41.
24. Spivak H, Abdelmelek MF, Beltran OR, Ng AW, Kitahama S. Long-term outcomes of laparoscopic adjustable gastric banding and laparoscopic Roux-en-Y gastric bypass in the United States. Surg Endosc. 2012;26(7):1909–19.
25. Adams S, Salhab M, Hussain Z, Miller G, Leveson S. Preoperatively determinable factors predictive of diabetes mellitus remission following Roux-en-Y gastric bypass: a review of the literature. Acta Diabetol. 2013;50(4):475–8.
26. Kim S, Richards WO. Long-term follow-up of the metabolic profiles in obese patients with type 2 diabetes mellitus after Roux-en-Y gastric bypass. Ann Surg. 2010;251(6):1049–55.
27. Schauer PR, Kashyap SR, Wolski K, Brethauer SA, Kirwan JP, Pothier CE, et al. Bariatric surgery versus intensive medical therapy in obese patients with diabetes. N Engl J Med. 2012;366(17):1567–76.
28. Burcelin R, Serino M, Chabo C, Blasco-Baque V, Amar J. Gut microbiota and diabetes: from pathogenesis to therapeutic perspective. Acta Diabetol. 2011;48(4):257–73.

29. Amar J, Serino M, Lange C, Chabo C, Iacovoni J, Mondot S, et al. Involvement of tissue bacteria in the onset of diabetes in humans: evidence for a concept. Diabetologia. 2011;54(12):3055–61.

30. Ishida RK, Faintuch J, Paula AMR, Risttori CA, Silva SN, Gomes ES, et al. Microbial flora of the stomach after gastric bypass for morbid obesity. Obes Surg. 2007;17(6):752–8.

31. Dixon JB, le Roux CW, Rubino F, Zimmet P. Bariatric surgery for type 2 diabetes. Lancet. 2012;379(9833):2300–11.

32. Pournaras DJ, Osborne A, Hawkins SC, Vincent RP, Mahon D, Ewings P, et al. Remission of type 2 diabetes after gastric bypass and banding: mechanisms and 2 year outcomes. Ann Surg. 2010;252(6):966–71.

33. Thaler JP, Cummings DE. Minireview: hormonal and metabolic mechanisms of diabetes remission after gastrointestinal surgery. Endocrinology. 2009;150(6):2518–25.

34. Vetter ML, Ritter S, Wadden TA, Sarwer DB. Comparison of bariatric surgical procedures for diabetes remission: efficacy and mechanisms. Diabetes Spectr Publ Am Diabetes Assoc. 2012;25(4):200–10.

35. Kelley DE, Wing R, Buonocore C, Sturis J, Polonsky K, Fitzsimmons M. Relative effects of calorie restriction and weight loss in noninsulin-dependent diabetes mellitus. J Clin Endocrinol Metab. 1993;77(5):1287–93.

36. Gumbs AA, Modlin IM, Ballantyne GH. Changes in insulin resistance following bariatric surgery: role of caloric restriction and weight loss. Obes Surg. 2005;15(4):462–73.

37. Cummings DE, Overduin J, Shannon MH, Foster-Schubert KE. 2004 ABS Consensus Conference. Hormonal mechanisms of weight loss and diabetes resolution after bariatric surgery. Surg Obes Relat Dis Off J Am Soc Bariatr Surg. 2005;1(3):358–68.

38. Kashyap SR, Daud S, Kelly KR, Gastaldelli A, Win H, Brethauer S, et al. Acute effects of gastric bypass versus gastric restrictive surgery on beta-cell function and insulinotropic hormones in severely obese patients with type 2 diabetes. Int J Obes. 2010;34(3):462–71.

39. Laferrère B, Heshka S, Wang K, Khan Y, McGinty J, Teixeira J, et al. Incretin levels and effect are markedly enhanced 1 month after Roux-en-Y gastric bypass surgery in obese patients with type 2 diabetes. Diabetes Care. 2007;30(7):1709–16.

40. Hayes MT, Hunt LA, Foo J, Tychinskaya Y, Stubbs RS. A model for predicting the resolution of type 2 diabetes in severely obese subjects following Roux-en Y gastric bypass surgery. Obes Surg. 2011;21(7):910–6.

41. Maciejewski ML, Livingston EH, Kahwati LC, Henderson WG, Kavee AL, Arterburn DE. Discontinuation of diabetes and lipid-lowering medications after bariatric surgery at Veterans Affairs medical centers. Surg Obes Relat Dis Off J Am Soc Bariatr Surg. 2010;6(6):601–7.

42. Chikunguwo SM, Wolfe LG, Dodson P, Meador JG, Baugh N, Clore JN, et al. Analysis of factors associated with durable remission of diabetes after Roux-en-Y gastric bypass. Surg Obes Relat Dis Off J Am Soc Bariatr Surg. 2010;6(3):254–9.

43. Hamza N, Abbas MH, Darwish A, Shafeek Z, New J, Ammori BJ. Predictors of remission of type 2 diabetes mellitus after laparoscopic gastric banding and bypass. Surg Obes Relat Dis Off J Am Soc Bariatr Surg. 2011;7(6):691–6.

44. Benraouane F, Litwin SE. Reductions in cardiovascular risk after bariatric surgery. Curr Opin Cardiol. 2011;26(6):555–61.

45. Nguyen NT, Varela E, Sabio A, Tran C-L, Stamos M, Wilson SE. Resolution of hyperlipidemia after laparoscopic Roux-en-Y gastric bypass. J Am Coll Surg. 2006;203(1):24–9.

46. DeMaria EJ, Pate V, Warthen M, Winegar DA. Baseline data from American Society for Metabolic and Bariatric surgery-designated bariatric surgery centers of excellence using the bariatric outcomes longitudinal database. Surg Obes Relat Dis Off J Am Soc Bariatr Surg. 2010;6(4):347–55.

47. DeMaria EJ, Murr M, Byrne TK, Blackstone R, Grant JP, Budak A, et al. Validation of the obesity surgery mortality risk score in a multicenter study proves it stratifies mortality risk in patients undergoing gastric bypass for morbid obesity. Ann Surg. 2007;246(4):578–82; (discussion 583-584).

48. Flum DR, Salem L, Elrod JAB, Dellinger EP, Cheadle A, Chan L. Early mortality among Medicare beneficiaries undergoing bariatric surgical procedures. JAMA J Am Med Assoc. 2005;294(15):1903–8.

49. Mason EE, Renquist KE, Huang Y-H, Jamal M, Samuel I. Causes of 30-day bariatric surgery mortality: with emphasis on bypass obstruction. Obes Surg. 2007;17(1):9–14.

50. Fridman A, Moon R, Cozacov Y, Ampudia C, Lo Menzo E, Szomstein S, et al. Procedure-related morbidity in bariatric surgery: a retrospective short- and mid-term follow-up of a single institution of the American college of surgeons bariatric surgery centers of excellence. J Am Coll Surg. 2013;217(4):614–20.

51. Abasbassi M, Pottel H, Deylgat B, Vansteenkiste F, Van Rooy F, Devriendt D, et al. Small bowel obstruction after antecolic antegastric laparoscopic Roux-en-Y gastric bypass without division of small bowel mesentery: a single-centre, 7-year review. Obes Surg. 2011;21(12):1822–7.

52. Higa K, Ho T, Tercero F, Yunus T, Boone KB. Laparoscopic Roux-en-Y gastric bypass: 10-year follow-up. Surg Obes Relat Dis Off J Am Soc Bariatr Surg. 2011;7(4):516–25.

53. Cho M, Pinto D, Carrodeguas L, Lascano C, Soto F, Whipple O, et al. Frequency and management of internal hernias after laparoscopic antecolic antegastric Roux-en-Y gastric bypass without division of the small bowel mesentery or closure of mesenteric defects: review of 1400 consecutive cases. Surg Obes Relat Dis Off J Am Soc Bariatr Surg. 2006;2(2):87–91.

54. Gumbs AA, Duffy AJ, Bell RL. Incidence and management of marginal ulceration after laparoscopic Roux-Y gastric bypass. Surg Obes Relat Dis Off J Am Soc Bariatr Surg. 2006;2(4):460–3.

55. Siilin H, Wanders A, Gustavsson S, Sundbom M. The proximal gastric pouch invariably contains acid-producing parietal cells in Roux-en-Y gastric bypass. Obes Surg. 2005;15(6):771–7.

56. Garrido AB Jr, Rossi M, Lima SE Jr, Brenner AS, Gomes CAR Jr. Early marginal ulcer following Roux-en-Y gastric bypass under proton pump inhibitor treatment: prospective multicentric study. Arq Gastroenterol. 2010;47(2):130–4.

57. Scheffel O, Daskalakis M, Weiner RA. Two important criteria for reducing the risk of postoperative ulcers at the gastrojejunostomy site after gastric bypass: patient compliance and type of gastric bypass. Obes Facts. 2011;4(Suppl 1):39–41.

58. Carrodeguas L, Szomstein S, Soto F, Whipple O, Simpfendorfer C, Gonzalvo JP, et al. Management of gastrogastric fistulas after divided Roux-en-Y gastric bypass surgery for morbid obesity: analysis of 1292 consecutive patients and review of literature. Surg Obes Relat Dis Off J Am Soc Bariatr Surg. 2005;1(5):467–74.

59. Rasmussen JJ, Fuller W, Ali MR. Marginal ulceration after laparoscopic gastric bypass: an analysis of predisposing factors in 260 patients. Surg Endosc. 2007;21(7):1090–4.

60. Patel S, Szomstein S, Rosenthal RJ. Reasons and outcomes of reoperative bariatric surgery for failed and complicated procedures (excluding adjustable gastric banding). Obes Surg. 2011;21(8):1209–19.

61. Kruseman M, Leimgruber A, Zumbach F, Golay A. Dietary, weight, and psychological changes among patients with obesity, 8 years after gastric bypass. J Am Diet Assoc. 2010;110(4):527–34.

62. Himpens J, Coromina L, Verbrugghe A, Cadière G-B. Outcomes of revisional procedures for insufficient weight loss or weight regain after Roux-en-Y gastric bypass. Obes Surg. 2012;22(11):1746–54.

63. Tack J, Arts J, Caenepeel P, De Wulf D, Bisschops R. Pathophysiology, diagnosis and management of postoperative dumping syndrome. Nat Rev Gastroenterol Hepatol. 2009;6(10):583–90.

64. Mechanick JI, Youdim A, Jones DB. Clinical practice guidelines for the perioperative, nutritional, metabolic and nonsurgical support of the bariatric surgery patient-2013 update. Endo Prac. 2013;19(2):e1–e36.

65. Brolin RE, Bradley LJ, Wilson AC, Cody RP. Lipid risk profile and weight stability after gastric restrictive operations for morbid obesity. J Gastrointest Surg Off J Soc Surg Aliment Tract. 2000;4(5):464–9.

66. Brolin RE, Leung M. Survey of vitamin and mineral supplementation after gastric bypass and biliopancreatic diversion for morbid obesity. Obes Surg. 1999;9(2):150–4.
67. Elliot K. Nutritional considerations after bariatric surgery. Crit Care Nurs Q. 2003;26(2):133–8.
68. Gudzune KA, Huizinga MM, Chang H-Y, Asamoah V, Gadgil M, Clark JM. Screening and diagnosis of micronutrient deficiencies before and after bariatric surgery. Obes Surg. 2013;23(10):1581–9.
69. Bloomberg RD, Fleishman A, Nalle JE, Herron DM, Kini S. Nutritional deficiencies following bariatric surgery: what have we learned? Obes Surg. 2005;15(2):145–54.

Chapter 8
Sleeve Gastrectomy: Procedure and Outcomes

Allison M. Barrett and Miguel A. Burch

Introduction

Sleeve gastrectomy involves dividing the stomach along the lesser curvature, excising the majority of the antrum and body, and leaving the remaining stomach as a long narrow tube. The procedure is purely restrictive, reducing the volume of the stomach by about 90 % [1]. It differs from gastric bypass in that there is no anastomosis and there is no malabsorptive component to the procedure. It is not reversible.

The sleeve gastrectomy was initially described as the first step in a biliopancreatic diversion with duodenal switch (BPD/DS) [2]. In the super-obese, morbidity rates were very high from this procedure, so surgeons experimented with performing the operation in two stages, with sleeve gastrectomy first, followed later by BPD/DS. Early data showed that laparoscopic sleeve gastrectomy resulted in significant weight loss and resolution of comorbidities without the need for further intervention [3]. With this new information, surgeons began to perform sleeve gastrectomy as a stand-alone operation.

There has been a trend toward increasing use of sleeve gastrectomy as a primary bariatric operation, with decrease in usage of both gastric bypass and gastric band.

M. A. Burch (✉)
Minimally Invasive Surgery, Cedars-Sinai Medical Center,
Los Angeles, CA, USA
e-mail: Miguel.burch@cshs.org

A. M. Barrett
Department of Surgery, North Shore-LIJ Hospital System, Manhasset, NY, USA

© Springer Science+Business Media New York 2015
A. Youdim (ed.), *The Clinician's Guide to the Treatment of Obesity,*
Endocrine Updates, DOI 10.1007/978-1-4939-2146-1_8

From 2008 to 2012, the use of sleeve gastrectomy as a percentage of all bariatric surgeries increased from 0.8% in 2008 to 36% in 2012, while gastric banding decreased from 23% in 2008 to 4% in 2012 [4].

Patient Selection and Preoperative Preparation

Indications

The indications for all bariatric surgery procedures were established by the National Institutes of Health and published as a consensus statement in 1991 [5]. Indications for sleeve gastrectomy are similar to other weight loss surgeries. Most insurers will cover sleeve gastrectomy for patients with body mass index (BMI) greater than 35, at least one obesity-related comorbidity, and documentation of failed attempts at weight loss by nonsurgical measures. The Centers for Medicare and Medicaid Services allowed for local coverage determination by Medicare networks. This has allowed for variable coverage under Medicare with some local networks limiting coverage by age.

Contraindications

The presence of severe gastroesophageal reflux disease (GERD) is considered by some to be a relative contraindication to sleeve gastrectomy, as reflux may worsen temporarily after surgery. This is thought to be due to higher pressure within the gastric conduit. Yehoshua et al. found that the volume of the gastric sleeve averages 129 ml, which represents approximately 10% of the preoperative gastric volume of 1500 ml. The pressure in the sleeve with full distension averages 43 mmHg, compared to a pressure of 34 mmHg with full distention of the native stomach. Therefore, very small volumes added to the gastric lumen result in significant increases in intraluminal pressure, creating a sensation of early satiety [1]. This is thought to contribute to postoperative gastroesophageal reflux, which is therefore considered by some to be a contraindication to sleeve gastrectomy. Tai et al. found an increase in GERD symptoms from 12.1% preoperatively to 47% at 1 year postoperatively [6].

However, some reports show an improvement in reflux symptoms after sleeve gastrectomy. Patients found to have a hernia at the esophageal hiatus at the time of bariatric operation are six times more likely to have reported preoperative GERD. With proper hiatus hernia repair and appropriate position of the sleeve without rotation, Daes et al. determined that postoperative reflux was rare, even in those with preoperative reflux [7]. They saw a drop in the rate of GERD from 49.2% preoperatively to 1.5% at 12 months postoperatively. It is unclear why there is such a stark difference in postoperative GERD rates in the literature, but it may be related to operative technique and appropriate crural closure [8].

In patients with severe reflux symptoms preoperatively, workup may include endoscopy, barium swallow and manometry to assess for intrinsic esophageal dysmotility, abnormal lower esophageal sphincter pressure, presence of a hiatus hernia, and *Helicobacter pylori* infection. If lower esophageal sphincter pressure is below normal at baseline, sleeve gastrectomy is likely to worsen reflux symptoms. Many surgeons obtain an endoscopy in all patients prior to sleeve gastrectomy or gastric bypass, as the proportion of abnormal findings is high and may change decision making [9]. For example, Barrett's esophagus is considered an absolute contraindication to sleeve gastrectomy by our group.

Management of Medical Comorbidities

Medical comorbidities should be optimized prior to surgery, but there are few that are absolute contraindications. Recent reports suggest that bariatric surgery can be performed safely in patients with chronic liver disease with good liver function and no varices [10], as well as in patients with congestive heart failure with ventricular assist devices [11]. Poor glycemic control predicts poor wound healing in diabetics, and measures should be taken to lower blood sugar preoperatively. Goals should include hemoglobin A1c less than 7.0% or significantly improving with optimal medical management [12]. Tobacco users are encouraged to quit, as smokers are more likely to develop peptic ulcer disease [13].

Procedure

The procedure is performed laparoscopically, typically with five to six ports. The greater omentum is divided from the greater curvature of the stomach using an electrocautery or ultrasonic scalpel. This is carried superiorly to the left diaphragmatic crus, which is freed from the stomach and esophagus. If a hiatal hernia is present, the esophagus is dissected circumferentially to ensure adequate intra-abdominal length. The hernia is repaired by closing the crura with nonabsorbable sutures. An endoscope, bougie, or other sizing device is then placed in to the stomach from the mouth by the anesthesiologist or an assistant. Sizing devices for sleeve gastrectomy range from 32 F (10.6 mm) or higher, depending on surgeon preference. A surgical stapler is used to divide the stomach at a distance up to 6 cm from the pylorus, serially stapling up the stomach, hugging the sizer with the stapler, until the left crus is reached (Fig. 8.1). The freed portion of the stomach is removed from the operative field and sent for pathologic analysis. The sleeve staple line can be reinforced using manufactured buttress material, additional sutures, or omentum. Most surgeons perform a leak test by clamping the distal end of the stomach and insufflating the lumen with air or methylene blue. A drain may be left in the surgical field [7] (Figs. 8.2 and 8.3).

Fig. 8.1 A surgical stapler
is used to divide the stomach
from a point just proximal to
the pylorus up to the esophageal hiatus. Note the bougie
within the gastric lumen
and the stapler dividing just
lateral to it. (Adapted from
[36])

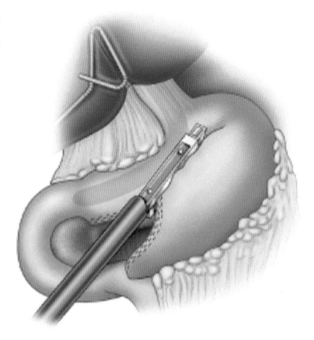

Fig. 8.2 The completed
sleeve gastrectomy. (Adapted
from [36])

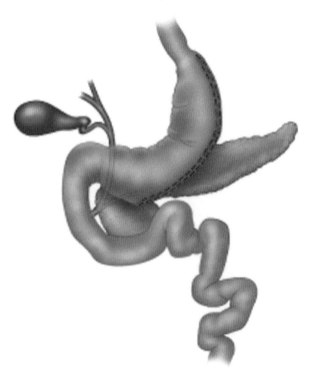

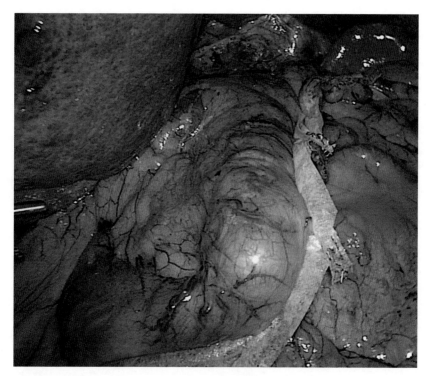

Fig. 8.3 Intraoperative view of completed sleeve gastrectomy, with manufactured buttress material used along the staple line. (Courtesy: Cedars-Sinai Medical Center)

Postoperative Management

Early

In-Hospital Care

Immediate postoperative care includes monitoring of vital signs, urine output, and pain. Inpatient staff assess for signs of dehydration, bleeding, sepsis, pulmonary embolism, and deep venous thrombosis. In some centers, postoperative esophagram swallow study is routinely performed to assess the staple line prior to initiating a diet. Others perform esophagram selectively. Though there is no data specifically on the use of routine imaging studies following sleeve gastrectomy, we can draw a corollary from the gastric bypass literature in which research suggests there is no need for imaging unless clinically indicated [14] (Fig. 8.4).

Fig. 8.4 Normal upper gastrointestinal soluble contrast study following sleeve gastrectomy. There is a radiopaque drain seen overlying the stomach as well as several clips surrounding the sleeve gastrectomy. (Courtesy: Cedars-Sinai Medical Center)

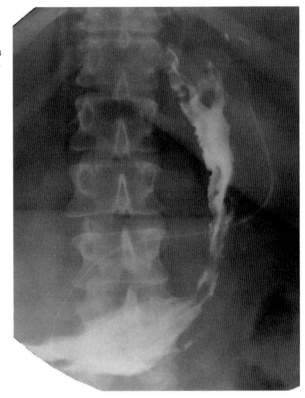

Dietary Progression

Dietary progression begins with a sugar-free liquid diet on postoperative day 1–2. This consists of sugar-free juices, broth, protein shakes, and gelatin. This diet continues for the first 1–2 weeks, then progresses over the following 4–5 weeks from pureed to soft foods. Regular diet is usually reached around 6 weeks after surgery [15] (Table 8.1).

Table 8.1 Postoperative dietary progression following sleeve gastrectomy. (Adapted from [15])

Time postoperatively	Week 1–2	Week 3–4	Week 5	Week 6 and maintenance
Texture	Liquid	Pureed	Soft solid	Solid
Acceptable foods	Thin broth, juice, skim milk, sugar-free gelatin, protein shakes	Pudding, oatmeal, yogurt, and pureed meats, fruits, and vegetables	Cooked vegetables, canned fruits, moist cooked meats, soft noodles	Whole grains, tender meats, raw and cooked vegetables and fruits

Dry or more fibrous foods do not pass easily through the sleeve. Items such as chicken or raw vegetables, if not chewed well, will be regurgitated. Patients are advised to chew their food thoroughly and wait between bites. At mealtime, protein-based foods should be prioritized, with carbohydrate- or fat-rich foods later in the meal. This will ensure that protein malnutrition does not develop. Liquids, especially carbonated ones, should be avoided during meals, as they fill up space in the small sleeve. To avoid daytime hunger, protein-based snacks should be taken in small amounts between meals.

Dehydration is common in the early postoperative period due to the small volume of the sleeve. The patient must be persistent in drinking liquids throughout the day to ensure adequate hydration. As postoperative gastric edema decreases, the capacity of the sleeve becomes larger and dehydration less common.

Late

Micronutrient supplementation is advised for all bariatric surgery patients [16, 17], though little has been published on specific postoperative deficiencies in sleeve gastrectomy patients. Consensus guidelines recommend supplementation with a multivitamin, calcium with vitamin D, folic acid, elemental iron, and vitamin B12, with regular monitoring of micronutrient levels postoperatively [12]. Vitamin B12 deficiency is thought to be due to insufficient production of intrinsic factor and inadequate B12 intake, while iron absorption may be affected by alterations in acid production [15]. Thiamine deficiency resulting in Wernicke's encephalopathy has been described in case reports following sleeve gastrectomy [18] (Table 8.2).

Regular postoperative visits to the surgeon and dietician are designed to recognize complications such as nutritional deficiencies, but also to help eliminate poor dietary choices and avoid weight regain. Visits occur every 3 months for the first year, then annually thereafter. Many bariatric centers host regular seminars for their postoperative patients to encourage good dietary habits.

Table 8.2 Recommended daily vitamin intake following sleeve gastrectomy. (Adapted from [15])

Supplement	Recommended daily amount	Timing	Laboratory tests to follow
Chewable multivitamin	One	Take with meal, protein drink, or milk to improve tolerance	Thiamine, folate, zinc, copper, vitamin A, B6, E, K
Chewable or liquid calcium with vitamin D	1000–1500 mg calcium 400–800 mg vitamin D	Do not take with iron to improve absorption	Vitamin D, PTH, calcium, phosphorous
Sublingual B12	500 µg	Take with MVI	Vitamin B12
Chewable elemental iron	325 mg	Do not take with calcium to improve absorption	Ferritin, iron, total iron-binding capacity, CBC

PTH parathyroid hormone, *MVI* multivitamin, *CBC* complete blood count

Outcomes

Weight Loss

Weight loss is rapid following surgery. In the bariatric literature, weight goals are measured as the percent of excess weight lost (%EWL). This measurement takes in to account the starting body weight, current body weight, and ideal body weight. At 12 months postoperatively, average %EWL is between 55 and 75% [19–21], but has been reported as high as 84.8% [22]. Peak weight loss is seen between 12 and 24 months (average 18 months) after surgery, with some patients experiencing an increase in weight thereafter. Braghetto et al. reported weight regain in 30% of patients at 5 years postoperatively, with average %EWL of 57.3 [22]. Bohdjalian found similar results, with 19% of patients regaining weight and %EWL falling to 55.0% at 5 years [23]. This was corroborated by a review of the published data by Gagner et al. [24] (Table 8.3).

Weight regain may be a result of dilation of the sleeve over time, which results in less restriction. Patients find that they can eat larger volumes of food several years after surgery. While this may be the natural history of the sleeve gastrectomy, it can likely be prevented by avoiding carbonated liquids and mixing of solids and liquids, both of which stretch the pouch over time. Emphasis should be placed on prevention; however should medical management and counseling fail, surgical revision as a salvage maneuver remains an option. Revision from sleeve gastrectomy to gastric bypass addresses both weight regain and reflux disease [25]. Resizing or narrowing of the sleeve has also been described [26], as well as placement of an adjustable gastric band around the sleeve [27].

Effect on Comorbidities

Sleeve gastrectomy has proven to be very effective treatment for obesity-related comorbidities. Most studies report resolution or improvement of diabetes, hyperten-

Table 8.3 Percent excess weight loss (%EWL) at 12, 24, and 36 months following sleeve gastrectomy

Article	%EWL 12 months	%EWL 24 months	%EWL 36 months
Braghetto [22]	84.8		71.5
Yaghoubian [19]	72.0		
Carlin [20]	60	60	56
Himpens [34]	57.7		66
Bohdjalian [23]	57.5	60.3	60.0
Pequignot [28]	54.2	57.7	
Eisenberg [21]		61	

sion, and hyperlipidemia in greater than 60 % of patients at 3–5-year follow-up [20, 22, 28]. Pequignot et al. found that comorbidities continued to improve between years 1 and 2 after surgery, despite no change in %EWL. In multivariate analysis, preoperative elevated systolic blood pressure was the only negative predictive factor for resolution of metabolic syndrome [28]. Studies report resolution of diabetes in 70–100 % of patients [22].

Complications

Early

Surgical complications can be divided into early (occurring within 30 days of surgery) or late. The overall early complication rate following sleeve gastrectomy is 5.7 %, according to the 2009 Consensus Summit on Sleeve Gastrectomy [24]. Early complication rates are very similar between gastric bypass and sleeve gastrectomy [20].

Of the early complications, staple-line leak is perhaps the most serious, although very rare. Leakage of gastric contents through the staple line and in to the peritoneal cavity can result in profound sepsis and death. Sakran et al. found an overall leak rate of 1.2 % in patients undergoing primary sleeve gastrectomy. Leaks were diagnosed at a median time of 7 days postoperatively and required reoperation in 61.4 %. Other techniques for management included percutaneous drainage, endoscopic clip placement, and endoscopic stent placement. The most common site of leak was at the proximal staple line (75 %). Median time to closure was 40 days, ranging from 2 to 270 days. In those with prolonged leak refractory to conservative approaches, total gastrectomy was used for salvage. Four patients died, for an overall mortality of 9.1 % from leak [29]. A meta-analysis of sleeve gastrectomy outcomes found that leak was more common with smaller bougie size [30].

Early diagnosis of a staple-line leak is imperative to prevent sepsis and death. The patient may first complain of increasing abdominal pain, especially in the left upper quadrant, and may have dyspnea, tachycardia, and poor oxygenation. Leukocytosis, fever, and low urine output are common. Computed tomography (CT) scan is very sensitive for diagnosing leaks, as oral contrast given immediately prior to imaging may be seen extravasating from the staple line. If there is a large fluid collection in the left upper quadrant but no obvious leakage of oral contrast, the patient should still be treated as a leak until proven otherwise. Priority should be placed on resuscitation with intravenous fluids, broad-spectrum antibiotic coverage, and gaining control of the leak by percutaneous drainage, endoscopic stenting, or reoperation (Fig. 8.5).

Early strictures or obstruction occur in 1 % [24]. This may be secondary to narrowed sleeve caliber from small bougie size, intramural hematoma, or torsion of the sleeve. Early strictures may benefit from endoscopic dilation or placement of a stent, but reoperation for conversion to a gastric bypass may be necessary [28, 31–33] (Fig. 8.6).

Fig. 8.5 Sleeve gastrectomy leak seen on CT scan 4 weeks postoperatively in a 35-year-old male. The *red* arrow indicates a pocket of free air with surrounding fluid and inflammation adjacent to the sleeve gastrectomy staple line. This patient was managed with percutaneous drainage and endoscopic stent placement. *CT* computed tomography. (Courtesy: Cedars-Sinai Medical Center)

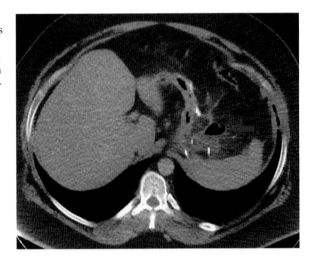

Fig. 8.6 Upper GI study demonstrating complete obstruction of the sleeve gastrectomy 2 weeks postoperatively. This patient went on to develop a leak from the staple line and was managed with percutaneous drainage and endoscopic stent placement. *GI* gastrointestinal. (Courtesy: Cedars-Sinai Medical Center)

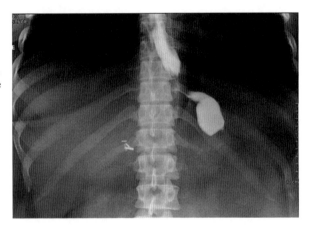

Hemorrhage requiring intervention occurs in 1–2%. In the University of Chile series, the most common site of bleeding was from the staple line, which was controlled laparoscopically with sutures, while three patients presented with laparoscopic port-site bleeding [22]. Other early complications include deep venous thrombosis and pulmonary embolism (0–0.3%). Overall surgical mortality is approximately 0–0.9% [22, 24].

Late

Gallstone formation can occur secondary to rapid weight loss from any bariatric surgery. This can result in symptomatic cholelithiasis, choledocholithiasis with cholangitis, or gallstone pancreatitis. Li et al. found that the type of bariatric operation performed was not a predictor of development of symptomatic cholelithiasis, but rather the total amount of weight loss compared to preoperative weight. On average, 7.8% of patients developed symptomatic cholelithiasis following bariatric surgery at an average of 10.2 months postoperatively [32].

Reflux disease is a common preoperative complaint of bariatric patients, and there is inconclusive data on whether sleeve gastrectomy improves or worsens this process. Braghetto et al. found a 27% rate of symptomatic reflux following sleeve gastrectomy, with 15.5% of those demonstrating esophagitis on endoscopy, while Daes et al. had a rate of only 1.5% [7]. Reflux may have a bimodal distribution postoperatively, according to Himpens et al., who found an increased rate of GERD at 1 year postoperatively (22%), which decreased to 3% at 3 years, then rose again to 21% at 6 years [34, 35]. Manometry postoperatively in a subset of patients reporting reflux has shown decreased lower esophageal sphincter pressure [22]. In patients whose reflux disease worsens following sleeve gastrectomy, surgeons should consider revision to a gastric bypass procedure if medical management fails [32].

Late reoperation, performed most commonly for intractable reflux or weight regain, is required in 5% of sleeve gastrectomy patients, compared to a rate of 2–16% following gastric bypass and 10–39% following gastric band [22].

Conclusions

Sleeve gastrectomy is an effective bariatric procedure, with outcomes similar to gastric bypass with respect to weight loss and comorbidity resolution, but a lower rate of complications and need for late reoperation. Complications specific to sleeve gastrectomy include obstruction of the sleeve and may include worsening of GERD. Weight regain is possible, but nutritional deficiencies are likely less common than following gastric bypass.

References

1. Yehoshua RT, Eidelman LA, Stein M, et al. Laparoscopic sleeve gastrectomy: volume and pressure assessment. Obes Surg. 2008;18:1083–8.
2. Ren CJ, Patterson E, Gagner M. Early results of laparoscopic biliopancreatic diversion with duodenal switch: a case series of 40 consecutive patients. Obes Surg. 2000;10:514–23.
3. Silecchia G, Boru C, Pecchia A, et al. Effectiveness of laparoscopic sleeve gastrectomy (first stage of biliopancreatic diversion with duodenal switch) on co-morbidities in super-obese high-risk patients. Obes Surg. 2006;16:1138–44.
4. Nguyen NT, Nguyen B, Gebhart A, Hohmann S. Changes in the makeup of bariatric surgery: a national increase in use of laparoscopic sleeve gastrectomy. JACS. 2013;216(2):252–57.
5. Gastrointestinal surgery for severe obesity. NIH Consens Statement. 1991;9(1):1–20.
6. Tai CM, Huang CK, Lee YC, Chang CY, Lee CT, Lin JT. Increase in gastroesophageal reflux disease symptoms and erosive esophagitis 1 year after laparoscopic sleeve gastrectomy among obese adults. Surg Endosc. 2013;27:1260–6.

7. Daes J, Jimenez ME, Said N, Daza JC, Dennis R. Laparoscopic sleeve gastrectomy: symptoms of gastroesophageal reflux can be reduced by changes in surgical technique. Obes Surg. 2012;22:1874–79.

8. Elazary R, Phillips EH, Cunneen S, Burch MA. Comments on "Increase in gastroesophageal reflux disease symptoms and erosive esophagitis 1 year after laparoscopic sleeve gastrectomy among obese adults." Surg Endosc. 2013;27:3935–36.

9. Munoz R, Ibanez L, Salines J, et al. Importance of routine preoperative upper GI endoscopy: why all patients should be evaluated? Obes Surg. 2009;19:427–31.

10. Weingarten TN, Swain JM, Kendrick ML, et al. Nonalcoholic steatohepatitis (NASH) does not increase complications after laparoscopic bariatric surgery. Obes Surg. 2011;21:1714–20.

11. Caceres M, Czer LSC, Esmailian F, Ramzy D, Moriguchi J. Bariatric surgery in severe obesity and end-stage heart failure with mechanical circulatory support as a bridge to successful heart transplantation: a case report. Trans Proc. 2013;45(2):798–99.

12. Mechanick JI, Kushner RF, Sugerman HJ, et al. Executive summary of the recommendations of the American Association of Clinical Endocrinologists, the Obesity Society, and American Society for Metabolic & Bariatric Surgery: medical guidelines for clinical practice for the perioperative nutritional, metabolic, and nonsurgical support of the bariatric surgery patient. Endocr Pract. 2008;14(3):319–36.

13. Maity P, Biswas K, Roy S, Banerjee RK, Bandyopadhyay U. Smoking and the pathogenesis of gastroduodenal ulcer: recent mechanistic update. Molec Cell Biochem. 2003;253:329–38.

14. Lyass S, Khalili TM, Cunneen S, et al. Radiological studies after laparoscopic Roux-en-Y gastric bypass: routine or selective? Am Surg. 2004;70(10):918–21.

15. Snyder-Marlow G, Taylor D, Lenhard MJ. Nutrition care for patients undergoing laparoscopic sleeve gastrectomy for weight loss. J Am Diet Assoc. 2010;110(4):600–7.

16. Miller AD, Smith KM. Medication and nutrient administration considerations after bariatric surgery. Am J Health-Syst Pharm. 2006;63:1852–7.

17. Heber D, Greenway FL, Kaplan LM, Livingston E, Salvador J, Still C. Endocrine and nutritional management of the post-bariatric surgery patient: an Endocrine Society clinical practice guideline. J Clin Endocrinol Metab. 2010;95(11):4823–43.

18. Moize V, Ibarzabal A, Dalmau BS, et al. Nystagmus: an uncommon neurological manifestation of thiamine deficiency as a serious complication of sleeve gastrectomy. Nut Clin Prac. 2012;27(6):788–92.

19. Yaghoubian A, Tolan A, Stabile BE, et al. Laparoscopic roux-en-y gastric bypass and sleeve gastrectomy achieve comparable weight loss at 1 year. Am Surg. 2012;78:1325–8.

20. Carlin AM, Zeni TM, English WJ, et al. The comparative effectiveness of sleeve gastrectomy, gastric bypass, and adjustable gastric banding procedures for the treatment of morbid obesity. Ann Surg. 2013;257(5):791–7.

21. Eisenberg D, Bellatorre A, Bellatorre N. Sleeve gastrectomy as a stand-alone bariatric operation for severe, morbid, and super obesity. J Soc Laprosc Endosc Surg. 2013;17:63–7.

22. Braghetto I, Csendes A, Lanzarini E, Papapietro K, Carcamo C, Molina JC. Is laparoscopic sleeve gastrectomy an acceptable primary bariatric procedure in obese patients? Early and 5-year postoperative results. Surg Laparosc Endosc Percutan Tech. 2012;22(6):479–86.

23. Bohdjalian A, Langer FB, Shakeri-Leidenmuhler S, et al. Sleeve Gastrectomy as sole and definitive bariatric procedure: 5-year results for weight loss and ghrelin. Obes Surg. 2010;20(5):535–40.

24. Gagner M, Deitel M, Kalberer TL, et al. The second international consensus summit for sleeve gastrectomy. Surg Obes Relat Dis. 2009;5:476–85.

25. Langer FB, Bohdjalian A, Shakeri-Leidenmuhler S, Schoppman SF, Zacherl J, Prager G. Conversion from sleeve gastrectomy to roux-en-y gastric bypass: indications and outcome. Obes Surg. 2010;20(7):835–40.

26. Ianelli A, Schneck AS, Noel P, Amor IB, Krawczykowski D, Gugenheim J. Re-sleeve gastrectomy for failed laparoscopic sleeve gastrectomy: a feasibility study. Obes Surg. 2011;21(7):832–83.

27. Greenstein AJ, Jacob BP. Placement of a laparoscopic adjustable gastric band after failed sleeve gastrectomy. Surg Obes Rel Dis. 2008;4(4):556–8
28. Pequignot A, Dhahri A, Verhaeghe P, Desailloud R, Lalau JD, Regimbeau JM. Efficiency of laparoscopic sleeve gastrectomy on metabolic syndrome disorders: two years results. J Visc Surg. 2012;149:e350–5.
29. Sakran N, Goitein D, Raziel A, et al. Gastric leaks after sleeve gastrectomy: a multicenter experience with 2834 patients. Surg Endosc. 2013;27:240–5.
30. Parikh M, Issa R, McCrillis A, Saunders JK, Ude-Welcome A, Gagner M. Surgical strategies that may decrease leak after laparoscopic sleeve gastrectomy. Ann Surg. 2013;257(2):231–7.
31. Bellorin O, Lieb J, Szomstein S, Rosenthal RJ. Laparoscopic conversion of sleeve gastrectomy to Roux-en-Y gastric bypass for acute gastric outlet obstruction after laparoscopic sleeve gastrectomy for morbid obesity. Surg Obes Rel Dis. 2010;6(5):566–8.
32. Li VKM, Pulido N, Fajnwaks P, Szomstein S, Rosenthal R. Predictors of gallstone formation after bariatric surgery: a multivariate analysis of risk factors comparing gastric bypass, gastric banding, and sleeve gastrectomy. Surg Endosc. 2009;23:1640–4.
33. Abdemur A. Fendrich I. Rosenthal R. Laparoscopic conversion of laparoscopic sleeve gastrectomy to gastric bypass for intractable gastroesophageal reflux disease. Surg Obes Rel Dis. 2012;8(5):654.
34. Himpens J, Dapri G, Cadiere GB. A prospective randomized study between laparoscopic gastric banding and laparoscopic isolated sleeve gastrectomy: results after 1 and 3 years. Obes Surg. 2006;16:1450–56.
35. Himpens J, Dobbeleir J, Peeters G. Long-term results of laparoscopic sleeve gastrectomy for obesity. Ann Surg. 2010;252(2):319–24.
36. Sherman V, Brethauer SA, Chand B, Schauer PR. Laparoscopic sleeve gastrectomy. In: Schauer PR, Schirmer BD, Brethauer SA, editors. Minimally invasive bariatric surgery. New York: Springer, 2007. pp. 173–78.

Chapter 9
Laparoscopic Adjustable Gastric Banding: Procedure and Outcomes

Brandice Durkan and Monali Misra

History

The gastric band was originally designed as a nonadjustable device placed on the upper aspect of the stomach to allow restriction of intake of food, with the ultimate goal of early satiety and weight loss. Unfortunately, as patients lose weight, a loss of restriction was noted, which affected the end goal of weight loss. This prompted the need to develop a band with the ability to be adjusted to different levels of restriction as required by the patient. Fortunately in the mid 1980s, this device was created and performed with favorable results [1, 2]. In the early 1990s, the laparoscopic version of the adjustable gastric band was created, allowing a minimally invasive, safe option for significant, durable weight loss [3–5].

The gastric band was originally placed lower on the stomach, using a perigastric dissection. This choice for initial placement contributed to unacceptable rates of gastric herniation which is also referred to as slippage or prolapse (10–15%) [6]. This can occur early or much later in the patient's surgical course. Early prolapse usually leads to severe obstructive symptoms while late prolapses can be either chronic or acute in presentation. When chronic, one finds progressive enlargement of the pouch, which leads to the appearance of chronically worsening obstructive symptoms of heartburn, reflux, and vomiting.

In order to lower the high gastric herniation rate, a new surgical method termed the pars flaccida technique was developed. This technique had been determined

M. Misra (✉) · B. Durkan
Department of Surgery, Cedars Sinai Medical Center,
Los Angeles, CA, USA
e-mail: drmonamisra@gmail.com

B. Durkan
e-mail: brandice.durkan@cshs.org

© Springer Science+Business Media New York 2015
A. Youdim (ed.), *The Clinician's Guide to the Treatment of Obesity*,
Endocrine Updates, DOI 10.1007/978-1-4939-2146-1_9

to be as effective as the perigastric approach in generating substantial weight loss, improved health, and quality of life and has been shown to be significantly less associated with early and late prolapse [7].

Technique

Typically, the adjustable gastric band is placed laparoscopically using 4–6 small incisions. The key points of the operation include creating a retrogastric tunnel extending from the lower medial aspect of the right crus of the diaphragm toward the angle of His. This is best created under direct visualization. Gentle and careful blind passage of a blunt instrument is also performed by some surgeons, but significant experience of the anatomy is needed. Great care must be taken to avoid injuring the posterior wall of the stomach with this maneuver. This is especially important in patients with preexisting hiatal hernias.

The band is then prepared with sterile saline and then placed into the abdomen via the 15 mm port. The end-tag of the band is then brought up to meet the now retrogastric grasper or specially designed band passer and is pulled through (Fig. 9.1a–c). The band tubing is then grasped and the band is retracted into appropriate position (Fig. 9.2). The band is then locked into position (Fig. 9.3a–c). Permanent suture is employed to secure the band in place by creating an anterior gastro-gastric fundoplication in order to prevent herniation of the stomach upward through the band (Figs. 9.4 and 9.5). The final position of the band should appear in a 2-to-8 angle for proper placement as referenced to the face of a clock.

The tubing is brought out through the abdominal wall. The distal end of the band tubing is then attached to the port. The port is fixed to the anterior fascia to allow it to remain flat against the fascia and prevent flipping of the port. The excess tubing is placed back into the abdomen.

Currently, there are two brands of adjustable gastric bands which are FDA approved for use in the USA. Both are equally safe and effective [8].

Mechanism of Action

The LAGB has been clearly shown to reduce energy intake [9, 10]. The mechanism of action was originally attributed to restriction; however, several studies have shown minimal to no delayed gastric emptying. If weight loss were due to generating enhanced difficulty in attaining desired meal size alone, strong evolutionary mechanisms to maintain energy balance would likely produce shortened post-meal satiety and resultant grazing between meals. The negligible delay in gastric emptying and prolonged satiety noted by LAGB patients suggests stronger additional mechanisms at work. Greater early satiation and a longer period of satiety appear to be essential to the ability of the band to produce sustained weight loss. This was

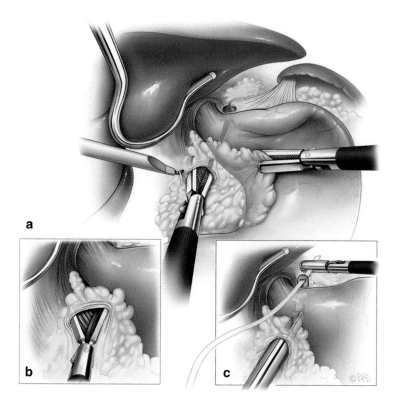

Fig. 9.1 a The retrogastric tunnel extends from the lower medial aspect of the *right crus* of the diaphragm toward the angle of His. **b** The tunnel is best created under direct visualization or by careful blind passage of a blunt instrument by surgeons with significant experience of the anatomy. **c** The end-tag of the band is brought up to meet the retrogastric grasper or band passer and is pulled through

demonstrated by a double-blind randomized, controlled trial with the band either correctly adjusted or empty. When the band was correctly adjusted, subjects were less hungry after a 12-h fast and found a small meal more satisfying [11]. Glucose, insulin, ghrelin, and leptin levels in this study did not vary between optimal and decreased, suboptimal restriction.

Esophageal motility has been shown to be well preserved in LAGB patients with a successful outcome. One study showed that varying the volume between optimal, 20 % under, and empty produced few changes in esophageal motility [12]. The authors also noted repetitive esophageal contractions in 40 % of swallows in optimally adjusted LAGB patients. Repetitive contractions appear to be of functional importance as they reflect the esophageal response to decreased bolus transport across the band.

Postoperative management is affected by achieving appropriately adjusted bands, carefully avoiding either a lack of restriction or excessive restriction with obstructive symptoms.

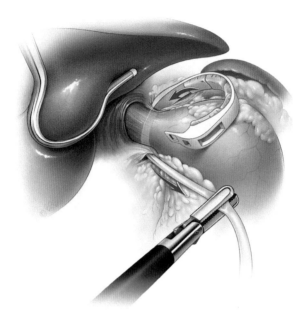

Fig. 9.2 The band tubing is then grasped and the band is retracted into appropriate position

Band Adjustments

Band adjustments are typically performed in the office with or without the aid of fluoroscopy. Prior to each band fill, a detailed history is required including current food choices, hunger between meals, portion sizes, symptoms of regurgitation, night cough, and any discomfort with eating should be noted. Patients need to comprehend the importance of early satiation and prolonged satiety in permitting 50% reduction in daily energy intake [13]. This may be accomplished by eating slowly and increasing the time spent for chewing to avoid obstructive symptoms. One bite of food should be chewed almost 20 times until mushy. Once swallowed, at least 30 s to a minute should pass before another small bite is placed into their mouth. The standard portion size is approximately 1–1.5 decks of cards (or the palm of your hand) consumed slowly over approximately 20–30 min. Patients are recommended to consume 3–4 small meals a day.

The band should be adjusted to the "green zone" based on symptomatology (Fig. 9.6). If patients are hungry between meals and needing larger portions, they are likely in the yellow zone and an adjustment to add fluid into the band is needed. If they are having good portion control with feelings of satisfaction and lack of hunger, they are in the green zone and no adjustment is needed. Lastly, if they are experiencing symptoms of regurgitation, discomfort while eating, or night cough, they are in the red zone and will require an adjustment to remove fluid from the band. Red zone

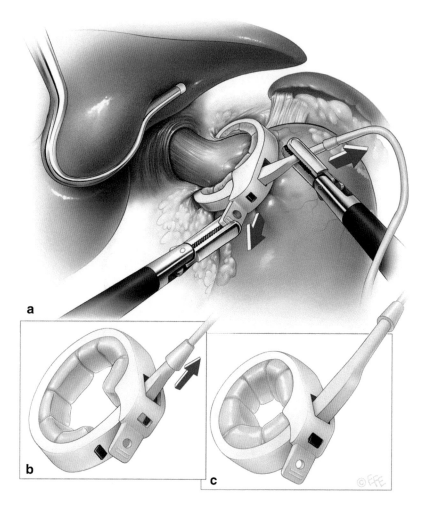

Fig. 9.3 a The band is then locked into position through the use of counter tension applied by graspers in the direction of the *arrows*. **b** The band is in the unlocked position and the *arrow* illustrates the force vector required to lock the band in place. **c** The band is now in the locked position

patients typically have poor weight loss and make poor food choices such as high calorie liquids as they are too tight and unable to tolerate healthy optimal foods.

Adjustments are performed using sterile technique. Often a small amount of lidocaine is used to numb the skin above the port. A Huber needle is always used to adjust the band as it has a beveled tip to prevent coring of the port with repeated adjustments. Saline fluid is either added or removed as needed. Patients are usually asked to drink a couple of glasses of water prior to leaving the office to ensure they are not too tight. Patients are typically asked to return for an adjustment when they are no longer in the green zone.

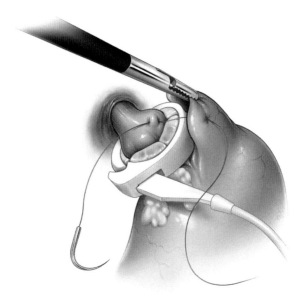

Fig. 9.4 An anterior gastro-gastric fundoplication is made in order to prevent herniation of the stomach through the band. Permanent suture is used to secure the band in place

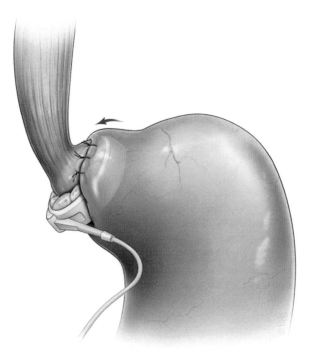

Fig. 9.5 The final position of the band should be from the 2 o'clock to 8 o'clock angle for proper placement

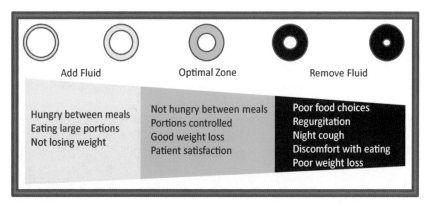

Fig. 9.6 The *green* zone chart allows patients to understand what a correctly adjusted band should feel like

Indications and Contraindications

Criteria for patient selection for weight loss surgery are based on guidelines of the National Institute of Health and national surgical societies. The American College of Surgeons, Society of Gastrointestinal Endoscopic Surgeons (SAGES) and The American Society of Bariatric Surgeons have all offered guidelines for patient selection.

The National Heart, Lung, and Blood Institute in cooperation with The National Institute of Diabetes and Digestive and Kidney Diseases of the National Institutes of Health (NIH) compiled recommendations on patient selection for bariatric surgery in 1998. This report updated the NIH Consensus Development Conference Statement of 1991. The 1998 recommendations were published as the Clinical Guidelines on the Identification, Evaluation, and Treatment of Overweight and Obesity in Adults: The Evidence Report [14]. The NIH made the recommendation that weight loss surgery is an option for carefully selected patients with clinically severe obesity (Body Mass Index > 40 or > 35 with comorbid conditions). This is after less invasive weight loss methods have failed and the patient remains at a high risk for obesity-related morbidity or mortality. The report also summarized available data regarding weight reduction after the age of 65. The potential benefits of weight reduction for daily functioning, decreased risk of future cardiovascular events, and the patient's motivation for weight reduction should be thoroughly evaluated. Any weight reduction program should minimize the likelihood of adverse effects on bone health and overall nutritional status in the older adult.

The America College of Surgeons published recommendations for "Recommendations for Facilities Performing Bariatric Surgery" (ST-34) [15]. They point out that bariatric surgical procedures are not for cosmesis, but for prevention of negative health consequences of morbid obesity. Patients must be committed to both the appropriate preoperative evaluation and the long-term postoperative medical management. Patients must have a full understanding of the potential complications of the procedure.

The American Society of Gastrointestinal Endoscopic Surgeons (SAGES) issued "The SAGES Guidelines for Laparoscopic and Conventional Surgical Treatment of Morbid Obesity." The specific criteria for surgical therapy are for people with a body mass index (BMI) of greater than 40 kg/m^2 or a BMI greater than 35 kg/m^2 with significant comorbidities, with evidence that dietary attempts at weight control have been ineffective.

The American Society of Bariatric Surgeons (ASBS) emphasize that surgical treatment should be offered to patients who are severely obese, well informed, motivated, and have acceptable operative risks. Anyone with psychopathology that jeopardizes an informed consent and cooperation with long-term follow-up may be poor surgical candidates. Central obesity and obesity-associated functional impairments such as musculoskeletal or neurologic or body size problems precluding or severely interfering with employment, family function, and ambulation may be best served by surgical treatment.

There are six categories defined by the NIH recommendations that assist in determining appropriateness for surgical weight loss: Age, BMI, family history of significant comorbid medical conditions related to morbid obesity, the development of significant comorbid health conditions related to morbid obesity, failure of established weight control programs to achieve sustained weight loss, and mental competence to give informed consent to participate in long-term follow-up programs.

Optimal age range for surgical intervention is between 18- and 65-years-old. Younger patients may be considered if they require rapid weight reduction for resolution of obesity-related life-threatening comorbid health conditions. For patients who are older than 65 years, the expectation of improved life expectancy or quality of life should outweigh the risk of surgery. Patients should have a body mass index >40 kg/m^2 or a body mass index >35 and <40 kg/m^2 with the presence of significant comorbid conditions related to morbid obesity.

According to the NIH, weight loss surgery is indicated for people with a high risk for obesity-associated morbidity or mortality. As such, surgery may be indicated in for a person with a strong family history of obesity-related health conditions. For patients who have already developed significant medical conditions related to morbid obesity, weight loss surgery may cure or significantly improve comorbid diseases and prevent their associated morbidity and mortality. Examples of significant medical conditions include diabetes mellitus, sleep apnea, high cholesterol, the metabolic syndrome, or infertility.

Surgical treatment of morbid obesity is appropriate only in patients in whom success with established weight loss programs seems unlikely. In order to qualify, patients must have made sustained efforts in organized weight loss programs over a substantial time period. Appropriate programs include a variety of commercial weight loss programs, caloric restriction diets directed by nutritionists, dieticians, or diabetes centers, or intense exercise programs directed by an exercise therapist or other qualified professional.

Patients must be mentally competent to give informed consent. Patients with a significant psychosis may not be able to adhere to the prolonged follow-up programs.

In 2011, the FDA approved the use of the lap band in patients with BMIs of 30–34.9 with one significant obesity-related comorbidity, or patients with BMIs of 35–39.9 with no comorbidities. This decision was made after review of studies showing the safety and efficacy of the lap band in lower BMI patients, providing durable weight loss and significant comorbidity improvement or resolution [16, 17]. Although currently insurance companies follow the original guidelines and have not adopted coverage of the lap band procedure at this lowered BMI, it is an option for patients requiring sustainable weight loss for comorbidity resolution or improvement, and will significantly impact comorbidity prevention.

Weight Loss Outcomes

Although weight loss after LAGB surgery is not as rapid as seen with Roux-Y-gastric bypass or sleeve gastrectomy, weight loss with the band is progressive over approximately 2 years and appears durable. One study demonstrated that after reaching peak weight loss at 2 years, there is a high degree of stability of the weight loss status through the next 13 years [18]. Randomized controlled trials have demonstrated LAGB to be superior to conventional nonsurgical weight-loss programs for sustained weight loss and diabetes management [19–21].

The first adjustable band was approved by the US Food and Drug Administration in 2001. As the LAGB has been available for use outside the USA since 1993, there are much longer follow-up durations. An Italian series has the longest follow-up and details of 1791 consecutive patients with a mean excess weight loss of 50 % 12 years after LAGB [19]. Procedures such as RYGB and sleeve gastrectomy have better early weight loss but usual partial weight regain 2–5 years after surgery [22, 23]. Although LAGB weight loss takes a longer course to reach a maximum, at 5 years LAGB patients achieve the comparable weight loss results of 55 % of excess weight loss versus 58 % with Gastric Bypass. [22].

Health Outcomes

Diabetes

The risk of developing type 2 diabetes increases with the degree and duration of obesity and is more common with a central weight distribution. The associated decrease in insulin sensitivity seen with central obesity correlates with impaired glucose tolerance, dyslipidemia, and systemic hypertension and increased cardiovascular risk. The beneficial effect of weight reduction on control of type 2 diabetes has been known for some time and studies have shown benefit even from modest weight reduction [24, 25].

At 2 years after placement of the lap band, 50 % of those with type 2 diabetes mellitus will no longer require diabetic therapy [21, 26]. The sooner the intervention to time of diabetic onset, the higher the remission rate, likely due to the maintained β-cell function [27]. The improvement in insulin sensitivity is correlated with weight loss, but improvement in β-cell function is not. The percentage of excess weight lost also affects the likelihood of remission of type 2 diabetes.

A randomized controlled study published by Dixon in 2008 clearly demonstrated the effectiveness of Lap band versus conventional medical therapy for diabetes resolution with 73 % versus 13 % resolution seen in the surgical group at 2 years [21].

The recent meta-analytic review of the two most commonly used LAGBs revealed a 60 % resolution of diabetes, and significant improvements of the other parameters of the metabolic syndrome, clearly demonstrating the effectiveness of this device in comorbidity resolution as well as weight loss [8].

Asthma/Sleep Apnea

Morbidly obese adults have a high rate of asthma, and major reductions in asthma severity occur after weight loss. This is likely due in part to the prevention of gastroesophageal reflux. One study examining the effect of LAGB on asthma symptoms found significant improvements in all aspects of asthma assessed. These included severity, daily impact, medications needed, hospitalization, sleep, and exercise [28].

Obesity-related sleep disorders improve markedly after weight loss. Waist circumference was the best clinical measure predicting observed sleep apnea [29]. Following the expected excess weight loss with band placement, there is a statistically significant improvement in habitual snoring, observed sleep, abnormal daytime sleepiness, and poor sleep quality.

A 93 % resolution of sleep apnea was shown in a study published in 2001, clearly demonstrating the continued benefits of comorbidity resolution of this safe, effective device [29].

Hypertension

Weight loss also modifies other significant cardiovascular risk factors. Hypertension is better controlled and fewer patients require antihypertensive medications following band placement [27]. Resolution of hypertension, defined as no longer requiring medications to remain normotensive, has been found in 68–74 % of lap band patients [27, 30].

These findings were once again demonstrated in the meta-analysis by Cunneen et al. revealing an average of 46–63 % resolution of hypertension with LAGB [8].

Gastroesophageal Reflux

The relationship between morbid obesity and gastroesophageal reflux disease (GERD) before and after LAGB placement remains controversial. It is commonly thought that obesity is an important factor for the development of GERD. Perhaps the chronic elevation in intra-abdominal pressure favors reflux [31]. Other studies have not found any correlation between obesity and gastroesophageal reflux symptoms and esophageal dysmotility [32]. At this time, most surgeons recommend and studies demonstrate an aggressive approach to hiatal hernia repair at the same time as LAGB placement. They believe that this significantly reduces the risk of development of GERD and improvement in GERD symptoms postoperatively. Dixon's paper clearly shows a 76% resolution and 14% improvement in GERD symptoms 2 years postop [33].

Complications

LAGB, as a surgery for obesity, carries lower procedural risks and is a shorter, less invasive operation when compared to RNYGB or sleeve gastrectomy. There is evidence to support that band placement may even be safely performed in an ambulatory care surgical center [34, 35]. LAGB surgery generally has a very low risk of mortality and morbidity. Mortality rates are in the range of 0.05% [36]. Despite the rarity of operative and early postoperative mortality, deaths attributed to pulmonary thromboembolism, vascular injury and resultant blood loss, and bowel perforation leading to sepsis have been reported. Data from the American College of Surgeons Bariatric Surgery Center Network (Table 9.1) shows the LAGB procedure to compare favorably to the gastric bypass and sleeve gastrectomy procedures in short- and medium-term follow-up.

Over the course of the laparoscopic adjustable band's history, there have been several changes that have led to a significant decrease in the need for revisional surgery. These may be mostly attributed to technical changes in the bands and adjustment systems, and better teaching of placement technique. Currently, the most common complication is dilatation of the proximal gastric pouch [36]. This is most likely due to overly tightening the LABG in attempts to achieve greater weight loss and poor follow-up. This eventually leads to either a portion of the stomach herniating above the band or a progressive stretching of the gastric wall. Both are associated with dysphagia and regurgitation, gastroesophageal reflux, obstruction, night cough, and poor eating behavior. Once the symptoms are identified and diagnosis

Table 9.1 Morbidity and mortality associated with LRYGB, LSG, and LAGB from the ACS-BSCN dataset. (Data from [37])

–	LRYGB	LSG	LAGB
30-day mortality (%)	0.14	0.11	0.05
1 year mortality (%)	0.34	0.21	0.08
30-day morbidity (%)	5.91	5.61	1.44
30-day readmission (%)	6.47	5.40	1.71
30-day reoperation/intervention (%)	5.02	2.97	0.92

LRYGB laparoscopic Roux-en-Y gastric bypass, *LSG* laparoscopic sleeve gastrectomy, *LAGB* laparoscopic adjustable gastric band confirmed on upper gastrointestinal imaging series, treatment involves laparoscopic repositioning or removal of the band. Findings of complete obstruction may become life threatening, and patients with such symptoms must be seen urgently by a bariatric surgeon [38]. Unfortunately, the recent reports of high degrees of long-term failure may be directly attributed to this poor follow-up.

Band erosion into the lumen of the stomach is a rare but potentially devastating complication of LAGB placement. Band erosion has an incidence of approximately 1.5 % and is lower in the hands of experienced surgeons [39]. The mean time from initial band placement to erosion is 12 months. Erosions usually do not present as surgical emergencies but as loss of action of the band.

Complications requiring reoperation are reported in 10–15 % of patients, and permanent removal of the band is infrequent; less than 5 % [40, 41]. These numbers have been decreasing since the advent of the band given improvements in band materials and adjustment techniques. Given that the band is made of synthetic material, band replacement due to material wear remains a possibility even for a correctly placed and maintained band system.

Postoperative Management

The success with LAGB begins prior to surgery. It is imperative that the patient understand that obesity is a chronic condition, and a commitment to follow-up is integral to successful postsurgical outcomes. At the completion of the surgical placement, no additional saline should be added. The initial addition of fluid most commonly occurs at the 4–6-week postoperative patient visit. Timely band adjustments support weight loss by helping patients avoid feeling symptoms associated with under or over filling. Band adjustments may be performed within an office visit. The use of fluoroscopy is helpful, especially in difficult patients. Patients generally require 4–10 adjustments in the first year and 1–3 during subsequent years [42]. Clear dietary recommendations are important immediately postoperative and in the long term. Only liquid intake is encouraged within the first 2 weeks after band placement. The anticipated intake during this time is approximated to be 800–1000 cal. Over the following 2–4 weeks, there is a transition phase from liquids to soft foods to solid food. A once-a-day multivitamin containing daily requirements of folic acid, vitamin B1, and vitamin B12 is recommended. In addition, other supplements, including calcium, vitamin D, and iron, may be added.

The LAGB allows for a sense of satiety and compliance with the following recommendations. Patients are typically encouraged to eat three to four small meals per day of high protein or complex carbohydrate, solid foods. Many patients experience difficulty with breads and red meat. Occasionally, there may be some difficulty with dry chicken, rice, and some types of vegetables. Patients are advised to eat slowly, stop when comfortable, and not snack between meals. There are to be no liquids with the meals, and most liquids should be calorie-free. Analysis of food intake with these specified rules indicated a daily consumption of between 800 and 1200 cal [42].

Generally, it is recommended that the LAGB patient be seen every 4–6 weeks during the first postoperative year and every 3–6 months for 2 additional years. After this period, yearly visits suffice depending on the need for adjustment. Associated comorbidities such as diabetes, hypertension, sleep apnea, and asthma should be monitored and therapy modified as needed. Plasma glucose, lipid profile, liver function tests, iron, vitamin B1, vitamin B12, and folate levels should be monitored. Communication with the patient's primary care provider is essential to managing these comorbid conditions. Postoperative care is continued for as long as the LAGB is in place and may represent a lifelong commitment.

It is clear that LAGB is a safe, effective solution to significant, sustainable weight loss as well as comorbidity resolution. It is also clear that patients receive long-term postoperative care to ensure the best outcomes.

Acknowledgment   A special thanks to Allergan Inc. for providing the Lap Band placement figures.

References

1. Hallberg D. Why the operation I prefer is adjustable gastric banding. Obes Surg. 1991;1:187–8.
2. Kuzmak LI. A review of seven years' experience with silicone gastric banding. Obes Surg. 1991;1:403–8.
3. Belachew M, Legrand M, Vincent V, Lismonde M, Le Docte N, Deschamps V. Laparoscopic adjustable gastric banding. World J Surg. 1998;22:955–63.
4. Flum DR, Belle SH, King WC, Wahed AS, Berk P, Chapman W, Pories W, Courcoulas A, McCloskey C, Mitchell J, Patterson E, Pomp A, Staten MA, Yanovski SZ, Thirlby R, Wolfe B. Perioperative safety in the longitudinal assessment of bariatric surgery. N Engl J Med. 2009;361:445–54.
5. DeMaria EJ, Pate V, Warthen M, Winegar DA. Baseline data from American society for metabolic and bariatric surgery-designated bariatric surgery centers of excellence using the bariatric outcomes longitudinal database. Surg Obes Relat Dis. 2010;6:347–55.
6. O'Brien PE, Dixon JB, Brown W, et al. The laparoscopic adjustable gastric band (Lap-Band): a prospective study of medium-term effects on weight, health and quality of life. Obes Surg. 2002;12:652–60.
7. O'Brien PE, Dixon JB, Laurie C, Anderson M. A prospective randomized trial of placement of the laparoscopic adjustable gastric band: comparison of the perigastric and pars flaccida pathways. Obes Surg. 2005;15:813–9.
8. Cunneen SA, Phillips E, Fielding G, Sledge I, Banel D, Estok R, Fahrbach K. Studies of the Swedish adjustable gastric band and Lap-Band®: a systematic review and meta-analysis. Surg Obes Relat Dis. 2008;4(2):174–85.
9. Lang T, Hauser R, Buddeberg C, Klaghofer R. Impact of gastric banding on eating behavior and weight. Obes Surg. 2002;12:100–7.
10. Busetto L, Valente P, Pisent C, Segato G, de Marchi F, Favretti F, Lise M, Enzi G. Eating pattern in the first year following adjustable silicone gastric banding (ASGB) for morbid obesity. Int J Obes Relat Metab Disord. 1996;20:539–46.
11. Dixon AFR, Dixon JB, O'Brien PE. Laparoscopic adjustable gastric banding induces prolonged satiety: a randomized blind crossover study. J Clin Endocrinol Metab. 2005;90(2):813–9.
12. Burton PR, Brown W, Laurie C, Richards M, Afkari S, Yap K, Korin A, Hebbard G, O'Brien PE. The effect of laparoscopic adjustable gastric bands on esophageal motility and the gastroesophageal junction: analysis using high-resolution video manometry. Obes Surg. 2009;19:905–14.

13. Colles SL, Dixon JB, O'Brien PE. Hunger control and regular physical activity facilitate weight loss after laparoscopic adjustable gastric banding. Obes Surg. 2008;18:833–40.
14. NIH Publication No. 98-4083. September 1998. National Institute of Health.
15. [ST-34] Recommendations for facilities performing bariatric surgery. Bull Am Coll Surg. 2000;85(9).
16. Michaelson R, Murphy DK, Gross TM, Whitcup SM, LAP-BAND Lower BMI Study Group. LAP-BAND for lower BMI: 2-year results from the multicenter pivotal study. Obesity (Silver Spring). 2013;21(6):1148–58.
17. Parikh M, Duncombe J, Fielding GA. Laproscopic adjustable gastric banding for patients with body mass index of < or =35 kg/m2. Surg Obes Relat Dis. 2006;2(5):518–22.
16. Burton PR, Yap K, Brown WA, et al. Changes in satiety, supra- and infraband transit, and gastric emptying following laparoscopic adjustable gastric banding: a prospective follow-up study. Obes Surg. 2011;21:217–23.
18. Favretti F, Segato G, Ashton D, Busetto L, De Luca M, Mazza M, Ceoloni A, Banzato O, Calo E, Enzi G. Laparoscopic adjustable gastric banding in 1791 consecutive obese patients: 12-year results. Obes Surg. 2007;17:168–75.
19. O'Brien PE, Dixon JB, Laurie C, Skinner S, Proietto J, McNeil J, Strauss B, Marks S, Schachter L, Chapman L, Anderson M. Treatmentof mild to moderate obesity with laparoscopic adjustable bandingor an intensive medical program: a randomized trial. Ann Intern Med. 2006;144:625–33.
21. Dixon JB, O'Brien PE, Playfair J, Chapman L, Schachter LM, Skinner S, Proietto J, Bailey M, Anderson M. Adjustable gastric banding and conventional therapy for type 2 diabetes: a randomized controlled trial. JAMA. 2008;299:316–23.
22. O'Brien PE, McPhail T, Chaston TB, Dixon JB. Systematic review of medium-term weight loss after bariatric operations. Obes Surg. 2006;16:1032–40.
23. Himpens J, Dobbeleir J, Peeters G. Long-term results of laparoscopic sleeve gastrectomy for obesity. Ann Surg. 2010;252:319–24.
24. Newburgh L. Control of hyperglycaemia of obese "diabetics" by weight reduction. Ann Intern Med. 1942;17:935–42.
25. Eriksson KF, Lindgarde F. Prevention of type 2 (non-insulin-dependent) diabetes mellitus by diet and physical exercise: the 6-year Malmo feasibility study. Diabetologia. 1991;34:891–8.
26. Buchwald H, Estok R, Fahrbach K, Banel D, Jensen MD, Pories WJ, Bantle JP, Sledge I. Weight and type 2 diabetes after bariatric surgery: systematic review and meta-analysis. Am J Med. 2009;122:248–56.e5.
27. Dixon JB, O'Brien P. Health outcomes of severely obese type 2 diabetic subjects 1 year after laparoscopic adjustable gastric banding. Diabetes Care. 2002;25:358–63.
28. Dixon JB, Chapman L, O'Brien P. Marked improvement in asthma after Lap-Band surgery for morbid obesity. Obes Surg. 1999;9(4):385–9.
29. Dixon JB, Schachter LM, O'Brien PE. Sleep disturbance and obesity. Arch Intern Med. 2001;161(1):102–6.
30. Jaime Ponce, MD; Beverly Haynes, RN; Steven Paynter, MD; Richard Fromm, MD; Brooke Lindsey, RN; Amanda Shafer, PA-C; Eric Manahan, MD; Christopher Sutterfield, MD. Effect of Lap-Band®-induced weight loss on type 2 diabetes mellitus and hypertension. Obes Surg. 2004;14:1335–42.
31. Fisher BL, Pennathur A, Mutnick JL, et al. Obesity correlates with gastroesophageal reflux. Dig Dis Sci. 1999;44:2290–4.
32. Korenkov M, Kohler L, Yucel N, Grass G, Sauerland S, Lempa M, Troidl H. Esophageal motility and reflux symptoms before and after bariatric surgery. Obes Surg. 2002;12:72–76
33. Dixon JB, O'Brien PE. Gastroesophageal reflux in obesity: the effect of Lap-Band placement. Obes Surg. 1999;9(6):527–31.
34. Cobourn C, Mumford D, Chapman MA, Wells L. Laparoscopic gastric banding is safe in outpatient surgical centers. Obes Surg. 2010;20:415–22.
35. Watkins BM, Ahroni JH, Michaelson R, Montgomery KF, Abrams RE, Erlitz MD, Scurlock JE. Laparoscopic adjustable gastric banding in an ambulatory surgery center. Surg Obes Relat Dis. 2008;4(suppl):S56–S62.

36. Brown WA, Burton PR, Anderson M, Korin A, Dixon JB, Hebbard G, O'Brien PE. Symmetrical pouch dilatation after laparoscopic adjustable gastric banding: incidence and management. Obes Surg. 2008;18:1104–8.
37. Hutter MM, Schirmer BD, Jones DB, et al. First report from the American College of Surgeons Bariatric Surgery Center Network: laparoscopic sleeve gastrectomy has morbidity and effectiveness positioned between the band and the bypass. Ann Surg 2011;254(3):410–20.
38. Kirshtein B, Lantsberg L, Mizrahi S, Avinoach E. Bariatric emergencies for non-bariatric surgeons: complications of laparoscopic gastric banding. Obes Surg. 2010;20:1468–78.
39. Egberts K, Brown WA, O'Brien PE. Systematic review of erosion after laparoscopic adjustable gastric banding. Obes Surg. 2011;21:1272–9.
40. Chevallier JM, Zinzindohoue F, Douard R, et al. Complications after laparoscopic adjustable gastric banding for morbid obesity: experience with 1000 patients over 7 years. Obes Surg. 2004;14:407–14.
41. Lyass S, Cunneen SA, Hagiike M, Misra M, Burch M, Khalili TM, Furman G, Phillips EH. Device-related reoperations after laparoscopic adjustable gastric banding. Am Surg. 2005;71:738–43.
42. Favretti F, O'Brien PE, Dixon JB. Patient management after LAP-BAND placement. Am J Surg. 2002;184:38S–41S.

Chapter 10
Perioperative Care of the Surgical Patient

Patchaya Boonchaya-Anant, Amanda G. Powell and
Caroline M. Apovian

Introduction

The prevalence of obesity has been increasing in adults over the past 30 years. In the USA, it is estimated that 35 % of adults are obese [1]. Obesity is a risk factor for metabolic complications such as insulin resistance, type 2 diabetes, nonalcoholic fatty liver disease, dyslipidemia and hypertension and can lead to morbidities including atherosclerosis and cardiovascular disease. Treatment of obesity includes behavioral modification, pharmacotherapy, and bariatric surgery. Bariatric surgery is the most effective treatment for obesity and can reduce mortality and obesity-related comorbid conditions in severely obese patients [2, 3]. There has been an increase in the number of bariatric surgeries performed since the introduction of minimally invasive surgery with an estimated 113,000 cases performed currently per year [4].

C. M. Apovian (✉) · A. G. Powell
Department of Medicine, Section of Endocrinology, Diabetes and Nutrition, Boston University School of Medicine, Boston Medical Center, 88 East Newton Street, Robinson 4400, Boston, MA 02118, USA
e-mail: caroline.apovian@bmc.org

A. G. Powell
e-mail: amanda.powell@lahey.org

P. Boonchaya-Anant
King Chulalongkorn Memorial Hospital, Division of Endocrinology and Metabolism, Department of Medicine, Chulalongkorn University, Thai Red Cross Society, 1873 Rama 4 Rd, Pathum Wan, Bangkok 10330, Thailand
e-mail: b_patchaya@yahoo.com

© Springer Science+Business Media New York 2015
A. Youdim (ed.), *The Clinician's Guide to the Treatment of Obesity,*
Endocrine Updates, DOI 10.1007/978-1-4939-2146-1_10

Appropriate Candidates for Bariatric Surgery

The 1991 NIH Consensus Development Conference Panel and the National Heart, Lung, and Blood Institute guideline recommended bariatric surgery in patients if they are morbidly obese (BMI >40 or ≥35 kg/m² with comorbidities), have failed attempts at diet and exercise, are motivated and well informed, and are free of significant psychological disease [5]. There are no absolute contraindications to bariatric surgery. Relative contraindications to surgery may include severe heart failure, unstable coronary artery disease, end-stage lung disease, active cancer diagnosis/ treatment, cirrhosis with portal hypertension, uncontrolled drug or alcohol dependency, and severely impaired intellectual capacity [6]. Practitioners must decide if a patient demonstrates adequate understanding of the procedure and motivation to comply with follow-up care. This includes an understanding of the complications of bariatric surgery, and the need for postoperative medical and nutritional visits. It is crucial to engage the entire team caring for the patient when making the final decision so as to ensure the safest and most optimal outcome for the patient.

Preoperative Evaluation

A multidisciplinary team, including a medical practitioner, nutritionist, mental health professional, and surgeon, should be involved in the evaluation of patients undergoing bariatric surgery. The goal of the evaluation is to ensure proper candidate selection, reduce surgical risks, and optimize postoperative outcomes.

History and Physical Examination; Comorbidities, Weight Loss History

Patient evaluation prior to bariatric surgery should be comprehensive, and include the obesity-related comorbidities, possible treatable underlying causes of obesity, weight loss history, psychosocial history, and physical exam. The detailed weight history includes patterns of weight gain and loss, as well as prior weight loss attempts with dietary and medical therapies. Most patients who present for the evaluation of bariatric surgery have a history of extensive dieting. The physician should also review the patient's compliance with prior medical therapies. Commitment to medical follow-up is an important component in eligibility for bariatric surgery, as it is critical to monitor for nutritional deficiencies and ensure optimal long-term weight loss [7, 8].

Screening for Causes of Obesity

Secondary causes of obesity can be screened mostly by a good history and physical examination. Obesity is associated with increased thyroid stimulating hormone (TSH) levels and subclinical hypothyroidism [9]. Hypothyroidism is more common in obesity than normal weight individuals and can cause weight gain but it is usually not the sole cause of obesity. High-risk patients including patients with history of autoimmune disease, history of neck radiation or thyroid surgery, family history of thyroid disease, or an abnormal thyroid examination should be screened with a TSH level and treated with levothyroxine accordingly [10]. Prevalence of Cushing's syndrome (CS) in morbidly obese patients was found to be 0.6% [11]. Routine screening for CS is not recommended and caution should be made since screening tests can give false positive results in overweight/obese subjects [12, 13]. Some clinical signs such as purplish striae, proximal muscle weakness, and osteopenia may be a clue for further work up. In a case with clinical features of Cushing's syndrome, the overnight dexamethasone suppression test is a choice for screening in the obese population since it gives fewer false positive rate than the 24 h free urinary cortisol test [14].

Screening for Obesity-Related Comorbidities

The goal of this evaluation is reduce operative risk and optimize postsurgical outcomes. Common obesity-related comorbidities include type 2 diabetes, hypertension, dyslipidemia, obstructive sleep apnea (OSA), and nonalcoholic fatty liver disease (NAFLD) [15]. The physical examination should be comprehensive, and include calculation of BMI, measurement of blood pressure, heart rate, height, weight, and also waist circumference. Routine preoperative tests should include fasting blood glucose, lipid panel, kidney function, liver function test, urinary analysis, prothrombin time/INR, and complete blood count.

Cardiovascular risks should be assessed based on individual coronary risk factors, physical exercise capacity, and symptoms of unstable cardiac disease. A baseline electrocardiogram (EKG) is recommended to screen for ischemia and prior infarction. Patients with existing heart disease may require extensive evaluation by cardiologists. Preoperative stress tests should be considered on patients with known heart disease, those older than 55, patients who have had diabetes for more than 10 years, and those with atypical chest pain. EKG should be performed in patients with congestive heart failure or suspected pulmonary hypertension [16]. Prophylactic beta-blockers should be considered in moderate- to high-risk patients, including those with two or more cardiac risk factors. Major risk factors include a prior history of heart disease, heart failure, cerebrovascular disease, insulin-dependent diabetes, and chronic renal insufficiency [17, 18].

The extent of preoperative pulmonary evaluation varies between institutions. Chest X-rays should be considered as part of the evaluation [19]. OSA is quite common in obese patients with prevalence up to 80% in men [20]. Moderate to severe

OSA is associated with an increased risk of adverse outcomes [21] and mortality [22, 23]. Screening should include symptoms of OSA such as daytime sleepiness, decreased concentration, snoring, gasping/choking at night, and morning head-aches. If sleep apnea is suspected, the patient should be referred for polysomnogra-phy. Standard treatment with continuous positive airway pressure (CPAP) is recom-mended prior to surgery. There is an evidence that the use of CPAP prior to surgery reduces postoperative pulmonary complications [24].

Obesity itself and rapid weight loss following bariatric surgery increase the risk for gallstone formation and gallbladder disease. NAFLD is estimated to oc-cur in 70–80% of the obese population [25, 26] and is one of the leading causes of chronic liver disease. Routine abdominal ultrasound may be considered since it is the most cost-effective and noninvasive study to evaluate gallstone and fatty liver. Many obese patients will have asymptomatic elevations of liver enzymes due to NAFLD but viral hepatitis screen is needed to exclude other causes. Patients with evidence of liver dysfunction should have a liver biopsy done at the time of surgery to determine the extent of hepatic damage and the prognosis. Routine screening for *Helicobactor pylori* (*H. pylori*) may be considered in high-prevalence areas. If screening test with *H. pylori* antibody is positive, treatment with antibiotics, and the urea breath test to confirm eradication are recommended [27]. Some evidences suggested that screening and treatment of *H. pylori* infection reduced postoperative marginal ulcers [28, 29].

Obesity is a risk factor for venous thromboembolism. Perioperative venous thromboembolism remains an important complication of bariatric surgery. Routine evaluation with Doppler ultrasound is not recommended but diligent perioperative prophylaxis is critical. Unfractionated heparin, 5000 IU subcutaneously, or low molecular weight heparin therapy should be initiated shortly (within 30–120 min) before bariatric surgery and repeated every 8–12 h postoperatively until the patient is fully mobile [30]. Patients with history of deep venous thrombosis or cor pulmo-nale should have further diagnostic tests but whether they should be considered for prophylactic inferior vena cava (IVC) filter placement remains controversial since placement of an IVC filter may lead to additional complications [31–33].

Obesity and weight change increase the risk of gout. Gout attacks can be precipi-tated by rapid weight loss. Patients with history of gout should be considered for prophylactic treatment. Bariatric surgery is associated with bone loss [34, 35], but obese persons generally have higher bone mass to begin with despite higher preva-lence of vitamin D deficiency. There are insufficient data to recommend routine preoperative dual-energy X-ray absorptiometry (DXA) but may be considered in patients with risk factors or postmenopausal women [36].

Baseline Nutrient Screening

Routine nutrient screening includes iron studies, folate level, vitamin B12 level, and 25-vitamin D. Thiamine levels are recommended in adolescents prior to surgery

Table 10.1 Preoperative laboratory testing prior to weight loss surgery

Complete blood count
Fasting glucose (and hemoglobin A1C if diabetic)
Basic metabolic panel including kidney function
Liver function tests
Lipid panel
Urinary analysis
Prothrombin time/INR
TSH
B12, iron studies, folate, 25-vitamin D (and Thiamine level in adolescents)
Electrocardiogram, chest X-ray
In some patients: *H. pylori* screening, gallbladder ultrasound, polysomnography, fat-soluble vitamins (A and E)

TSH thyroid stimulating hormone

[37]. Patients undergoing malabsorptive procedures may be considered for extensive tests such as measurement of fat-soluble vitamins (vitamin A and E) [38]. The prevalence of vitamin D deficiency and insufficiency is high in obese population and vitamin D deficiency should be corrected prior to surgery [39] (Table 10.1).

Clinical Nutrition Evaluation and Psychosocial-Behavioral Evaluation

Patients should be evaluated for existing knowledge regarding healthy diet and exercise habits. The patient should demonstrate appropriate insight into the causes and consequences of obesity, and an understanding of the adjustments that will need to be made after surgery. A dietitian will be needed to prepare the patient for the postoperative nutritional guidelines.

The practitioner should look for evidence of an eating disorder or other psychiatric condition. This should include questions targeted at untreated depression, personality disorders, and substance abuse. It is estimated that more than 50% of patients referred for bariatric surgery have a psychiatric disorder [40]. Patients with history or suspected psychiatric illness, substance abuse, or dependence, should undergo a formal mental health evaluation prior to surgery [19]. Binge eating disorder and night eating syndrome are quite common in obese patients [41]. Patients should be educated for nutritional and behavioral changes before and after bariatric surgery. Bulimia nervosa is rare but should be considered a contraindication to bariatric surgery.

Roux-en-Y gastric bypass (RYGB) and sleeve gastrectomy increase the rate of alcohol absorption and blood alcohol concentration [42, 43]. Patients should be advised about alcohol consumption. Some evidence suggested that bariatric surgery candidates have an increased risk of alcohol use disorder after surgery [44, 45]. Screening and assessment preoperatively is appropriate.

Tobacco smoking was found to be associated with increased risk of pneumonia and postoperative marginal ulcers [46]. Patients should be advised about smoking cessation. Smoking should be stopped at least 8 weeks prior to surgery. Obesity is associated with increased risk of malignancies and mortality from cancer [47–49]. Patients should undergo age- and risk-appropriated cancer screening prior to bariatric surgery.

Pregnancy should be avoided 12–24 months postoperatively [50]. Patients should be advised about contraception since their fertility status might be improved after weight loss [51, 52]. Close monitoring is needed in patients who become pregnant after bariatric surgery for appropriate weight gain, nutritional supplements, and fetal health monitoring [53]. Patients taking hormone therapies that increase the risk of thrombotic complications should be advised to discontinue this medication. Premenopausal women should stop oral contraceptive pills 6 weeks before surgery, and postmenopausal women on hormone replacement therapy should be tapered off the medication 4–6 weeks before surgery [19]. These medications should not be restarted until at least 90 days after surgery.

Preoperative Weight Loss and Glycemic Control

Preoperative weight loss is recommended, if possible. Weight loss of 5% of excess body weight or 10% of total weight is associated with reduced liver volume and shortened operative time [54–56]. Whether preoperative weight loss has an impact on long-term outcomes such as postoperative weight loss and resolution of comorbidities is still unclear [57–60]. There is a concern that patients who are unable to lose some amount of weight prior to bariatric surgery will be unable to comply with medical advice and the necessary dietary restrictions after surgery. Such patients should be evaluated on a case-by-case basis to determine if proceeding to bariatric surgery is appropriate [59].

Preoperative glycemic control in patients with diabetes should include medical nutrition therapy, physical activity, and medication adjustment as recommended by the American Diabetes Association. Glycemic targets include hemoglobin A1c of $<7.0\%$, preprandial capillary plasma glucose of 70–130 mg/dl and peak postprandial capillary plasma glucose of <180 mg/dl [61]. Less-stringent targets for hemoglobin A1c may be considered in patients with advanced microvascular and macrovascular complications, long duration of diabetes, and those who are at risk of hypoglycemia [62]. Poor preoperative glycemic control is associated with postoperative hyperglycemia and less weight loss [63], and postoperative hyperglycemia is an independent risk factor for surgical site infection [64, 65].

Immediate Postoperative Management

Prevention and Recognition of Complications

There has been an increase in the number of bariatric procedures performed in the USA over the past 10 years. With improvement in surgical techniques and surgical experience, the 30-day inpatient mortality rate has declined to about 0.09–0.3% [21, 66, 67]. The major complication rates following bariatric surgery are approximately 5–10% and most common are venous thromboembolism and respiratory complications [68]. Patients who are at high risk for postoperative myocardial infarction should be monitored in an intensive care setting. High-risk features include age > 50, history of congestive heart failure, myocardial infarction, OSA, venous thromboembolism, metabolic syndrome, chronic respiratory failure, and pulmonary hypertension [69, 70].

Pulmonary embolism is by far the most common cause of mortality after bariatric surgery. Increased risk is seen in patients with a BMI > 60, severe venous stasis disease, and obesity hypoventilation syndrome [71]. Prophylaxis against deep venous thrombosis is recommended for all patients. Most physicians employ intermittent compression stockings or subcutaneous unfractionated heparin or low molecular weight heparin as mentioned in the previous section. Post hospital discharge, extended thromboprophylaxis may be considered depending on patient's risk factors, activity level and risk of bleeding [72], and may help in reducing the incidence of venous thromboembolism after hospital discharge [73].

Pneumonia or aspiration can occur in 0.14–2.6% of patients [68, 74]. Pulmonary complications can be prevented by use of incentive spirometry, early ambulation, and adequate pain control [75]. Studies have shown that CPAP can be used safely and does not cause an increased anastomotic leak rate [76]. CPAP can be used if clinically indicated and can improve oxygenation and reduce the rate of intubation [77].

Another serious postoperative complication is anastomotic or staple line leak. Leaks are the second most common cause of death following bariatric surgery, and account for 38% of deaths after laparoscopic gastric bypass, and 12.5% of deaths after open bypass [74]. Anastomotic leaks can lead to sepsis, organ failure, and death, and may be difficult to diagnose. The presence of tachycardia of > 120 beats/min, tachypnea, fever, or abdominal pain should prompt an evaluation [78, 79]. In the clinically stable patient, upper GI study or computed tomography may be considered for initial evaluation. Less severe cases can be managed with antibiotics and drainage; however, reoperation is necessary in some cases [80].

Rhabdomyolysis is a potential complication of surgical procedures in morbidly obese patients. Risks include BMI > 55 kg/m^2, prolonged operative time, and diabetic status [81–83]. Prevention can be implemented by adequate padding at pressure points and screening CK levels in high-risk patients [84].

Surgical site infections are another concern after bariatric surgery. They are more common after open procedures than those done laparoscopically (an incidence of 7% vs. 3%) [74, 85]. Patients should be managed with prophylactic antibiotics and drainage as needed. While wound infections rarely cause death, they cause signifi-

Table 10.2 Postoperative diet stages

Diet stage	Length of time	Fluids/food	Example
Stage 1	1 day	Begin sips of water	1 fluid oz. water per hour
Stage 2	1 day	Sugar-free clear liquid diet	32 fluid oz. per day (1 quart)
		Noncarbonated; no caffeine	Water, broth, Crystal Light
Stage 3	2–3 weeks	Full liquids; high protein drinks	48–64 + fluid oz. per day
			Nonfat Lactaid 100 milk
			Nonfat, no-added sugar soy-milk fortified with calcium
			Plain nonfat yogurt; Greek yogurt
Stage 4	4 weeks	Soft protein foods	4–6 small meals per day
		Soft, moist, diced, ground or pureed protein	Eggs, ground meats, poultry, fish, cottage cheese, fat-free cheese, yogurt
Stage 5	Ongoing	High-protein solid foods	60+ g of protein per day
		Low-fat, sugar-free food	Plus fruits and vegetables
			Always eat protein first

cant morbidity and increase the length of hospital stay. Hyperglycemia is one of the risk factors for surgical site infection [86] and attempt should be made to control postoperative hyperglycemia.

Diet and Nutritional Support

Nutritional support after bariatric surgery is designed to ensure adequate hydration, promote wound healing, preserve lean body mass, and minimize GI distress. Careful counseling by a dietitian is critical for success. Usually, a protocol-derived nutritional program can be started within 24 h after surgery but the diet progression should be discussed with the surgeon and guided by the dietitian. The general progression of a patient's diet after surgery includes five stages over two months after surgery. Patients will advance through stages 1 and 2 to stage 3 while in the hospital and will continue on stage 3 at home before being advanced to stages 4 and 5 after post op evaluation by their physician. The diet is advanced from only liquids to high-protein soft solids and then eventually to low-fat high-protein solid foods over the course of 2 months. Details of postoperative diet stages are in Table 10.2. Protein intake should be assessed and guided by the dietitian. Minimum protein intake of 60–90 g per day should be achieved to avoid loss of lean body mass [87, 88]. Protein intake is usually inadequate in the first 2 months after surgery; therefore, protein supplements such as protein powder are often advised to achieve optimal protein intake.

There are some general principles to help patients adjust to digestion with their new anatomy. Patients should chew food very thoroughly to facilitate swallowing

Table 10.3 Suggested routine postoperative nutritional supplements

Supplement	For purely restrictive procedure, e.g., LAGB	For malabsorptive procedure, e.g., LRYGB
Multivitamin plus mineral	1 tab daily	2 tabs daily
Calcium citrate	1200–1500 mg of elemental calcium per day, divided doses	1200–1500 mg of elemental calcium per day, divided doses
Vitamin D		3000 IU per day or more
Vitamin B12		Oral crystalline B12 350 mcg per day Or 1000 mcg intramuscularly every 1–3 months Or 500 mcg intranasally every week
Folate		400 mcg per day in multivitamins
Iron		Ferrous fumarate 325 mg twice per day for menstruating women

LAGB laparoscopic adjustable gastric banding; *LRYGB* laparoscopic Roux-en-Y gastric bypass

and prevent vomiting. During the progression through early food stages, patients should not drink liquids at the same time as they are eating their regular small meals. It is common for patients to have difficulty tolerating several types of food during the first several months after surgery, most commonly dry meats, breads, pasta, milk, and nuts. Patients should keep a food log to help identify food intolerances and monitor compliance. Protein should be consumed at the onset of the meal and carbohydrate should come from nutrient-dense complex carbohydrates to avoid Dumping syndrome [89]. Dumping syndrome can occur after the Roux-en-Y gastric bypass due to the loss of the physiologic sphincter at the stomach outlet. If the patient consumes a bolus of high sugar or high fat food, its arrival into the small intestine will cause a release of gut hormones and an influx of intraluminal fluid. The patient may experience nausea, diarrhea, flushing, and palpitations. This syndrome can usually be managed with nutritional counseling.

Routine vitamin supplementation will vary from patient to patient, with the most important determinant being the type of surgery performed. Though the laparoscopic adjustable gastric banding does not generally cause vitamin or mineral malabsorption, the variety and amount of food intake are restricted. It is recommended to take a multivitamin to meet daily requirements for both vitamins and minerals. Those undergoing Roux-en-Y gastric bypass, biliopancreatic diversion or biliopancreatic with duodenal switch are at greater risk for nutritional deficiencies [90]. Routine nutrient supplementation is shown in Table 10.3.

All patients should be encouraged to consume 1–2 multivitamins per day after surgery depending on the type of procedure performed. Patients may initially tolerate two chewable children's tablet more easily during the first 1–2 months after surgery. Most clinicians recommend routine supplementation with 1200–1500 mg of calcium per day. Calcium citrate tablets may be better absorbed than calcium carbonate tablets due to decrease in stomach acid. Most calcium tablets also contain vitamin D but this may not provide adequate supplementation. At least 3000 IU of vitamin D is required to get 25-vitamin D levels >30 ng/ml. Some patients may require a much higher dose of vitamin D to achieve this level. It is estimated that 30–50 % of patients might develop B12 deficiency after gastric bypass if not supplemented beyond a multivitamin [91, 92]. Treatment with oral crystalline B12 at doses of at least 350 mcg per day has been shown to maintain normal plasma B12 levels [93]. Subcutaneous or intramuscular injections may be used in patients not responding to oral therapy. A multivitamin containing folate will generally provide sufficient folic acid after surgery [94]. Iron deficiency after gastric bypass is quite common especially in premenopausal women. Additional ferrous fumarate supplementation with 325 mg twice per day may be needed in menstruating women [95]. Vitamin C may also be used to facilitate absorption.

Early Post-op Medication Management

During the immediate postoperative period, obesity-related comorbidities may change dramatically and it is important to monitor closely. In addition, patients undergoing Roux-en-Y gastric bypass or other malabsorptive procedures may have a change in the bioavailability of a particular drug depending on its site of absorption. For example, extended release formulations should be changed to immediate release and given in the crushed form.

Postoperative Blood Glucose Control and Medications Adjustment

After bariatric surgery, patients demonstrate a dramatic change in insulin sensitivity and glucose tolerance. In the immediate postoperative period, the patient's medications may need to undergo significant adjustment. Insulin secretagogues (sulfonylureas and meglitinides) should be discontinued and insulin dosage should be reduced due to risk of hypoglycemia. Insulin therapy can be used in hospitalized patients to obtain a premeal blood glucose target of less than 140 mg/dl and random blood glucose of less than 180 mg/dl [96]. Metformin may be used postoperatively once patient is able to tolerate fluids and diet but caution should be made in patients with reduced glomerular filtration rate (GFR) [97, 98]. Patients who are on insulin therapy are encouraged to monitor their blood sugar at home at least 3–4 times a day. The dosage of insulin should be titrated depending on patients' blood sugar level. Recently, a simple scoring system (DiaRem score) has been developed as a tool to help predict the likelihood of diabetes remission after Roux-en-Y gastric bypass surgery by using four clinical parameters: insulin use, age, HbA1c concentration, and type of antidiabetic drugs [99].

Antihypertensive medications should be adjusted during perioperative period. Diuretics and angiotensin converting enzyme inhibitors should be withheld 24 h before surgery due to the risk of hypovolemia and electrolyte imbalance. They can be slowly restarted if clinically indicated. Beta-blockers should be continued throughout, if possible. Stopping beta-blockers abruptly may lead to withdrawal syndrome with tachycardia and rebound hypertension [100]. Beta-blockers have potential adverse metabolic effects on lipids and insulin sensitivity and can cause weight gain in some patients [101]. If a beta-blocker is no longer indicated, practitioner should consider tapering it off and switching to other antihypertensive agents.

Long-term Follow-Up After Bariatric Surgery

Initial Follow-Up and Weight Loss

The timing of visits with the medical practitioner depends upon the type of surgery, as well as the patient's comorbidities and overall health. Initial follow-up would be at 2–6 weeks after surgery and then every 3–6 months interval [19, 102]. Patients with serious comorbidities or complications should be seen more frequently. After the first year, visits may be spaced out to every 6–12 months. All patients should be reminded that they must visit a medical practitioner at least annually to monitor for complications and nutritional deficiencies.

Generally, patients are able to start a walking exercise program within 1 week. Most patients should not do more vigorous exercise than walking until 6–12 weeks. Patients are encouraged to gradually increase their physical activity to a minimum of 150 min per week and to a goal of 300 min per week for aerobic physical activity, plus strength training 2–3 times per week [103].

Nutritional Status

It is recommended that patients be routinely screened for micronutrient deficiencies at 3, 6, and 12 months after surgery, and annually thereafter [19]. Suggested laboratory monitoring is shown in Table 10.4. Patients consuming a multivitamin after bariatric surgery generally maintain adequate levels of fat-soluble vitamins. There is currently insufficient evidence to support routine screening for essential fatty acid, vitamin E, or K deficiencies. Screening for vitamin A deficiency may be indicated in patients who have undergone a malabsorptive procedure and presenting with ocular symptoms.

Anemia should prompt an evaluation for nutritional deficiencies. Iron deficiency is common after bariatric surgery. Contributing factors include low intake of red meat, bypass of the duodenum and proximal jejunum where most of the absorption occurs, and a decrease in gastric acid needed for adequate iron absorption. Patients who remain iron deficient despite oral supplementation should undergo a work-up for gastrointestinal (GI) blood loss (including marginal ulceration), and be consid-

Table 10.4 Suggested postoperative laboratory monitoring

	1 month	3 months	6 months	12 months	Annually
CBC/plt	X	X	X	X	X
BMP	X	X	X	X	X
LFTs	X	X	X	X	X
Glucose	X	X	X	X	X
Lipids		X	X	X	X
Iron studies/ vitamin B12/ folate		X	X	X	X
25-vitamin D			X	X	X
iPTH/ Calcium/ALP			X	X	X
Vitamin B1		Optional	Optional	Optional	
Zinc			Optional	Optional	
Vitamin A				Optional	

BMP basic metabolic panel including kidney function; *LFTs* liver function tests; *iPTH* intact parathyroid hormone; *ALP* alkaline phosphatase, *CBC* complete blood count

ered for intravenous (IV) iron therapy. Serum ferritin is the most sensitive marker of early iron deficiency [104] and should be included in routine screening.

Vitamin B12 deficiencies can occur after bariatric surgery procedures that bypass the lower stomach. The initiation of vitamin B12 supplementation within 6 months postoperatively is important. Signs and symptoms of vitamin B12 deficiency are pernicious anemia, neuropathy, depression, and dementia. When assessing B12 deficiency, levels of homocysteine and methylmalonic acid should also be obtained as these are more sensitive markers of B12 deficiency [105]. Treatment with oral crystalline B12 at 1000 mcg daily or B12 500 mcg intranasal weekly is recommended. If B12 sufficiency cannot be maintained by oral or intranasal routes, intramuscular or subcutaneous B12 1000 mcg every month to 1000–3000 mcg every 6–12 months is indicated.

Multivitamin supplements providing 400 mcg/day folate can effectively prevent the development of folate deficiency after bariatric surgery. Routine supplementation is recommended especially in women of childbearing age to reduce the risk of fetal neural tube defects.

Thiamine deficiency can occur as a result of bypass of the jejunum, where thiamine is primarily absorbed. Thiamine deficiency after gastric bypass is rare but should be considered in patients who have persistent vomiting or inadequate nutrient intake and it can occur around 6 weeks to 3 months after surgery. Empiric treatment should be considered in patients with rapid weight loss, intractable vomiting, alcohol use, neuropathy, encephalopathy or congestive heart failure. Early recognition and treatment is important to prevent devastating complications such as Wernicke–Korsakoff syndrome. Parenteral supplementation with thiamine 100 mg per day should be initiated in the patient with active neurological symptoms. Severe cases should be treated with IV thiamine 500 mg per day for 3–5 days, followed by 250 mg per day until resolution of symptoms [106–108]. After 7–14 days, one can switch to an oral supplement of 10 mg per day.

Oral calcium and vitamin D supplements are important for bone health and to prevent secondary hyperparathyroidism. Vitamin D malabsorption occurs after bariatric surgery and in some patients the doses of vitamin D supplement may need to be as high as 50,000 units 1–3 times weekly. Following bariatric surgery, there is a significant increase in markers of bone turnover associated with a decrease in bone mass and the degree of loss of bone mineral density is associated with the amount of weight loss [109]. Possible mechanisms are skeletal unloading and secondary hyperparathyroidism [35]. Because of the complexity of calcium and vitamin D regulation, it is recommended that several parameters of bone health be monitored, including parathyroid hormone, total calcium, albumin, 25-OH vitamin D, 24-h urine calcium and bone-specific alkaline phosphatase levels. Dual-energy X-ray absorptiometry (DXA) is indicated to monitor for osteoporosis at 2-year intervals especially in high risk groups such as postmenopausal women.

Some bariatric patients have been documented to have low levels of selenium, zinc, and copper. Of these, zinc deficiency may be the most common, particularly after malabsorptive procedure. Symptoms of zinc deficiency include impaired immune function, hair loss, pica, and rash. Unfortunately, zinc deficiency is difficult to diagnose as serum levels represent <0.1 % of total zinc stores, and during periods of inflammation this level will be artificially low due to increased zinc uptake in the liver [110]. Practitioners should rely on the clinical picture and laboratory data to assess the need for supplemental zinc. Oral Zinc supplement of 15–20 mg per day or up to 60 mg per day in the setting of malabsorption is advised [111].

Clinically relevant deficiencies of selenium and copper are poorly studied and seem to be rare. Symptoms of copper deficiency such as peripheral neuropathy and myelopathy are often indistinguishable from those occurring with vitamin B_{12} deficiency. Low plasma copper concentration and ceruloplasmin activity can be helpful to make the diagnosis. Treatment with IV copper of 2.4 mg daily for 6 days, followed by weekly intravenous copper of 2.4 mg combined with oral supplementation of 8 mg copper/daily until normal copper levels in blood are achieved was suggested [50].

Despite routine multivitamins and minerals supplementation, nutritional deficiencies can still occur. This could be due to baseline nutritional status, adherence to supplementation, adequacy of dietary intake, and type of bariatric surgery [112]. Thiamine deficiency can occur as early as 2–3 months postoperative in patients with frequent vomiting. Iron deficiency and vitamin B12 deficiency can be seen at 6 and 12 months, respectively. Copper deficiency can be seen at 24 months following gastric bypass surgery [113]. A small study has shown reduced Zinc concentration at 12–18 months after gastric bypass surgery [114].

Medical Management of Comorbidities and Medication Adjustment

During routine follow-up visits, the practitioner should assess for resolution or improvement of patients' comorbidities. Bariatric surgery has been shown to dramatically improve diabetes [115, 116] and more than 70% of patients will be normoglycemic off medication 2 years after surgery [117]. Patients who were taking insulin prior to surgery should have their basal insulin dosage decreased by half and discontinued for low sugars. Patients taking prandial insulin should not resume this practice until postprandial glucose values rise above 150 mg/dl. The most important factor in assuring safety is frequent monitoring, and patients should check their blood sugar 3–4 times daily and if needed discuss these values several times per week with their clinician. Because of the risk of future diabetes, patients who have been weaned off all of their medications should be checked at regular intervals for recurrent hyperglycemia. It is unclear if patients who have had resolution of their diabetes should continue other aspects of preventative diabetic care.

Hypertension improves variably after bariatric surgery, but approximately 30% of patients with prior hypertension will not require medication at 2 years postoperative [117]. The reduction in blood pressure can be seen as early as 1 week postoperative [118]. Antihypertensive medications should be adjusted and patients' blood pressure should be monitored periodically. Use of diuretics should be cautious due to risk for dehydration and electrolyte abnormalities.

After bariatric surgery, patients can anticipate an improvement in total cholesterol, triglycerides, and HDL as early as 3 months postoperatively [119]. In the 6 months following surgery, a reduction of more than 15% of total cholesterol and a triglyceride reduction of more than 50% can be observed [120]. Patients should then have their cholesterol levels measured 3 months postoperatively and rechecked periodically. Statin use may be continued depending on patient's cardiovascular risk factors and lipid level goals [121].

Patients with NAFLD generally see improvement following bariatric surgery. Weight loss after bariatric surgery in obese patients will decrease the grade of steatosis, hepatic inflammation, and even the fibrosis [122–124]. Patients with history of transaminitis should be followed with liver function tests periodically to ensure that the levels fall into normal range.

Over 75% of patients with OSA can expect resolution or improvement of their disease following bariatric surgery [125]. At this time, there are no standing recommendations for discontinuation of CPAP therapy after bariatric surgery. However, it may be reasonable to seek repeat polysomnography after the patient has achieved 30% loss of excess body weight [126].

Psychiatric medications may need to be continued postoperatively and the need for medications reassessed in conjunction with a psychiatrist. Weight loss after bariatric surgery increases fertility. Hormonal methods such as oral contraceptive pills may be less effective due to malabsorption and changes in sex hormone binding globulins [127]. Alternative methods should be discussed with a gynecologist.

Weight-based dosing medications should be adjusted according to rapid changes in patient's body weight postoperatively. In patients with hypothyroidism, dosage of levothyroxine replacement is related to the amount of lean body mass [128]. As the patient is losing weight after gastric bypass surgery, levothyroxine dosage should be decreased and TSH should be monitored every 2–3 months.

Complications After Bariatric Surgery

During the first 30 days after surgery, complications are usually related to the operative procedure. Patients experiencing severe vomiting, wound infections, and blood clots should be referred back to the surgical team. Complications beyond the first month will be discussed in more detail below.

Vomiting after bariatric surgery is multifactorial and occurs in most patients for the first several months. Patients will have to adjust to new eating habits with their new smaller stomach pouch. In our center, patients presenting to the emergency room with vomiting after bariatric surgery receive 100 mg of thiamine, 1 mg of folate, and 10 cc of liquid multivitamin in normal saline to prevent Wernicke–Korsakoff syndrome. Patients who continue to have severe vomiting, or persistent vomiting for longer than 6 months should undergo further work-up for obstruction, ulceration, stenosis, or dysmotility. Patients with bloating, abdominal pain and bleeding should be evaluated for marginal ulceration. If uncomplicated, marginal ulceration can usually be managed medically. Nonsteroidal anti-inflammatory drugs should not be used after bariatric surgery due to risk of ulcers. Gastric dumping occurs initially in patients who have had a Roux-en-Y gastric bypass from bypassing the gastric pylorus so food and nutrients will enter small intestine rapidly [129]. Abdominal pain and cramping, nausea, diarrhea, light-headedness, flushing, tachycardia, and syncope are symptoms indicative of dumping. Postprandial or reactive hypoglycemia can be part of "late dumping symptoms" due to rapid glucose absorption stimulating incretins and insulin secretion. Symptoms usually will be less prominent over time and patients are advised to eating small frequent meals, avoiding simple sugars, and increasing fiber and protein intake [130]. Postgastric bypass noninsulinoma pancreatogenous hypoglycemia syndrome (NIPHS) is very rare but several cases have been reported [131, 132]. If hypoglycemia persists despite dietary modification, patient should be referred to an endocrinologist for further evaluation.

Intestinal bacterial overgrowth is uncommon but can occur after biliopancreatic diversion. Symptoms are nonspecific. Sometimes patients presented with diarrhea, malabsorption, or thiamine deficiency [133, 134]. Treatment includes oral antibiotics and probiotics [135]. Incisional hernias can occur after bariatric surgery particularly in those patients who have undergone open surgical procedures. If the patient is asymptomatic, it is usually recommended that surgical repair be deferred until maximal weight loss has been achieved. In contrast, internal hernias are more common after laparoscopic surgery and can be difficult to diagnose due to altered gastrointestinal tract anatomy. These patients will often complain of postprandial abdominal pain, nausea, and vomiting. When an internal hernia is suspected, patients should be referred back to the surgeon for diagnostic imaging and possible exploratory surgery [136, 137]. Internal hernia is considered surgical emergency since delay in diagnosis can cause morbidity and death.

Gallstones can develop in 28% of patients after bariatric surgery [138, 139]. Patients who presented with right upper quadrant abdominal pain should have imaging test with an ultrasound. Several studies have suggested that prophylactic cholecystectomy with bariatric surgery may be reasonable to prevent gallstone-related complications [140, 141]. Ursodeoxycholic acid 300–1200 mg/day divided doses can decrease gallstone formation in patients who have not had a cholecystectomy [142]. Patients who have had malabsorptive procedures are at risk for renal oxalate stones because of impaired oxalate binding in the small intestine. These patients should consume a moderate calcium diet, avoid dehydration, limit dietary oxalate, and adhere with low fat diet. Patients should have periodic urine testing for calcium, oxalate and citrate, and careful monitoring of calcium and vitamin D status.

Although rare, some patients have been hospitalized with persistent vomiting, weakness, and hyporeflexia after bariatric surgery. This syndrome is known as acute post-gastric reduction surgery (APGARS) neuropathy, and remains poorly understood. Nutritional deficiencies were thought to play a role in pathogenesis. When suspected, these patients should undergo testing for vitamin deficiencies, especially B12, copper, and thiamine, as this has been linked to the syndrome [50, 143].

Hair loss commonly occurs in 3–6 months following surgery. The most common form is telogen effluvium, and two risk factors are major surgery and rapid weight loss. Patients should be reassured that this should reverse with time and weight stabilization.

In general, most patients will have improved psychological functioning after surgery. However, a subset of patients will experience difficulties adjusting to their new lifestyles and changing interpersonal relationships. The clinician should periodically screen for this and refer to a mental health professional as needed.

Inadequate Weight Loss and Weight Regain

Patients will often lose up to a half to one pound per day for the first 3 months after surgery. Maximal weight loss after gastric bypass usually occurs between 12 and 18 months after bariatric surgery, but may be more gradual in patients after laparoscopic gastric banding. In general, bariatric surgery is considered successful if the patient loses more than 50% of their excess body weight. During the period of rapid weight loss, it is common for patients to complain of fatigue, hair loss, and cold intolerance. After patients achieve peak weight loss, there is usually a period of weight stabilization, followed by gradual weight regain. Significant weight regain is defined as weight regain of ≥ 15% of total weight loss and this can occur in about 15% of patients [144].

When a patient complains of weight regain or failure to lose weight, the practitioner should evaluate for patient's adherence to lifestyle modification, medications associated with weight gain, development of maladaptive eating behaviors, psychological complications, and imaging studies of the gastrointestinal tract [19]. Due to improved surgical techniques, ruptured staple line, anastomotic dilation, and formation of fistula are now rare causes of weight regain but still can occur in about 2–5% of patients [145, 146]. Binge eating disorder and grazing can be causes of inadequate weight loss and weight regain. Practitioners should document weight patterns and carefully review patients' dietary habits. Nutritional management with low glycemic load with 45% of carbohydrates, 35% of protein (80 g for women and 100 g for men) and 20% of fat, three servings of dairy products, and a supplement of soluble fibers (15 g/day) was found to be helpful [147]. When weight regain is severe and uncontrolled, pharmacological therapy or revisional bariatric surgery should be considered but with a careful decision by a multidisciplinary team.

Pregnancy

Pregnancy should be avoided 12–24 months postoperatively [50]. Obesity is associated with subfertility status due to oligo-ovulation or anovulation. Patient's fertility status usually improves after weight loss with bariatric surgery. Patients should be compliant with micronutrient intake even at preconception state to reduce risks of early pregnancy loss and fetal neural tube defect. Folic acid, vitamin B12, and other micronutrients are very important and should be monitored closely. Obstetricians should be aware of potential complications such as internal hernias from increased intra-abdominal pressure during pregnancy [148]. Patients may present with nausea, vomiting, and abdominal pain. If suspected, a surgical exploration should not be delayed to avoid maternal and/or fetal death.

Evidence has shown that women who have had bariatric surgery may have lower rates of obesity-related pregnancy complications such as gestational diabetes and hypertensive disorders compared to obese women who had pregnancies before their bariatric procedures [149]. This could result from improvement of their obesity-related comorbidities after weight loss from bariatric surgery. In a cohort, bariatric surgery did not increase the risk of congenital malformation [150]. Risk of fetal macrosomia is lower in obese women [151], but risk of low birth weight and intrauterine growth retardation might be higher [152]. Overall, pregnancy after bariatric surgery seems to be safe but patients should be monitored closely by multidisciplinary team including, obstetrician, nutritionist, and bariatric surgeon.

Body Contouring Surgery

Excess skin after massive weight loss can cause impaired quality of life, skin infection, and impaired mobility. Some patients may report poor self-esteem and difficulty adjusting to their new bodies. Body contouring surgery after gastric bypass surgery was found to improve patient's satisfaction and quality of life [153, 154]. Most frequent procedures offered were abdominoplasty and breast reduction/mastopexy. The rate of complications of body contouring after massive weight loss is quite high at 26% including wound dehiscence, wound infection, hematoma, and tissue necrosis [155]. Body contouring surgery is recommended 18–24 months after bariatric surgery to ensure that weight loss has stabilized. Patients who had stable weight for 3 months that is close to normal were found to have lower risk of complications after body contouring surgery [156].

Conclusion

There has been much promising evidence and research in obesity and bariatric surgery over the past 10 years. Bariatric surgery has shown to reduce mortality and obesity-related comorbid conditions. Careful pre- and postoperative assessment by a multidisciplinary team is crucial to optimize patient outcomes.

Acknowledgment The authors would like to acknowledge Wendy Anderson, registered dietitian at Boston Medical Center, for her suggestions contributing to this chapter.

References

1. Flegal KM, Carroll MD, Kit BK, Ogden CL. Prevalence of obesity and trends in the distribution of body mass index among US adults, 1999–2010. JAMA. 2012;307(5):491–7. Epub 2012/01/19.
2. Christou NV, Sampalis JS, Liberman M, Look D, Auger S, McLean AP, et al. Surgery decreases long-term mortality, morbidity, and health care use in morbidly obese patients. Ann Surg. 2004;240(3):416–23. discussion 23–4. Epub 2004/08/21.
3. Sjostrom L . Bariatric surgery and reduction in morbidity and mortality: experiences from the SOS study. Int J Obes (Lond). 2008;32(Suppl 7):93–7. Epub 2009/01/16.
4. Livingston EH. The incidence of bariatric surgery has plateaued in the U.S. Am J Surg. 2010;200(3):378–85. Epub 2010/04/23.
5. NIH conference. Gastrointestinal surgery for severe obesity. Consensus development conference panel. Ann Intern Med. 1991;115(12):956–61. Epub 1991/12/15.
6. SAGES. Guideline for clinical application of laparoscopic bariatric surgery. Surg Endosc. 2008;22(10):2281–300. Epub 2008/09/16.
7. Harper J, Madan AK, Ternovits CA, Tichansky DS. What happens to patients who do not follow-up after bariatric surgery? Am Surg. 2007;73(2):181–4. Epub 2007/02/20.
8. Shen R, Dugay G, Rajaram K, Cabrera I, Siegel N, Ren CJ. Impact of patient follow-up on weight loss after bariatric surgery. Obes Surg. 2004;14(4):514–9. Epub 2004/05/08.
9. Moulin de Moraes CM, Mancini MC, de Melo ME, Figueiredo DA, Villares SM, Rascovski A, et al. Prevalence of subclinical hypothyroidism in a morbidly obese population and improvement after weight loss induced by Roux-en-Y gastric bypass. Obes Surg. 2005;15(9):1287–91. Epub 2005/11/02.

10. Garber JR, Cobin RH, Gharib H, Hennessey JV, Klein I, Mechanick JI, et al. Clinical practice guidelines for hypothyroidism in adults: cosponsored by the American Association of Clinical Endocrinologists and the American Thyroid Association. Endocr Pract Off J Am Coll Endocrinol Am Assoc Clin Endocrinol. 2012;18(6):988–1028. Epub 2012/12/19.

11. Jankovic D, Wolf P, Anderwald CH, Winhofer Y, Promintzer-Schifferl M, Hofer A, et al. Prevalence of endocrine disorders in morbidly obese patients and the effects of bariatric surgery on endocrine and metabolic parameters. Obes Surg. 2012;22(1):62–9. Epub 2011/11/05.

12. Baid SK, Rubino D, Sinaii N, Ramsey S, Frank A, Nieman LK. Specificity of screening tests for Cushing's syndrome in an overweight and obese population. J Clin Endocrinol Metab. 2009;94(10):3857–64. Epub 2009/07/16.

13. Sahin SB, Sezgin H, Ayaz T, Uslu Gur E, Ilkkilic K. Routine Screening for Cushing's syndrome is not required in patients presenting with obesity. ISRN Endocrinol. 2013;2013:321063. Epub 2013/07/11.

14. Ness-Abramof R, Nabriski D, Apovian CM, Niven M, Weiss E, Shapiro MS, et al. Overnight dexamethasone suppression test: a reliable screen for Cushing's syndrome in the obese. Obes Res. 2002;10(12):1217–21. Epub 2002/12/20.

15. Bray GA. Medical consequences of obesity. J Clin Endocrinol Metab. 2004;89(6):2583–9. Epub 2004/06/08.

16. Tavares Ida S, Sousa AC, Menezes Filho RS, Aguiar-Oliveira MH, Barreto-Filho JA, Brito AF, et al. Left ventricular diastolic function in morbidly obese patients in the preoperative for bariatric surgery. Arq Bras de Cardiol. 2012;98(4):300–6. Epub 2012/03/28.

17. Kwon S, Thompson R, Florence M, Maier R, McIntyre L, Rogers T, et al. Beta-blocker continuation after noncardiac surgery: a report from the surgical care and outcomes assessment program. Arch Surg. 2012;147(5):467–73. Epub 2012/01/18.

18. Auerbach A, Goldman L. Assessing and reducing the cardiac risk of noncardiac surgery. Circulation. 2006;113(10):1361–76. Epub 2006/03/15.

19. Mechanick JI, Youdim A, Jones DB, Garvey WT, Hurley DL, McMahon MM, et al. Clinical practice guidelines for the perioperative nutritional, metabolic, and nonsurgical support of the bariatric surgery patient–2013 update: cosponsored by American Association of Clinical Endocrinologists, the Obesity Society, and American Society for Metabolic & Bariatric Surgery. Obesity (Silver Spring). 2013;21(Suppl 1):1–27. Epub 2013/04/03.

20. Daltro C, Gregorio PB, Alves E, Abreu M, Bomfim D, Chicourel MH, et al. Prevalence and severity of sleep apnea in a group of morbidly obese patients. Obes Surg. 2007;17(6):809–14. Epub 2007/09/21.

21. Flum DR, Belle SH, King WC, Wahed AS, Berk P, Chapman W, et al. Perioperative safety in the longitudinal assessment of bariatric surgery. N Engl J Med. 2009;361(5):445–54. Epub 2009/07/31.

22. Marshall NS, Wong KK, Liu PY, Cullen SR, Knuiman MW, Grunstein RR. Sleep apnea as an independent risk factor for all-cause mortality: the Busselton Health Study. Sleep. 2008;31(8):1079–85. Epub 2008/08/22.

23. Ge X, Han F, Huang Y, Zhang Y, Yang T, Bai C, et al. Is obstructive sleep apnea associated with cardiovascular and all-cause mortality? PloS ONE. 2013;8(7):e69432. Epub 2013/08/13.

24. Abbas Q, Arjomand F, Kumar M, Contreras J, Shahzad S, Jinnur P, Ahmad M, Tiwary T, Ali Rana, Vasudevan P. Occlusive Sleep Apnea (OSA) Screening and Preemptive Continuous Positive Airway Pressure (CPAP)/Bilevel Positive Airway Pressure (BiPAP) Application is effective in reducing post bariatric surgery pulmonary complications. Chest. 10/24/122012. p 1065A.

25. Sanyal AJ. AGA technical review on nonalcoholic fatty liver disease. Gastroenterology. 2002;123(5):1705–25. Epub 2002/10/31.

26. Wu J, You J, Yerian L, Shiba A, Schauer PR, Sessler DI. Prevalence of liver steatosis and fibrosis and the diagnostic accuracy of ultrasound in bariatric surgery patients. Obes Surg. 2012;22(2):240–7. Epub 2011/09/09.

27. Malfertheiner P, Megraud F, O'Morain CA, Atherton J, Axon AT, Bazzoli F, et al. Management of Helicobacter pylori infection–the Maastricht IV/Florence Consensus Report. Gut. 2012;61(5):646–64. Epub 2012/04/12.

28. Hartin CW, Jr., ReMine DS, Lucktong TA. Preoperative bariatric screening and treatment of Helicobacter pylori. Surg Endosc. 2009;23(11):2531–4. Epub 2009/05/16.

29. Schirmer B, Erenoglu C, Miller A. Flexible endoscopy in the management of patients undergoing Roux-en-Y gastric bypass. Obes Surg. 2002;12(5):634–8. Epub 2002/11/27.

30. Ogunnaike BO, Jones SB, Jones DB, Provost D, Whitten CW. Anesthetic considerations for bariatric surgery. Anesth Analg. 2002;95(6):1793–805. Epub 2002/11/29.

31. Birkmeyer NJ, Share D, Baser O, Carlin AM, Finks JF, Pesta CM, et al. Preoperative placement of inferior vena cava filters and outcomes after gastric bypass surgery. Ann Surg. 2010;252(2):313–8. Epub 2010/07/14.

32. Keeling WB, Haines K, Stone PA, Armstrong PA, Murr MM, Shames ML. Current indications for preoperative inferior vena cava filter insertion in patients undergoing surgery for morbid obesity. Obes Surg. 2005;15(7):1009–12. Epub 2005/08/18.

33. Atluri P, Raper SE. Factor V Leiden and postoperative deep vein thrombosis in patients undergoing open Roux-en-Y gastric bypass surgery. Obesity Surg. 2005;15(4):561–4. Epub 2005/06/11.

34. Vilarrasa N, San Jose P, Garcia I, Gomez-Vaquero C, Miras PM, de Gordejuela AG, et al. Evaluation of bone mineral density loss in morbidly obese women after gastric bypass: 3-year follow-up. Obes Surg. 2011;21(4):465–72. Epub 2010/12/29.

35. Stein EM, Carrelli A, Young P, Bucovsky M, Zhang C, Schrope B, et al. Bariatric surgery results in cortical bone loss. J Clin Endocrinol Metab. 2013;98(2):541–9. Epub 2013/01/09.

36. Miller PD. Guidelines for the diagnosis of osteoporosis: T-scores vs fractures. Rev Endocr Metab disord. 2006;7(1–2):75–89. Epub 2006/12/23.

37. Fullmer MA, Abrams SH, Hrovat K, Mooney L, Scheimann AO, Hillman JB, et al. Nutritional strategy for adolescents undergoing bariatric surgery: report of a working group of the Nutrition Committee of NASPGHAN/NACHRI. J Pediatr Gastroenterol Nutr. 2012;54(1):125–35. Epub 2011/08/23.

38. Brolin RE. Gastric bypass. Surg Clin North Am. 2001;81(5):1077–95. Epub 2001/10/09.

39. Goldner WS, Stoner JA, Thompson J, Taylor K, Larson L, Erickson J, et al. Prevalence of vitamin D insufficiency and deficiency in morbidly obese patients: a comparison with nonobese controls. Obesity Surg. 2008;18(2):145–50. Epub 2008/01/05.

40. Sarwer DB, Cohn NI, Gibbons LM, Magee L, Crerand CE, Raper SE, et al. Psychiatric diagnoses and psychiatric treatment among bariatric surgery candidates. Obesity Surg. 2004;14(9):1148–56. Epub 2004/11/06.

41. Kinzl JF, Maier C, Bosch A. [Morbidly obese patients: psychopathology and eating disorders—Results of a preoperative evaluation]. Neuropsychiatr (Klinik, Diagnostik, Therapie und Rehabilitation: Organ der Gesellschaft Osterreichischer Nervenarzte und Psychiater). 2012;26(4):159–65. Epub 2012/11/28. Morbid adipose Patienten: Psychopathologie und Esstorungen: Ergebnisse einer praoperativen Evaluation.

42. Klockhoff H, Naslund I, Jones AW. Faster absorption of ethanol and higher peak concentration in women after gastric bypass surgery. Br J Clin Pharmacol. 2002;54(6):587–91. Epub 2002/12/21.

43. Maluenda F, Csendes A, De Aretxabala X, Poniachik J, Salvo K, Delgado I, et al. Alcohol absorption modification after a laparoscopic sleeve gastrectomy due to obesity. Obesity Surg. 2010;20(6):744–8. Epub 2010/04/02.

44. Heinberg LJ, Ashton K, Coughlin J. Alcohol and bariatric surgery: review and suggested recommendations for assessment and management. Surg Obes Relat Dis Off J Am Soc Bariatr Surg. 2012;8(3):357–63. Epub 2012/03/20.

45. Kudsi OY, Huskey K, Grove S, Blackburn G, Jones DB, Wee CC. Prevalence of preoperative alcohol abuse among patients seeking weight-loss surgery. Surgical Endosc. 2013;27(4):1093–7. Epub 2012/10/12.

46. Felix EL, Kettelle J, Mobley E, Swartz D. Perforated marginal ulcers after laparoscopic gastric bypass. Surg Endosc. 2008;22(10):2128–32. Epub 2008/06/17.

47. Carroll KK. Obesity as a risk factor for certain types of cancer. Lipids. 1998;33(11):1055–9. Epub 1998/12/31.

48. Bergstrom A, Pisani P, Tenet V, Wolk A, Adami HO. Overweight as an avoidable cause of cancer in Europe. Int J Cancer. 2001;91(3):421–30. Epub 2001/02/15.

49. Calle EE, Rodriguez C, Walker-Thurmond K, Thun MJ. Overweight, obesity, and mortality from cancer in a prospectively studied cohort of U.S. adults. N Engl J Med. 2003;348(17):1625–38. Epub 2003/04/25.

50. Griffith DP, Liff DA, Ziegler TR, Esper GJ, Winton EF. Acquired copper deficiency: a potentially serious and preventable complication following gastric bypass surgery. Obesity (Silver Spring). 2009;17(4):827–31. Epub 2009/01/17.

51. Deitel M, Stone E, Kassam HA, Wilk EJ, Sutherland DJ. Gynecologic-obstetric changes after loss of massive excess weight following bariatric surgery. J Am Coll Nutr. 1988;7(2):147–53. Epub 1988/04/01.

52. Marceau P, Kaufman D, Biron S, Hould FS, Lebel S, Marceau S, et al. Outcome of pregnancies after biliopancreatic diversion. Obes Surg. 2004;14(3):318–24. Epub 2004/04/10.

53. Magdaleno R, Jr., Pereira BG, Chaim EA, Turato ER. Pregnancy after bariatric surgery: a current view of maternal, obstetrical and perinatal challenges. Arch Gynecol Obstet. 2012;285(3):559–66. Epub 2011/12/30.

54. Fris RJ. Preoperative low energy diet diminishes liver size. Obes Surg. 2004;14(9):1165–70. Epub 2004/11/06.

55. Alvarado R, Alami RS, Hsu G, Safadi BY, Sanchez BR, Morton JM, et al. The impact of preoperative weight loss in patients undergoing laparoscopic Roux-en-Y gastric bypass. Obes Surg. 2005;15(9):1282–6. Epub 2005/11/02.

56. Edholm D, Kullberg J, Haenni A, Karlsson FA, Ahlstrom A, Hedberg J, et al. Preoperative 4-week low-calorie diet reduces liver volume and intrahepatic fat, and facilitates laparoscopic gastric bypass in morbidly obese. Obes Surg. 2011;21(3):345–50. Epub 2010/12/25.

57. Alami RS, Morton JM, Schuster R, Lie J, Sanchez BR, Peters A, et al. Is there a benefit to preoperative weight loss in gastric bypass patients? A prospective randomized trial. Surg Obes Rel Dis Off J Am Soc Bariatr Surg. 2007;3(2):141–5; discussion 5–6. Epub 2007/03/03.

58. Livhits M, Mercado C, Yermilov I, Parikh JA, Dutson E, Mehran A, et al. Does weight loss immediately before bariatric surgery improve outcomes: a systematic review. Surg Obes Rel Dis Off J Am Soc Bariatr Surg. 2009;5(6):713–21. Epub 2009/11/03.

59. Becouarn G, Topart P, Ritz P. Weight loss prior to bariatric surgery is not a pre-requisite of excess weight loss outcomes in obese patients. Obes Surg. 2010;20(5):574–7. Epub 2010/02/23.

60. Cassie S, Menezes C, Birch DW, Shi X, Karmali S. Effect of preoperative weight loss in bariatric surgical patients: a systematic review. Surg Obes Rel Dis Off J Am Soc Bariatr Surg. 2011;7(6):760–7; discussion 7. Epub 2011/10/08.

61. American Diabetes Association. Standards of medical care in diabetes–2013. Diabetes Care. 2013;36(Suppl 1):11–66. Epub 2013/01/04.

62. Inzucchi SE, Bergenstal RM, Buse JB, Diamant M, Ferrannini E, Nauck M, et al. Management of hyperglycemia in type 2 diabetes: a patient-centered approach: position statement of the American Diabetes Association (ADA) and the European Association for the Study of Diabetes (EASD). Diabetes care. 2012;35(6):1364–79. Epub 2012/04/21.

63. Perna M, Romagnuolo J, Morgan K, Byrne TK, Baker M. Preoperative hemoglobin A1c and postoperative glucose control in outcomes after gastric bypass for obesity. Surg Obes Rel Dis Off J Am Soc Bariatr Surg. 2012;8(6):685–90. Epub 2011/10/11.

64. Pomposelli JJ, Baxter JK, 3rd, Babineau TJ, Pomfret EA, Driscoll DF, Forse RA, et al. Early postoperative glucose control predicts nosocomial infection rate in diabetic patients. JPEN J Parenter Enteral Nutr. 1998;22(2):77–81. Epub 1998/04/07.

65. Ata A, Lee J, Bestle SL, Desemone J, Stain SC. Postoperative hyperglycemia and surgical site infection in general surgery patients. Arch Surg. 2010;145(9):858–64. Epub 2010/09/22.

66. Maggard MA, Shugarman LR, Suttorp M, Maglione M, Sugerman HJ, Livingston EH, et al. Meta-analysis: surgical treatment of obesity. Ann Intern Med. 2005;142(7):547–59. Epub 2005/04/06.

67. DeMaria EJ, Pate V, Warthen M, Winegar DA. Baseline data from American Society for Metabolic and Bariatric Surgery-designated Bariatric Surgery Centers of Excellence using the Bariatric Outcomes Longitudinal Database. Surg Obes Rel Dis Off J Am Soc Bariatr Surg. 2010;6(4):347–55. Epub 2010/02/24.

68. Livingston EH. Procedure incidence and in-hospital complication rates of bariatric surgery in the United States. Am J Surg. 2004;188(2):105–10. Epub 2004/07/14.

69. Levi D, Goodman ER, Patel M, Savransky Y. Critical care of the obese and bariatric surgical patient. Crit Care Clin. 2003;19(1):11–32. Epub 2003/04/12.

70. Mukherjee D, Eagle KA. Perioperative cardiac assessment for noncardiac surgery: eight steps to the best possible outcome. Circulation. 2003;107(22):2771–4. Epub 2003/06/11.

71. Sapala JA, Wood MH, Schuhknecht MP, Sapala MA. Fatal pulmonary embolism after bariatric operations for morbid obesity: a 24-year retrospective analysis. Obes Surg. 2003;13(6):819–25. Epub 2004/01/24.

72. Magee CJ, Barry J, Javed S, Macadam R, Kerrigan D. Extended thromboprophylaxis reduces incidence of postoperative venous thromboembolism in laparoscopic bariatric surgery. Surg Obes Rel Dis Off J Am Soc Bariatr Surg. 2010;6(3):322–5. Epub 2010/06/01.

73. Raftopoulos I, Martindale C, Cronin A, Steinberg J. The effect of extended post-discharge chemical thromboprophylaxis on venous thromboembolism rates after bariatric surgery: a prospective comparison trial. Surg Endosc. 2008;22(11):2384–91. Epub 2008/07/16.

74. Podnos YD, Jimenez JC, Wilson SE, Stevens CM, Nguyen NT. Complications after laparoscopic gastric bypass: a review of 3464 cases. Arch Surg. 2003;138(9):957–61. Epub 2003/09/10.

75. Lawrence VA, Cornell JE, Smetana GW. Strategies to reduce postoperative pulmonary complications after noncardiothoracic surgery: systematic review for the American College of Physicians. Ann Intern Med. 2006;144(8):596–608. Epub 2006/04/19.

76. Ramirez A, Lalor PF, Szomstein S, Rosenthal RJ. Continuous positive airway pressure in immediate postoperative period after laparoscopic Roux-en-Y gastric bypass: is it safe? Surg Obes Relat Dis. 2009;5(5):544–6. Epub 2009/07/31.

77. Chiumello D, Chevallard G, Gregoretti C. Non-invasive ventilation in postoperative patients: a systematic review. Intensive Care Med. 2011;37(6):918–29. Epub 2011/03/23.

78. Hamilton EC, Sims TL, Hamilton TT, Mullican MA, Jones DB, Provost DA. Clinical predictors of leak after laparoscopic Roux-en-Y gastric bypass for morbid obesity. Surg Endosc. 2003;17(5):679–84. Epub 2003/03/06.

79. Bellorin O, Abdemur A, Sucandy I, Szomstein S, Rosenthal RJ. Understanding the significance, reasons and patterns of abnormal vital signs after gastric bypass for morbid obesity. Obes Surg. 2011;21(6):707–13. Epub 2010/06/29.

80. Griffith PS, Birch DW, Sharma AM, Karmali S. Managing complications associated with laparoscopic Roux-en-Y gastric bypass for morbid obesity. Can J Surg (J Can de Chir). 2012;55(5):329–36. Epub 2012/08/03.

81. Lagandre S, Arnalsteen L, Vallet B, Robin E, Jany T, Onraed B, et al. Predictive factors for rhabdomyolysis after bariatric surgery. Obes Surg. 2006;16(10):1365–70. Epub 2006/10/25.

82. de Oliveira LD, Diniz MT de Fatima HSDM, Savassi-Rocha AL, Camargos ST, Cardoso F. Rhabdomyolysis after bariatric surgery by Roux-en-Y gastric bypass: a prospective study. Obes Surg. 2009;19(8):1102–7. Epub 2008/12/20.

83. Chakravartty S, Sarma DR, Patel AG. Rhabdomyolysis in bariatric surgery: a systematic review. Obes Surg. 2013;23(8):1333–40. Epub 2013/04/09.

84. Wool DB, Lemmens HJ, Brodsky JB, Solomon H, Chong KP, Morton JM. Intraoperative fluid replacement and postoperative creatine phosphokinase levels in laparoscopic bariatric patients. Obes Surg. 2010;20(6):698–701. Epub 2010/03/04.

85. Shabanzadeh DM, Sorensen LT. Laparoscopic surgery compared with open surgery decreases surgical site infection in obese patients: a systematic review and meta-analysis. Ann Surg. 2012;256(6):934–45. Epub 2012/10/31.

86. Ruiz-Tovar J, Oller I, Llavero C, Arroyo A, Munoz JL, Calero A, et al. Pre-operative and early post-operative factors associated with surgical site infection after laparoscopic sleeve gastrectomy. Surg Infect. 2013;14(4):369–73. Epub 2013/05/31.

87. Faria SL, Faria OP, Buffington C, de Almeida Cardeal M, Ito MK. Dietary protein intake and bariatric surgery patients: a review. Obes Surg. 2011;21(11):1798–805. Epub 2011/05/19.

88. Raftopoulos I, Bernstein B, O'Hara K, Ruby JA, Chhatrala R, Carty J. Protein intake compliance of morbidly obese patients undergoing bariatric surgery and its effect on weight loss and biochemical parameters. Surg Obes Relat Dis. 2011;7(6):733–42. Epub 2011/09/20.

89. Moize VL, Pi-Sunyer X, Mochari H, Vidal J. Nutritional pyramid for post-gastric bypass patients. Obes Surg. 2010;20(8):1133–41. Epub 2010/04/20.

90. Malone M. Recommended nutritional supplements for bariatric surgery patients. Ann Pharmacother. 2008;42(12):1851–8. Epub 2008/11/20.

91. Provenzale D, Reinhold RB, Golner B, Irwin V, Dallal GE, Papathanasopoulos N, et al. Evidence for diminished B12 absorption after gastric bypass: oral supplementation does not prevent low plasma B12 levels in bypass patients. J Am Coll Nutr. 1992;11(1):29–35. Epub 1992/02/01.

92. Aarts EO, van Wageningen B, Janssen IM, Berends FJ. Prevalence of anemia and related deficiencies in the first year following laparoscopic gastric bypass for morbid obesity. J Obes. 2012;2012:193705. Epub 2012/04/24.

93. Rhode BM, Arseneau P, Cooper BA, Katz M, Gilfix BM, MacLean LD. Vitamin B–12 deficiency after gastric surgery for obesity. Am J Clin Nutr. 1996;63(1):103–9. Epub 1996/01/01.

94. Brolin RE, Gorman JH, Gorman RC, Petschenik AJ, Bradley LJ, Kenler HA, et al. Are vitamin B12 and folate deficiency clinically important after roux-en-Y gastric bypass? J Gastrointest Surg. 1998;2(5):436–42. Epub 1998/12/08.

95. Brolin RE, Gorman JH, Gorman RC, Petschenik AJ, Bradley LB, Kenler HA, et al. Prophylactic iron supplementation after Roux-en-Y gastric bypass: a prospective, double-blind, randomized study. Arch Surg. 1998;133(7):740–4. Epub 1998/08/04.

96. Umpierrez GE, Hellman R, Korytkowski MT, Kosiborod M, Maynard GA, Montori VM, et al. Management of hyperglycemia in hospitalized patients in non-critical care setting: an endocrine society clinical practice guideline. J Clin Endocrinol Metab. 2012;97(1):16–38. Epub 2012/01/10.

97. Aberle J, Reining F, Dannheim V, Flitsch J, Klinge A, Mann O. Metformin after bariatric surgery—an acid problem. Exp Clin Endocrinol Diabetes (Off J Ger Soc Endocrinol [and] Ger Diabetes Asso). 2012;120(3):152–3. Epub 2011/09/15.

98. Padwal RS, Gabr RQ, Sharma AM, Langkaas LA, Birch DW, Karmali S, et al. Effect of gastric bypass surgery on the absorption and bioavailability of metformin. Diabetes Care. 2011;34(6):1295–300. Epub 2011/04/12.

99. Still CD, Wood GC, Benotti P, Petrick AT, Gabrielsen J, Strodel WE, et al. Preoperative prediction of type 2 diabetes remission after Roux-en-Y gastric bypass surgery: a retrospective cohort study. Lancet Diabetes Endocrinol. 2013.

100. Houston MC. Abrupt cessation of treatment in hypertension: consideration of clinical features, mechanisms, prevention and management of the discontinuation syndrome. Am Heart J. 1981;102(3 Pt 1):415–30. Epub 1981/09/01.

101. Pischon T, Sharma AM. Use of beta-blockers in obesity hypertension: potential role of weight gain. Obes Rev. 2001;2(4):275–80. Epub 2002/07/18.

102. Heber D, Greenway FL, Kaplan LM, Livingston E, Salvador J, Still C. Endocrine and nutritional management of the post-bariatric surgery patient: an endocrine society clinical practice guideline. J Clin Endocrinol Metabol. 2010;95(11):4823–43. Epub 2010/11/06.

103. Garber CE, Blissmer B, Deschenes MR, Franklin BA, Lamonte MJ, Lee IM, et al. American College of Sports Medicine position stand. Quantity and quality of exercise for developing and maintaining cardiorespiratory, musculoskeletal, and neuromotor fitness in apparently healthy adults: guidance for prescribing exercise. Med Sci Sports Exerc. 2011;43(7):1334–59. Epub 2011/06/23.

104. Guyatt GH, Oxman AD, Ali M, Willan A, McIlroy W, Patterson C. Laboratory diagnosis of iron-deficiency anemia: an overview. J Gen Intern Med. 1992;7(2):145–53. Epub 1992/03/01.

105. Sumner AE, Chin MM, Abrahm JL, Berry GT, Gracely EJ, Allen RH, et al. Elevated meth-ylmalonic acid and total homocysteine levels show high prevalence of vitamin B12 defi-ciency after gastric surgery. Ann Intern Med. 1996;124(5):469–76. Epub 1996/03/01.

106. Chaves LC, Faintuch J, Kahwage S, Alencar Fde A. A cluster of polyneuropathy and Wernicke-Korsakoff syndrome in a bariatric unit. Obes Surg. 2002;12(3):328–34. Epub 2002/06/27.

107. Saltzman E, Philip Karl J. Nutrient deficiencies after gastric bypass surgery. Annu Rev Nutr. 2013;33:183–203. Epub 2013/05/07.

108. Sechi G. Prognosis and therapy of Wernicke's encephalopathy after obesity surgery. Am J Gastroenterol. 2008;103(12):3219. Epub 2008/12/18.

109. Fleischer J, Stein EM, Bessler M, Della Badia M, Restuccia N, Olivero-Rivera L, et al. The decline in hip bone density after gastric bypass surgery is associated with extent of weight loss. J Clin Endocrinol Metab. 2008;93(10):3735–40. Epub 2008/07/24.

110. King JC, Shames DM, Woodhouse LR. Zinc homeostasis in humans. J Nutr. 2000;130(5S Suppl):1360S–6S. Epub 2000/05/10.

111. Salle A, Demarsy D, Poirier AL, Lelievre B, Topart P, Guilloteau G, et al. Zinc defi-ciency: a frequent and underestimated complication after bariatric surgery. Obes Surg. 2010;20(12):1660–70. Epub 2010/08/14.

112. Gasteyger C, Suter M, Gaillard RC, Giusti V. Nutritional deficiencies after Roux-en-Y gas-tric bypass for morbid obesity often cannot be prevented by standard multivitamin supple-mentation. Am J Clin Nutr. 2008;87(5):1128–33. Epub 2008/05/13.

113. Gletsu-Miller N, Broderius M, Frediani JK, Zhao VM, Griffith DP, Davis SS, Jr., et al. Incidence and prevalence of copper deficiency following roux-en-y gastric bypass surgery. Int J Obes (Lond). 2012;36(3):328–35. Epub 2011/08/31.

114. Ruz M, Carrasco F, Rojas P, Codoceo J, Inostroza J, Basfi-fer K, et al. Zinc absorption and zinc status are reduced after Roux-en-Y gastric bypass: a randomized study using 2 supple-ments. Am J Clin Nutr. 2011;94(4):1004–11. Epub 2011/08/26.

115. Jimenez A, Casamitjana R, Flores L, Viaplana J, Corcelles R, Lacy A, et al. Long-term effects of sleeve gastrectomy and Roux-en-Y gastric bypass surgery on type 2 diabetes mellitus in morbidly obese subjects. Ann Surg. 2012;256(6):1023–9. Epub 2012/09/13.

116. Scott WR, Batterham RL. Roux-en-Y gastric bypass and laparoscopic sleeve gastrectomy: understanding weight loss and improvements in type 2 diabetes after bariatric surgery. Am J Physiol Reg Integr Comp Physiol. 2011;301(1):R15–27. Epub 2011/04/09.

117. Sjostrom L, Lindroos AK, Peltonen M, Torgerson J, Bouchard C, Carlsson B, et al. Life-style, diabetes, and cardiovascular risk factors 10 years after bariatric surgery. N Engl J Med. 2004;351(26):2683–93. Epub 2004/12/24.

118. Ahmed AR, Rickards G, Coniglio D, Xia Y, Johnson J, Boss T, et al. Laparoscopic Roux-en-Y gastric bypass and its early effect on blood pressure. Obes Surg. 2009;19(7):845–9. Epub 2008/09/02.

119. Nguyen NT, Varela E, Sabio A, Tran CL, Stamos M, Wilson SE. Resolution of hyperlip-idemia after laparoscopic Roux-en-Y gastric bypass. J Am Coll Surg. 2006;203(1):24–9. Epub 2006/06/27.

120. Brolin RE, Bradley LJ, Wilson AC, Cody RP. Lipid risk profile and weight stability after gastric restrictive operations for morbid obesity. J Gastrointest Surg Off J Soc Surg Aliment Tract. 2000;4(5):464–9. Epub 2000/11/15.

121. Stone NJ, Robinson JG, Lichtenstein AH, Bairey Merz CN, Blum CB, Eckel RH, et al. 2013 ACC/AHA guideline on the treatment of blood cholesterol to reduce atherosclerotic cardiovascular risk in adults: a report of the American College of Cardiology/American Heart Association Task Force on Practice Guidelines. J Am Coll Cardiol. 2014;63(25 Pt):2889–934.

122. Shaffer EA. Bariatric surgery: a promising solution for nonalcoholic steatohepatitis in the very obese. J Clin Gastroenterol. 2006;40(Suppl 1):44–50. Epub 2006/03/17.

123. Furuya CK, Jr., de Oliveira CP, de Mello ES, Faintuch J, Raskovski A, Matsuda M, et al. Effects of bariatric surgery on nonalcoholic fatty liver disease: preliminary findings after 2 years. J Gastroenterol Hepatol. 2007;22(4):510–4. Epub 2007/03/23.

124. Hafeez S, Ahmed MH. Bariatric surgery as potential treatment for nonalcoholic fatty liver disease: a future treatment by choice or by chance? J Obes. 2013;2013:839275. Epub 2013/02/23.

125. Sarkhosh K, Switzer NJ, El-Hadi M, Birch DW, Shi X, Karmali S. The impact of bariatric surgery on obstructive sleep apnea: a systematic review. Obes Surg. 2013;23(3):414–23. Epub 2013/01/10.

126. Ravesloot MJ, Hilgevoord AA, van Wagensveld BA, de Vries N. Assessment of the effect of bariatric surgery on obstructive sleep apnea at two postoperative intervals. Obes Surg. 2013. Epub 2013/07/17.

127. Sawaya RA, Jaffe J, Friedenberg L, Friedenberg FK. Vitamin, mineral, and drug absorption following bariatric surgery. Curr Drug Metab. 2012;13(9):1345–55. Epub 2012/07/04.

128. Santini F, Pinchera A, Marsili A, Ceccarini G, Castagna MG, Valeriano R, et al. Lean body mass is a major determinant of levothyroxine dosage in the treatment of thyroid diseases. J Clin Endocrinol Metab. 2005;90(1):124–7. Epub 2004/10/16.

129. Mallory GN, Macgregor AM, R and CS. The influence of dumping on weight loss after gastric restrictive surgery for morbid obesity. Obes Surg. 1996;6(6):474–8. Epub 1996/12/01.

130. Ukleja A. Dumping syndrome: pathophysiology and treatment. Nutr Clin Pract Off Publ Am Soc Parenter Enter Nutr. 2005;20(5):517–25. Epub 2005/10/07.

131. Service GJ, Thompson GB, Service FJ, Andrews JC, Collazo-Clavell ML, Lloyd RV. Hyperinsulinemic hypoglycemia with nesidioblastosis after gastric-bypass surgery. N Engl J Med. 2005;353(3):249–54. Epub 2005/07/22.

132. Ceppa EP, Ceppa DP, Omotosho PA, Dickerson JA, 2nd, Park CW, Portenier DD. Algorithm to diagnose etiology of hypoglycemia after Roux-en-Y gastric bypass for morbid obesity: case series and review of the literature. Surg Obes Relat Dis. 2012;8(5):641–7. Epub 2011/10/11. (official journal of the American Society for Bariatric Surgery)

133. Machado JD, Campos CS, Lopes Dah Silva C, Marques Suen VM, Barbosa Nonino-Borges C, Dos Santos JE, et al. Intestinal bacterial overgrowth after Roux-en-Y gastric bypass. Obes Surg. 2008;18(1):139–43. Epub 2007/12/18.

134. Lakhani SV, Shah HN, Alexander K, Finelli FC, Kirkpatrick JR, Koch TR. Small intestinal bacterial overgrowth and thiamine deficiency after Roux-en-Y gastric bypass surgery in obese patients. Nutr Res. 2008;28(5):293–8. Epub 2008/12/17.

135. Woodard GA, Encarnacion B, Downey JR, Peraza J, Chong K, Hernandez-Boussard T, et al. Probiotics improve outcomes after Roux-en-Y gastric bypass surgery: a prospective randomized trial. J Gastrointest Surg. 2009;13(7):1198–204. Epub 2009/04/22 (official journal of the Society for Surgery of the Alimentary Tract).

136. Garza E, Jr., Kuhn J, Arnold D, Nicholson W, Reddy S, McCarty T. Internal hernias after laparoscopic Roux-en-Y gastric bypass. Am J Surg. 2004;188(6):796–800. Epub 2004/12/28.

137. Husain S, Ahmed AR, Johnson J, Boss T, O'Malley W. Small-bowel obstruction after laparoscopic Roux-en-Y gastric bypass: etiology, diagnosis, and management. Arch Surg. 2007;142(10):988–93. Epub 2007/10/17.

138. Nagem R, Lazaro-da-Silva A. Cholecystolithiasis after gastric bypass: a clinical, biochemical, and ultrasonographic 3-year follow-up study. Obes Surg. 2012;22(10):1594–9. Epub 2012/07/07.

139. Nagem RG, Lazaro-da-Silva A, de Oliveira RM, Morato VG. Gallstone-related complications after Roux-en-Y gastric bypass: a prospective study. Hepatobiliary Pancreat Dis Int. 2012;11(6):630–5. Epub 2012/12/13. (HBPD INT).

140. Tarantino I, Warschkow R, Steffen T, Bisang P, Schultes B, Thurnheer M. Is routine cholecystectomy justified in severely obese patients undergoing a laparoscopic Roux-en-Y gastric bypass procedure? A comparative cohort study. Obes Surg. 2011;21(12):1870–8. Epub 2011/08/25.

141. Tucker ON, Fajnwaks P, Szomstein S, Rosenthal RJ. Is concomitant cholecystectomy necessary in obese patients undergoing laparoscopic gastric bypass surgery? Surg Endosc. 2008;22(11):2450–4. Epub 2008/02/22.

142. Uy MC, Talingdan-Te MC, Espinosa WZ, Daez ML, Ong JP. Ursodeoxycholic acid in the prevention of gallstone formation after bariatric surgery: a meta-analysis. Obes Surg. 2008;18(12):1532–8. Epub 2008/06/25.

143. Chang CG, Adams-Huet B, Provost DA. Acute post-gastric reduction surgery (APGARS) neuropathy. Obes Surg. 2004;14(2):182–9. Epub 2004/03/17.

144. Odom J, Zalesin KC, Washington TL, Miller WW, Hakmeh B, Zaremba DL, et al. Behavioral predictors of weight regain after bariatric surgery. Obes Surg. 2010;20(3):349–56. Epub 2009/06/26.

145. Fobi MA, Lee H, Igwe D, Jr., Felahy B, James E, Stanczyk M, et al. Revision of failed gastric bypass to distal Roux-en-Y gastric bypass: a review of 65 cases. Obes Surg. 2001;11(2):190–5. Epub 2001/05/17.

146. Carrodeguas L, Szomstein S, Soto F, Whipple O, Simpfendorfer C, Gonzalvo JP, et al. Management of gastrogastric fistulas after divided Roux-en-Y gastric bypass surgery for morbid obesity: analysis of 1,292 consecutive patients and review of literature. Surg Obes Relat Dis. 2005;1(5):467–74. Epub 2006/08/24. (official journal of the American Society for Bariatric Surgery).

147. Faria SL, de Oliveira Kelly E, Lins RD, Faria OP. Nutritional management of weight regain after bariatric surgery. Obes Surg. 2010;20(2):135–9. Epub 2008/06/26.

148. Kakarla N, Dailey C, Marino T, Shikora SA, Chelmow D. Pregnancy after gastric bypass surgery and internal hernia formation. Obstet Gynecol. 2005;105(5 Pt 2):1195–8. Epub 2005/05/03.

149. Abodeely A, Roye GD, Harrington DT, Cioffi WG. Pregnancy outcomes after bariatric surgery: maternal, fetal, and infant implications. Surg Obes Relat Dis. 2008;4(3):464–71. Epub 2007/11/03. (Official journal of the American Society for Bariatric Surgery).

150. Josefsson A, Bladh M, Wirehn AB, Sydsjo G. Risk for congenital malformations in offspring of women who have undergone bariatric surgery. A national cohort. BJOG. 2013. Epub 2013/08/10. (an international journal of obstetrics and gynaecology).

151. Shai D, Shoham-Vardi I, Amsalem D, Silverberg D, Levi I, Sheiner E. Pregnancy outcome of patients following bariatric surgery as compared with obese women: a population-based study. J Matern Fetal Neonatal Med. 2013. Epub 2013/06/19. (the official journal of the European Association of Perinatal Medicine, the Federation of Asia and Oceania Perinatal Societies, the International Society of Perinatal Obstet).

152. Kjaer MM, Lauenborg J, Breum BM, Nilas L. The risk of adverse pregnancy outcome after bariatric surgery: a nationwide register-based matched cohort study. Am J Obstet Gynecol. 2013;208(6):464 e1–5. Epub 2013/03/08.

153. van der Beek ES Te Riele W Specken TF Boerma D van Ramshorst B. The impact of reconstructive procedures following bariatric surgery on patient well-being and quality of life. Obes Surg. 2010;20(1):36–41. Epub 2009/08/19.

154. Modarressi A, Balague N, Huber O, Chilcott M, Pittet-Cuenod B. Plastic surgery after gastric bypass improves long-term quality of life. Obes Surg. 2013;23(1):24–30. Epub 2012/08/28.

155. de Kerviler S Husler R Banic A Constantinescu MA. Body contouring surgery following bariatric surgery and dietetically induced massive weight reduction: a risk analysis. Obes Surg. 2009;19(5):553–9. Epub 2008/08/30.

156. van der Beek ES van der Molen AM van Ramshorst B. Complications after body contouring surgery in post-bariatric patients: the importance of a stable weight close to normal. Obes Facts. 2011;4(1):61–6. Epub 2011/03/05.

Chapter 11
Surgical Complications of Weight Loss Surgery

Margaret E. Clark, Robert B. Lim, Souheil W. Adra and Daniel B. Jones

Introduction

When considering weight loss surgery (WLS), one must consider the potential benefits and risks of an operation. Studies by Wee et al. [1] have shown that many patients considering WLS expect their outcomes will be better than average and that many patients, despite extensive preoperative preparation and counseling, may not fully appreciate their risks of morbidity and mortality. Therefore, it is important that primary care providers (PCPs) consistently and accurately explain what can be achieved from WLS and that ultimate success requires a commitment to lifelong follow-up and lifestyle change. Moreover, the PCP should understand common postoperative complications so they can be diagnosed and managed early and

---

Disclaimer: The views expressed in this chapter are those of the authors and do not reflect the official policy or position of the Department of the Army, Department of Defense, or the US Government.

M. E. Clark (✉)
Department of General Surgery, Tripler Army Medical Center, 1 Jarrett White Rd, Honolulu, HI, 96859 USA
e-mail: margaret.e.clark34.mil@mail.mil

R. B. Lim
Department of Surgery, Tripler Army Medical Center, 1 Jarrett White Road, Honolulu, HI, 96859 USA
e-mail: Robert.b.lim.mil@mail.mil

S. W. Adra
Beth Israel Deaconess Medical Center, Harvard Medical School, Boston, MA, USA

D. B. Jones
Department of Surgery, Harvard Medical School, Beth Israel Deaconess Medical Center, Boston, MA, USA

© Springer Science+Business Media New York 2015   181
A. Youdim (ed.), *The Clinician's Guide to the Treatment of Obesity,*
Endocrine Updates, DOI 10.1007/978-1-4939-2146-1_11

appropriately, especially weight regain. This chapter discusses the complications of WLS that every practicing physician should be aware of.

Patient Selection

Not every patient is an ideal candidate for WLS. Most accredited bariatric programs have a multidisciplinary team including a bariatrician, social worker, nurse educator, psychologist, and a dietician as part of the preoperative assessment. Patients who are smoking tobacco, drinking alcohol, noncompliant or with uncontrolled psychological disorders are often not candidates for surgery. Furthermore, the team assesses whether candidates are prepared to make dietary and lifestyle modifications to maximize their outcomes and avoid preventable complications. Are candidates prepared to stop smoking, avoid nonsteroidal anti-inflammatory drugs (NSAIDS), curb drinking, limit their junk food, be very active in their nutritional choices, and increase their exercise? If a patient is a good candidate, then they should be appropriately counseled, and started on a pathway to successful weight loss.

Patients and PCPs should also be aware that while WLS is generally safe, complications can occur. The sentences should read. In a review from the Michigan Bariatric Surgical Collaborative published in 2011, 2.5% of patients experienced a serious complication. Significant risk factors for such complications included: a prior venous thrombotic event (VTE) with an odds ration (OR) of 1.9, poor functional status (OR=1.61), coronary artery disease (OR=1.53), age over 50 years (OR=1.38), pulmonary disease (OR=1.37), male gender (OR=1.26), smoking history (OR=1.20) and type of procedure, with the Biliopancreatic Diversion-Duodenal Switch (BPD-DS) (OR=9.68) and the open RYGB (OR=3.51) having the highest rates. [2].

It is very important to underline, at this point, that patients undergoing revisional surgery are generally viewed to represent a separate category with an increased risk for complications, especially leaks. Most reports list the rates of morbidity around 30%, with a major morbidity rate around 10%, a leak rate around 3.6%, and the rate of further operations around 8%. As more and more people have WLS, PCPs may see the need for more revisions. The long-term success of these revisions has yet to be determined and there are some surgical reasons that a revision may be needed. These are also discussed later [3–5].

Early Postoperative Complications

Death

Mortality is an uncommon complication after WLS, but must obviously be spoken of, and patients need to know the true risk. For the past 10 years, the Department of Health, insurance companies, and accreditation bodies have kept data on mortality

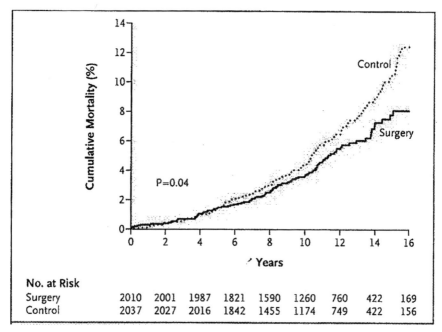

Fig. 11.1 Cumulative mortality for those patients undergoing weight loss surgery is significantly lower than a control group—patients received the customary nonsurgical treatment, ranging from lifestyle intervention and behavior medication to no treatment

after WLS. The mortality rate after the most common surgeries ranges from 0.09 to 1.2%. In 2010, the Bariatric Outcomes Longitudinal Database (BOLD) reported the outcome of almost 58,000 patients and found the 30-day mortality to be 0.09% [6]. AGB patients have the lowest mortality, followed by the SG, the RYGB and then the BPD-DS, which has the highest mortality, reported a 1.2%. [7]. Elderly patients (>65 years) may have mortality greater than 4% depending on their preoperative health status and the procedure selected [8]. No operation should be taken lightly and patients need to be appropriately counseled. That said, several excellent studies, including one published in the New England Journal of Medicine [9], has clearly demonstrated that patients who undergo WLS live much longer than patients who remain obese despite maximal medical therapy. (See Fig. 11.1)

Patients who are 100 pounds overweight and who have had a bariatric operation achieve superior weight loss, are healthier and live longer. It is reasonable for patients with a Body Mass Index (BMI) greater than 40 kg/m^2, or those with a BMI > 35 kg/m^2 with a weight related co-morbidity, or those with a BMI ranging from 30-34.9 kg/m^2 and either Type II Diabetes Mellitus or Dysmetabolic Syndrome X to be offered WLS, as the risk of not having an operation for exceeds the risk of undergoing an operation. The most common causes of death after bariatric surgery are from a pulmonary embolism (PE), sepsis most often due to an anastomotic leak, cardiac events such as a myocardial infarction, and respiratory failure.

Pulmonary Embolism

Obesity is a risk factor for deep venous thrombosis (DVT) and PE. The incidence of symptomatic PEs ranges from 0 to 5.4% [10]. Fifty percent of deaths in the perioperative period are caused by PE, making it the most common cause of death. The overall rate of in-hospital venous thrombotic event (VTE) was 0.17% with the highest rate observed in an open RYGB at 0.45%. [11]. While there is no standard for VTE prophylaxis perioperatively, many surgeons will use both chemoprophylaxis and mechanical prophylaxis via sequential compression devices (SCDs). Bariatric surgery candidates who are nonambulatory, have a history of venous stasis disorders, use hormonal therapy, have obesity hypoventilation syndrome, or have pulmonary hypertension are considered an even higher risk. Chemoprophylaxis is often given to these higher-risk patients for a longer duration like 3-6 weeks post operatively. Enoxaparin for a longer duration is often given to these higher-risk patients. In 2013, the American Society for Metabolic and Bariatric Surgery (ASMBS) published an updated position statement recommending perioperative VTE prophylaxis, but did not recommend a standardized dosing protocol [10]. There is support to use a combination of chemoprophylaxis and mechanical prophylaxis (SCDs), and though enoxaparin or heparin may be used, the highest-quality data suggest the use of enoxaparin.

Use of filters is controversial as the potential complications of inferior vena cava (IVC) filters are not insignificant and insertion and removal in super-obese patients may prove to be technically challenging for an interventionalist. A prospective clinical registry involving 20 Michigan hospitals accrued 6376 patients undergoing gastric bypass surgery between 2006 and 2008 [12]. IVC filter placement and complications within 30 days of surgery were analyzed in 542 gastric bypass patients (8.5%) who underwent preoperative IVC filter placement. In patients with IVC filters, they noticed an *increased* rates of postoperative VTE (1.7 vs. 0.5% $p=0.001$), death (1.0 vs. 0.2% $p=0.01$), and any complications (16.3 vs. 9.5% $p<0.001$). These complications included IVC thrombosis, filter migration, and embolization. Furthermore, the authors were unable to identify any patient subgroup for whom IVC filters were associated with improved outcomes.

Anastomotic Leaks

Leaks are the most dreaded complication and one of the most common causes of postoperative mortality.

During the operation, surgeons will inspect all staple lines, and may also inject methytlene blue saline, perform air insufflation, or perform endoscopy to assess for a leak. After an RYGB, a leak may occur at the gastrojejunostomy (GJ) (Fig. 11.2), jejunojejunostomy (JJ), or the staple line of the remnant stomach. A contrast swallow study might identify a leak at the GJ but miss other locations, and is unreliable for excluding a leak. Performing a computed tomography (CT) scan with oral

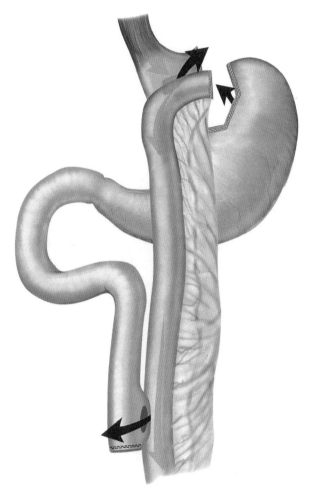

Fig. 11.2 Sites of potential leaks at the GJ, remnant stomach, and JJ; depicted by *blue arrows*. *GJ* gastojejunostomy, *JJ* jejunojejunostomy

contrast might identify free air, a fluid collection or extravasation of contrast. Early diagnosis is imperative. Tachycardia and respiratory compromise are early signs of a leak, signs that are present before hypotension, decreased urinary output, and abdominal pain. Another reported sign is a patient who has a "feeling of doom" [13]. Patients presenting postoperatively with shortness of breath are statistically more likely to have a leak than PE, and the surgeon should be promptly notified as a leak usually requires prompt return to the operating room for exploration. In the immediate postoperative period, an unexplained heart rate of greater than 120 beats/ min is a leak until proven otherwise, which might require reoperation, drains, and a gastric feeding tube. Delay in treatment is a common cause of death. Re-exploration would be warranted if an MI, PE, bleeding, atelectasis, hypovolemia, and pain (all potential causes of a postoperative tachycardia) are ruled out or treated and the patient remains tachycardic. A CT scan or swallow study may not be reliable to detect a small leak, leaving re-exploration as the only option for detection.

Leaks and perforations can also occur with an AGB, an SG, and a BPD-DS. With an SG and BPD-DS, a leak along the resected stomach can be very problematic as the narrow sleeve is a high-pressure zone. Once a leak is present, it tends to persist. This may be the reason, along with the long staple line, that the leak rate after an SG is the highest, up to 10 % [14], double the rate of leak after RYGB [6, 15]. While drainage alone may work to close the leak, sometimes an endoscopically placed stent or clip is required. If a leak after SG is associated with a distal obstruction, conversion to gastric bypass may be required to turn a high-pressure leak into a lower-pressure leak, thus giving the patient a better chance of healing.

Leaks can occur several weeks after the operation and providers must have a high index of suspicion for them so that they can attempt to diagnose them early. It is generally safer to reoperate to rule out a leak rather than allow it to become clinically obvious. By that time, the patient may already be suffering pulmonary, cardiac, and septic complications. Unfortunately, the diagnosis and management of intra-abdominal infections are more challenging in a morbidly obese patient, so a high index of suspicion is always warranted.

Cardiac Complications

Cardiac ischemic events are the second most common cause of perioperative death in bariatric surgery patients [16] accounting for 12.5–17.6 % of cases [17]. That said, cardiac events occur in <1 % of patients undergoing bariatric surgery [15]. Cardiovascular complications in the postoperative period decrease over time [18]. As many obese patients often have several comorbidities related to cardiac disease, a preoperative risk assessment should be considered in every patient.

Other Respiratory Complications

Bariatric surgery patients also have a spectrum of respiratory obstructive and restrictive pulmonary physiologies. Atelectasis is a common occurrence after WLS occurring in 8.4 % of patients [19]. In patients with obstructive sleep apnea (OSA), noninvasive ventilation was found to improve the lung function if started within 30 min after extubation in the recovery room [20]. Many patients seeking WLS will have OSA [21]. Patients who are untreated and chronically tired will gain weight. Furthermore, sedation and narcotics after surgery place the patient at high risk for respiratory compromise and death postoperatively. An OSA diagnosis should be actively sought prior to surgery and treated with continuous positive airway pressure (CPAP) if only to get patients comfortable using a mask they will require after the operation. WLS patients with OSA should continue to use their CPAP postoperatively, even on the first postoperative night.

Using the National Surgical Quality Improvement Program (NSQIP) database, the data for 32,889 patients between 2006 and 2008, were analyzed by Gupta et al. [22]. Postoperative pneumonia and postoperative respiratory failure accounted for mortality in 18.7% of cases. Length of stay in hospital and 30-day mortality are increased in those patients who develop postoperative pneumonia or respiratory failure. Preoperative risk factors for postoperative pneumonia were congestive heart failure (OR 5.3) and stroke (OR 4.1), as well as bleeding disorder, age > 50, chronic obstructive pulmonary disease, type of surgery, diabetes mellitus, anesthesia time, increasing weight, and smoking. Previous percutaneous coronary intervention (OR 2.8) and dyspnea at rest (OR 2.64) were the factors most strongly associated with postoperative respiratory failure. As such, all WLS candidates with these risk factors should have pulmonary function tests to evaluate their risk of postoperative pulmonary complications.

Chronic pulmonary complications may include recurrent aspiration pneumonia secondary to chronic reflux or vomiting. This could be seen with patients with stomal obstruction or stenosis [23], especially in patients with AGBs where a recent study reports a chronic respiratory complication rate of 1.4% [24].

Stenosis or Outlet Obstruction

Stenosis or an anastomotic stricture usually presents as vomiting, or the inability to tolerate oral intake. The stenosis may be severe enough that the patient cannot swallow his or her own secretions and saliva. This complication typically occurs in the first few months after the operation, with a median presentation at 46 days [25]. Strictures occurred significantly more frequently when a 21-mm versus a 25-mm circular stapler was used for the GJ anastomosis for an RYGB [25, 26]. The size of the stapler is one technical factor in the development of a stricture, as is tension on the anastomosis, or ischemia. Another factor is the patient and his or her ability to heal. The primary treatment for stricture is endoscopic balloon dilation, and sometimes more than one dilation may be required [25]. However, caution needs to be used with dilation as perforation or bleeding are two potential complications. Balloon dilation of the anastomosis should only be performed in experienced hands, with the bariatric surgeon who is knowledgeable and experienced in endoscopy— the best provider to treat a stricture. Repeat dilation may result in swelling of the anastomosis and make future dilations more difficult, and repeat dilations make operative intervention more likely [13]. It is recommended that within the first 3 weeks postoperatively dilation should not be performed, and instead the patient should be kept on a liquid diet, or even total parenteral nutrition if they cannot tolerate enough per os (PO) nutrition. However, if dilation is going to be performed in those few weeks a smaller balloon and lower pressure should be used [25].

Patients who have undergone an SG may also present with vomiting, dysphagia, and an inability to tolerate PO, due to narrowing and gastric outlet obstruction. This complication has been reported to occur in 0.7% of patients [27]. The ideal bougie size for construction of the sleeve has yet to be determined, currently ranging from 32 to 40 fr, and many surgeons currently use a 36-fr bougie [13]. Too small of a size may lead to narrowing and obstruction, but too large of a size may result in less weight loss. Treatment for these patients is also endoscopic dilation, unless the segment of narrowing is too long, in which case they may need repeat surgery and conversion to an RYGB.

Patients who have had an AGB may present with acute obstruction in the early period. This is usually due to bleeding underneath the band, or failure to remove the esophageal fat pad. In general, this can be managed by waiting for the edema to resolve after a few days or by surgical intervention to remove the hematoma or fat pad [28].

Late Postoperative Complications

Failure to Achieve Weight Loss or Weight Regain

Most patients lose weight after weight loss operations. In general, AGB patients can lose 30–70% excess weight loss (EWL) or 30–70 pounds of every hundred pounds above the ideal body weight (IBW). O'Brien et al. [29] showed a 47% EWL even out to 15 years after AGB (Fig. 11.3). After SG, patients typically lose more than 60% EWL [30], after RYGB 60–70% EWL [7, 31], and even more after BPD-DS. While there are metabolic, social, and behavioral reasons for failure to lose weight or to have weight regain, technical complications need to be considered.

After AGB, if the patient is eating high-calorie liquid foods such as ice cream and alcohol, they will not have appropriate postoperative weight loss, and may even continue to gain weight. These foods pass the band easily and can counter any weight loss efforts made by the patient. Alternatively, the band may not be achieving adequate restriction because it is not properly adjusted or because there is a leak in the tubing. If the band is not adequately restrictive then satiety is not achieved and larger portions of food are consumed. Using a Huber needle, the port can be accessed and the physician can determine the volume of fluid within the system and instill additional fluid into the band. If less fluid is withdrawn than expected, a leak may be present and the port or the band may need to be replaced. A leak may be due to fractured tubing, or at other times a slow leak can occur from a previous needle puncture. Overall, the band has a reoperation rate of up to 40% for complications such as leaks, band slips, band erosions, or failure to lose or sustain weight loss [29].

Even after a SG, a RYGB or a BPD-DS, patients may regain weight. Types of food eaten, amount of alcohol consumed, increasing portions or frequency of meals, decreasing exercise, and stress as it relates to eating and exercise should all be assessed by the PCP. It is important to encourage patients to have lifelong follow-up, and it is helpful for the patient to be monitored by registered dietitians, psychologists, bariatricians, and the operating surgeon. Having this lifelong follow-up can help prevent weight recidivism and also assist with identification of postoperative complications. The lowest weight on average is obtained 18 months after RYGB

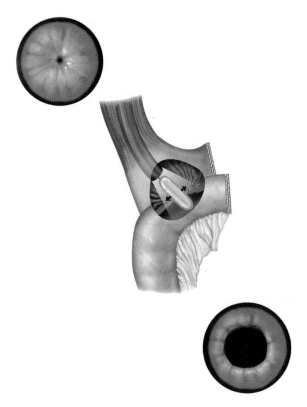

Fig. 11.3 Average weight loss over 15 years in surgery subgroups and controls not obtaining (no prof) or obtaining (prof) professional help

with weight regain becoming significant within 4 years after surgery [31]. A contrast study may be helpful to exclude a fistula from the pouch to the remnant stomach after RYGB or vertical banded gastroplasty, as a technical reason why patients may be able to eat much larger quantities of food than immediately after surgery. Of course, the stomach can also be stretched over time, but efforts to downsize the pouch have had poor results at achieving weight loss after postoperative weight gain. It remains to be seen if the SG results in sustained weight loss for more than 10 years. The overwhelming reason for weight regain after any operation is a failure to consistently live a healthy lifestyle that is conducive to sustained weight loss.

Too Much Weight Loss

This, too, can happen albeit infrequently. While anorexia and bulimic behaviors may be the cause, technical complications can also cause EWL. It can be very helpful to have a dietitian review the patient's food logs to help ensure they are getting adequate calorie intake. An AGB that is too tight and too restrictive may be easily corrected by withdrawing fluid from the band. Similarly, stenosis or obstruction that can occur after SG, RYGB, and BPD-DS can also cause excessive weight loss. An upper gastrointestinal (GI) series and a small bowel follow through or CT scan can also inform the surgeon if there is a stenosis or obstruction. Typically, weight loss will stop after a couple years as patients become accustomed to the restriction and instead begin to eat more often. The malabsorption component may also be overcome with time, though it is uncertain how much remains long term.

Persistent Vomiting

Vomiting can occur from eating too fast or too large of a portion, and all patients should be instructed to measure their portions, eat small bites, chew well, and eat slowly. If vomiting persists, something is wrong, and if left unaddressed can cause significant nutritional deficiencies. After an AGB, the band may be too tight and simply need to be adjusted. If this does not resolve the patient's nausea and vomiting, then the physician needs to consider that there is a prolapse, whereby the stomach below the band slides above the band, often obstructing the stoma and sometimes becoming a surgical emergency if the gastric blood supply is compromised. This can be diagnosed with an upper GI series or a CT scan and if it occurs, requires an operation to remove or replace the band.

After an SG, vomiting might occur if the sleeve has strictured, twisted, or was too narrow to begin with. This can be easily assessed by an upper GI series study by noting slow movement of contrast, or failure of contrast to progress. This can be treated with stenting or balloon dilation (Fig. 11.4) but may also require a revision to an RYGB.

After an RYGB or a BPD-DS, vomiting may occur if there is a stenosis of the GJ anastomosis. Often endoscopic dilation(s) can manage this complication, as mentioned earlier. The patient may first present with difficulty swallowing solid foods and then not be able to tolerate liquids as the anastomosis further narrows. Persistent vomiting again may rapidly cause a thiamine deficiency and requires supplementation. Thiamine levels should be checked and a thorough neurologic exam should be done if the patient endorses continued emesis. Other causes of vomiting may be a small bowel obstruction, from either adhesions or a hernia.

Abdominal Pain

Abdominal pain in a bariatric patient needs to be taken seriously, as they have not only the usual adult causes of abdominal pain but the cause of their abdominal pain may be due to a specific complication of their surgery as well. Abdominal pain may be difficult at times to diagnose in a bariatric patient given their rerouted anatomy, as well as the fact that these patients often have vague symptoms and an unreliable physical examination given their habitus. Unfortunately, sometimes bariatric

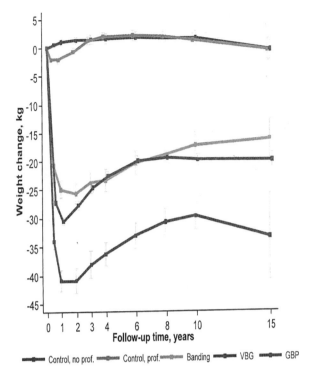

Fig. 11.4 Stenosis of the GJ, before and after treatment with balloon dilation. *GJ* gastojejunostomy

patients continue to have abdominal pain of unknown origin, even after extensive workup for defined causes.

Hernias

Hernias can occur at sites of previous incisions. Small port-site hernias may be difficult to diagnose without a CT scan and can cause significant pain for a patient. Hernias are more common with larger incisions such as laparotomy (open operation) or single incision laparoscopic surgery (SILS) whose smaller incisions can be up to 3–4 cm. A midline laparotomy in an obese patient has a 20–41 % chance of hernia development [32]. Port-site hernias should be repaired promptly given that the small size makes incarceration or strangulation more likely, whereas large incisional hernias may be best to delay repair until weight loss is achieved. This will lower the rate of a recurrent hernia. Mesh should be used during a definitive repair as it is more durable than sutures alone.

Another type of a hernia that often presents as abdominal pain is an internal hernia. When a retrocolic Roux limb is created, the Roux limb travels behind the colon up to the stomach pouch; and consequently, three potential spaces are created.

They are the opening of the transverse mesocolon that allows passage of the Roux limb, the space beneath the Roux limb but above the transverse mesocolon, also known as the Peterson's Defect, and the mesenteric defect of the J-J anastomosis. These defects must be closed with sutures, otherwise the openings in the mesentery allow the small bowel to herniate through the defect and cause a small bowel obstruction and pain. Additionally, after significant weight loss, the sutures that were used to close the potential hernia defects may loosen causing an internal hernia.

Patients may present with intermittent severe mid-abdominal pain. A CT scan should be obtained and may identify a "swirl sign." However, the hernia may not be visualized with a CT scan, especially if the hernia is self-reduced at the time of imaging. If after an extensive workup there is no other cause of abdominal pain, a surgeon may elect to explore in the operating room, as this is the definite way to determine if there is a hernia. As with any hernia, if the small bowel blood supply is compromised, the bowel can become ischemic and require emergent resection. Thus, an internal hernia can become a surgical emergency.

Marginal Ulcers

Another cause of abdominal pain may be an ulcer. Marginal ulcers usually are distal to the GJ anastomosis and result from gastric acid irritating the mucosa of the jejunum. Some surgeons will test all patients for *Helicobacter pylori* prior to surgery, and treat if positive. Schirmer et al. [33] found that 30.1 % of patients tested had *H. pylori*. They were treated and subsequently had a lower incidence of marginal ulcers, 2.4 versus 6.8 %. Ulcers can present with not only pain but also nausea, bleeding, or even perforation. Smoking, NSAIDs, and foreign bodies, such as sutures or staples, have both been linked to development of marginal ulcers. Patients can also have ulcers appear in their remnant stomach and duodenum. They may also present with pain, bleeding, or even perforation. At most institutions, patients are put on an H2-receptor blocker or proton-pump inhibitor postoperatively for a few weeks to months after an RYGB.

Obstruction

Obstruction has been said to occur on average from 0.3 to 7 months postoperatively, but Capella et al. [34] saw the majority of obstructions occurring between 6 and 24 months, and they may continue to occur years after surgery. Early obstructions occur within 6 weeks after the operation and are likely due to technical issues resulting in the internal hernias described above (Fig. 11.5). Adhesions are another potential cause of a small bowel obstruction. The incidence of obstruction after laparoscopic RYGB ranges anywhere from 0.2 to 9.7 % [13, 34]. Almost 20 % of patients who presented with obstruction had a second obstruction [34]. Patients who appear to have an obstruction caused by an adhesion may be given a trial of naso-

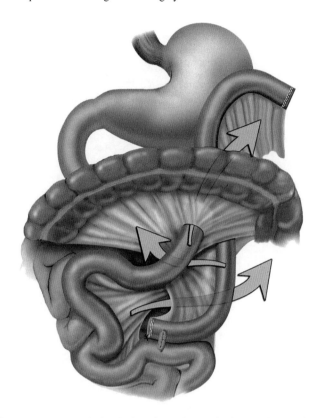

Fig. 11.5 Three *green arrows* depict the locations of potential internal hernias in a post-RYGB patient, often presenting as abdominal pain. *RYGB* Roux-en-Y gastric bypass

gastric decompression, but the nasogastric tube placement needs to be performed by an experienced provider and there should be consideration of placing it under fluoroscopic guidance due to the risk of perforation of the small gastric pouch which could be catastrophic [13]. Intussusception, though a rare cause of small bowel obstruction, may also present as with pain, nausea, and vomiting. Intussusception accounts for approximately 1 % of cases of small bowel obstruction [35]. This complication may develop several years after a RYGB and those patients who have lost more than 90 % EBW are at the highest risk [13, 35]. Intussusception that involves the JJ anastomosis should have the JJ anastomosis revised surgically. Although rare, intussusception needs to be considered given that it can lead to bowel ischemia and necrosis, and CT scan only has an accuracy of approximately 80 % in identifying this complication [36] and a normal scan does not rule out this diagnosis, as it also does not rule out an internal hernia.

Cholelithiasis

Weight loss increases a patient's risk of developing gallstones, and cholecystitis or cholelithiasis may be a cause of the patient's abdominal pain. The risk of symptomatic cholelithiasis after RYGB or SG is approximately 6% [37]. After gastric bypass, endoscopic retrograde cholangiopancreatography (ERCP) may not be possible given that the bowel is rerouted, so many surgeons have opted to perform a cholecystectomy at the time of the RYGB or BPD-DS. If the gallbladder is not removed, postoperative ursodiol given for 6 months after surgery can reduce the incidence to approximately 2% [32]. If the gallbladder has been removed, then other causes of right upper quadrant (RUQ) pain, like sphincter of Oddi dysfunction should be considered.

Malnutrition

Many patients who are obese are malnourished preoperatively (Table 11.1). Young women may need iron, and older women may need calcium supplements. B12 is another common deficiency in this population. Therefore, a nutritionist will usually assess all patients prior to a WLS. Patients are also educated about vitamin and mineral deficiencies that may occur after WLS such as B12, iron, calcium/vitamin D, folate, thiamine, vitamin A/E/K, copper, and zinc. Rate of weight loss and protein intake are also followed postoperatively as protein deficiency may be another complication of WLS if a patient is not compliant in ensuring proper intake. Sixty grams a day is recommended.

Many of the nutritional deficiencies can present as neurological problems, and those with thiamine deficiency can actually develop neurologic defects that are irreversible. Other neurologic presentations that need to be evaluated for nutritional deficiency include Wernicke–Korsakoff, paresthesias, peripheral neuropathies, ataxia, memory loss, and vision impairment. Wernicke encephalopathy and polyneuropathy caused by a thiamine deficiency most commonly present 2–3 months after surgery and most patients present with persistent vomiting [38]. If a WLS patient becomes an alcoholic postoperatively, then there needs to be an increased concern that they will develop a thiamine deficiency. Again, thiamine deficiencies should be suspected in patients with persistent vomiting and should be aggressively replenished, as a continued deficit can lead to permanent neurologic damage.

Other nutritional deficits may present as hypoglycemia or secondary hyperparathyroidism as well. If a patient presents with fractures, calcium levels should be checked. Hypocalcemia is a concern given that calcium is absorbed in the duodenum and proximal jejunum, making post-RYGB and BPD-DS patients at an increased risk.

A copper deficiency can also present with neurological complaints, often similarly to a B12 deficiency. Absorption of copper occurs in the stomach and proximal duodenum, so WLS patients are at an increased risk. Zinc supplementation can also

Table 11.1 Nutritional deficits, presentation, and recommended supplementation

Vitamin B12/folate	Weakness and fatigue (anemia), paresthesias, peripheral neuropathy-B12 not folate	B12- 350 µg/day Folate-400 µg/day
Iron	Weakness and fatigue (anemia), impaired thermoregulation, immune dysfunction, gastrointestinal disturbances, cognitive impairment, pica	650 mg/day—oral ferrous sulfate Vitamin C promotes absorption
Vitamin B1/thiamine	Wernicke–Korsakoff–ataxia, ophthalmoplegia, nystagmus, confusion	50–100 mg up to 3x/day
Calcium/vitamin D	Myalgias, arthralgias, weakness, fatigue	Calcium: 1.2–1.5 g/day Ergocalciferol:400 IU/day
Other fat-soluble vitamins: A,E, K	Vitamin A: night blindness	Without corneal changes:10,000–25,000 IU/day PO With corneal changes: 50,000–100,000 IU/day for 3 days IM
Zinc	Alopecia	MVI w/ zinc
Copper	Anemia, ataxia, optic neuropathy	1st week: 6 mg/day 2nd week: 4 mg/day followed by 2 mg/day
Protein	Excessive weight loss, diarrhea, marasmus	Total parenteral nutrition

IU International unit, *MVI w/zinc* multivitamin with zinc

prevent the absorption of copper as zinc competes with copper on the binding site of the same protein [39]. Iron deficiency is also common as it is absorbed in the duodenum and proximal jejunum, as well as the need for HCl to convert to Fe^{2+}. This deficiency occurs in 14–52 % of patients [40], and should especially be suspected in females of reproductive age.

Usually, vitamin deficiencies can usually be avoided with supplements but can occur even with supplementation. However, patients after RYGB and even more so after BPD-DS can get into trouble if they are not monitored closely and are not compliant with their supplements. Listed in Table 11.1 are the vitamin deficiencies, presentation, and recommended supplementation. Along with prescribing supplementations, patient's home medications should be adjusted, as RYGB and BPD-DS patients may not properly absorb sustained release, extended release, or enteric-coated medications.

For patients that present with malnutrition, simple oral replenishment is enough. If that fails or if the patient has difficulty maintaining a good nutritional status, then intravenous supplementation or even total parenteral nutrition can be given.

Dumping Syndrome

After gastric bypass, the bowel is rerouted such that a patient may experience cramps and diarrhea after eating simple sugars. Clinically significant dumping syndrome occurs in approximately 10% of patients [41]. Dumping syndrome can occur after RYGB and BPD-DS, but not after AGB and rarely after SG. There are two versions of dumping syndrome: early and late. Early dumping occurs 15–30 min after a meal. These patients endorse diarrhea, bloating, dizziness, nausea, flushing, and a rapid heart rate. The cause is thought to be how quickly hyperosmotic foods are introduced into the jejunum, due to the bypass of the rest of the stomach and ileum. The jejunum gets distended and has increased contractility along with increased intestinal fluids. Patients are at risk of becoming hypovolemic. Treatment is dietary change, to avoid sweet, acidic, or nutrient-rich drinks such as Gatorade. Patients should instead eat complex carbohydrates, high-fiber, and protein-rich foods, no different than what every bariatric patient should eat. Usually, early dumping is self-limited and will resolve in 7–12 weeks as the body adjusts to its postoperative state [41].

Late dumping occurs 2–3 h after a meal and is due to glucose absorption causing hyperglycemia, the release of glucagon-like peptide-1 (GLP-1) and gastric inhibitory polypeptide (GIP). This subsequently leads to an increased insulin response, hypoglycemia, and hypokalemia [41]. These patients present with diaphoresis, weakness, dizziness, and fatigue; they should make the same dietary modifications. Consultation with an endocrinologist may help to make the diagnosis and α-glucosidase inhibitors or somatostatin analogues may help to control the symptoms.

Hypoglycemia

Rarely after gastric bypass, a patient's sugar levels may drop causing another dumping-related complication that leads to symptoms of hypoglycemia, weakness, and even syncope. This can occur several years after surgery. This form of hypoglycemia is a hyperinsulinemic hypoglycemia which occurs due to pancreatic beta cell hypertrophy. This complication is also referred to as nesidioblastosis and if suspected an endocrinologist should be involved in the patient's care. Patients are advised to avoid sweets and eat more frequent small meals. Diet should be the first modification and works in approximately 50% of cases, but if patients continue to have symptoms then medical management can be tried, such as α-glucosidase inhibitors, such as acarbose and miglitol, that inhibit glucose absorption in the intestines. If all medications fail and a patient continues to have episodes of syncope, then a subtotal pancreatectomy to remove the hypertrophied beta cells may be considered. Increasing the restriction of the gastric pouch by revision or placement of a band in order to limit glucose intake has also been described for severe cases [13].

Psychiatric Complications

Alcoholism

Recent data show that gastric bypass patients are at increased risk for alcohol use disorders, especially in their second postoperative year [42]. Alcohol is quickly absorbed in the Roux limb, and after even a single glass of wine, the patient's blood alcohol level may exceed the legal limit. One in eight patients report consuming a least three drinks per typical drinking day, and one in six report "consumption at a hazardous level." [42] For all weight loss operations, alcohol can be a high source of calories and impede weight loss efforts or lead to weight regain. A high index of suspicion should be present to detect those patients and refer them for treatment of their alcohol use disorders.

Depression, Abuse, and Suicide

The psychological effects of WLS are as important as the physical and metabolic results. Obese patients have a high risk of psychiatric disorders, rates of 21–56 % axis I disorder, 22–32 % mood disorder, 20–29 % avoidant personality, and 15–24 % anxiety disorder [43]. Both axis I and axis II disorders have shown a significant reduction after WLS, but the patients with higher levels of shame preoperatively were at a significant increased risk of having a psychiatric disorder postoperatively [43].

While most patients are thrilled to lose weight, especially as their comorbid weight-related conditions go into remission, some patients can become more depressed. While the etiology of depression 6 months after gastric bypass is likely multifactorial, health-care providers should be mindful that while patients are getting thinner and healthier, depression may arise and need to be addressed. Bariatric patients are at increased risk for suicide postoperatively and should be screened during their follow-up visits. Sixty eight percent of suicides occur by 3 years postoperatively with possible etiologies being attributed to weight regain, especially at the time where close follow-up decreases [44]. Another etiology is undiagnosed or untreated preoperative psychological disorders.

Preoperatively, sexual abuse should also be screened for, as this abuse may be associated with poorer weight loss outcomes [45]. Alcohol addiction, psychiatric comorbidities, and low-income status are all associated with sexual abuse. Those patients with a history of sexual abuse are at a 40–60 % increased risk of having a BMI >35, and of those patients seeking bariatric care, a higher percentage have a reported history of abuse than the general population [45]. This is important to determine preoperatively, as identifying these patients may improve their chance of success by enabling counseling and other treatments to be given either prior to or after their WLS.

Posttraumatic stress disorder (PTSD) does not seem to affect weight loss after surgery, as veterans with PTSD were shown to have comparable weight loss to a control group without PTSD [46]. However, an advantage to screening for PTSD is that there is a significant association between PTSD and depression, as well as PTSD and other axis I disorders.

Excess Skin

If the patient is successful at weight loss, there may be excess skin in the arms, back, thighs, and abdomen. Sometimes skin breakdown and ulcers occur in the skin folds. While spandex, smaller bras and bigger cups, and form-fitting clothes can be helpful, many patients will desire body contouring operations. Unfortunately, many insurance companies do not cover these operations, and patients should be counseled prior to WLS that if they desire body contouring they will likely be paying out of pocket. Removal of this excess may assist with the patient's emotional well-being after WLS.

Indications for Reoperation

As stated before, many WLS patients may require a revision. Revision WLS has a higher complication rate and can be very difficult to perform. The most common indication for this is weight regain. While poor lifestyle choice is the most common reason for weight regain, there are some surgical reasons why a surgery may have failed to sustain significant weight loss. Still PCPs and patients should note that no matter what surgery is done or revised, without a proper diet, exercise plan and lifestyle, it is likely to fail. Revisions for failed weight loss should only be considered in patients who have be reevaluated by the entire weight loss team to help identify the barriers that led to weight regain and the inability to lose significant weight the first time.

One surgical reason that may lead to weight regain is the development of a fistula between the gastric pouch and the gastric remnant after an RYGB. Not only does this allow more food intake but the duodenum is no longer bypassed which may lead to a reversal of the hormonal changes that assisted in weight loss. Finally, the absorption of a patient with a gastro-gastric fistula (GGF) may be normal since food will go through the distal stomach, duodenum, and proximal jejunum. GGFs are also associated with marginal ulcers because the fistula allows the acid of the distal stomach to reflux and irritate the GJ anastomosis [47]. The marginal ulcer is not likely to heal completely without correction of the fistula.

Extreme malnutrition is another reason to consider a revision. If RYGB and BPD-DS patients fail intravenous replenishment then another option would be to reverse or shorten the length of the bypassing limb. This would provide more surface area in order to absorb the required nutrients.

Conclusion

Despite many potential complications, bariatric surgery remains a good option for weight loss and has been reported to be the most reliable way to achieve sustained weight loss [48]. Bariatric surgery also continues to show major impact in resolving comorbidities, especially type 2 diabetes [49]. WLS has been shown to correct hypertension and hyperlipidemia, along with reducing the chance of myocardial infarction, stroke, and cardiovascular-related deaths [18]. These health benefits have been shown to be independent of the amount of weight loss a patient achieves. It is important for any PCP to know the short- and long-term complications of WLS in order to properly diagnose and manage any and all complications a patient may encounter. All bariatric patients need to have lifelong care to include continued nutritional management and assistance in maintaining lifelong weight loss and a healthier lifestyle. Many of the complications can be prevented or discovered in a more timely fashion with proper follow-up.

References

1. Wee CC, Hamel MB, Apovian CM, et al. Expectations for weight loss and willingness to accept risk among patients seeking weight loss surgery. JAMA Surg. 2013;148:264–71.
2. Finks JF, Kole KL, Yenumula PR, et al. Predicting risk for serious complications with bariatric surgery: results from the michigan bariatric surgery collaborative. Ann Surg. 2011;254:633–40.
3. Fronza JS, Prystowsky JB, Hungness ES, Nagle AP. Revisional bariatric surgery at a single institution. Am J Surg. 2010;200:651–4.
4. Victorzon M. Revisional bariatric surgery by conversion to gastric bypass or sleeve—good short-term outcomes at higher risks. Obes Surg. 2012;22:29–33.
5. Hedberg J, Gustavsson S, Sundbom M. Long-term follow-up in patients undergoing open gastric bypass as a revisional operation for previous failed restrictive procedures. Surg Obes Relat Dis. 2012;8:696–701.
6. DeMaria EJ, Pate V, Warthen M, Winegar DA. Baseline data from American Society for Metabolic and Bariatric Surgery-designated Bariatric Surgery centers of excellence using the Bariatric outcomes longitudinal database. Surg Obes Relat Dis. 2010;6:347–55.
7. Nelson DW, Blair KS, Martin MJ. Analysis of obesity-related outcomes and bariatric failure rates with the duodenal switch vs gastric bypass for morbid obesity. Arch Surg. 2012;147:847–54.
8. Flum DR, Salem L, Elrod JA, et al. Early mortality among Medicare beneficiaries undergoing bariatric surgical procedures. JAMA. 2005;294:1903–8.
9. Sjostrom L, Narbro K, Sjostrom CD, et al. Effects of bariatric surgery on mortality in Swedish obese subjects. N Engl J Med. 2007;357:741–52.

10. American Society for Metabolic and Bariatric Surgery Clinical Issues Committee. ASMBS updated position statement on prophylactic measures to reduce the risk of venous thromboembolism in bariatric surgery patients. Surg Obes Relat Dis. 2013;9:493–7.

11. Masoomi H, Buchberg B, Reavis KM, et al. Factors predictive of venous thromboembolism in bariatric surgery. Am Surg. 2011;77:1403–6.

12. Birkmeyer NJ, Share D, Baser O, et al. Preoperative placement of inferior vena cava filters and outcomes after gastric bypass surgery. Ann Surg. 2010;252:313–8.

13. Lim RB, Blackburn GL, Jones DB. Benchmarking best practices in weight loss surgery. Curr Probl Surg. 2010;47:79–174.

14. Deitel M, Gagner M, Erickson AL, Crosby RD. Third international summit: current status of sleeve gastrectomy. Surg Obes Relat Dis. 2011;7:749–59.

15. Schneider BE, Villegas L, Blackburn GL, et al. Laparoscopic gastric bypass surgery: outcomes. J Laparoendosc Adv Surg Tech A. 2003;13:247–55.

16. Gagner M, Milone L, Yung E, et al. Causes of early mortality after laparoscopic adjustable gastric banding. J Am Coll Surg. 2008;206:664–9.

17. Morino M, Toppino M, Forestieri P, et al. Mortality after bariatric surgery: analysis of 13,871 morbidly obese patients from a national registry. Ann Surg. 2007;246:1002–7 (discussion 1007–9).

18. Sjostrom L, Peltonen M, Jacobson P, et al. Bariatric surgery and long-term cardiovascular events. JAMA. 2012;307:56–65.

19. Escalante-Tattersfield T, Tucker O, Fajnwaks P, et al. Incidence of deep vein thrombosis in morbidly obese patients undergoing laparoscopic Roux-en-Y gastric bypass. Surg Obes Relat Dis. 2008;4:126–30.

20. Neligan PJ, Malhotra G, Fraser M, et al. Noninvasive ventilation immediately after extubation improves lung function in morbidly obese patients with obstructive sleep apnea undergoing laparoscopic bariatric surgery. Anesth Analg. 2010;110:1360–5.

21. Dixon JB, Schachter LM, O'Brien PE, et al. Surgical vs conventional therapy for weight loss treatment of obstructive sleep apnea: a randomized controlled trial. JAMA. 2012;308:1142–9.

22. Gupta PK, Gupta H, Kaushik M, et al. Predictors of pulmonary complications after bariatric surgery. Surg Obes Relat Dis. 2012;8:574–81.

23. Alamoudi OS. Long-term pulmonary complications after laparoscopic adjustable gastric banding. Obes Surg. 2006;16:1685–8.

24. Avriel A, Warner E, Avinoach E, et al. Major respiratory adverse events after laparascopic gastric banding surgery for morbid obesity. Respir Med. 2012;106:1192–8.

25. Nguyen NT, Stevens CM, Wolfe BM. Incidence and outcome of anastomotic stricture after laparoscopic gastric bypass. J Gastrointest Surg. 2003;7(997):1003; discussion 1003.

26. Fisher BL, Atkinson JD, Cottam D. Incidence of gastroenterostomy stenosis in laparoscopic Roux-en-Y gastric bypass using 21- or 25-mm circular stapler: a randomized prospective blinded study. Surg Obes Relat Dis. 2007;3:176–9.

27. Lalor PF, Tucker ON, Szomstein S, Rosenthal RJ. Complications after laparoscopic sleeve gastrectomy. Surg Obes Relat Dis. 2008;4:33–8.

28. Spivak H, Favretti F. Avoiding postoperative complications with the LAP-BAND system. Am J Surg. 2002;184:31S–7S.

29. O'Brien PE, MacDonald L, Anderson M, et al. Long-term outcomes after bariatric surgery: fifteen-year follow-up of adjustable gastric banding and a systematic review of the bariatric surgical literature. Ann Surg. 2013;257:87–94.

30. Himpens J, Dapri G, Cadiere GB. A prospective randomized study between laparoscopic gastric banding and laparoscopic isolated sleeve gastrectomy: results after 1 and 3 years. Obes Surg. 2006;16:1450–6.

31. Magro DO, Geloneze B, Delfini R, et al. Long-term weight regain after gastric bypass: a 5-year prospective study. Obes Surg. 2008;18:648–51.

32. Sugerman HJ, Brewer WH, Shiffman ML, et al. A multicenter, placebo-controlled, randomized, double-blind, prospective trial of prophylactic ursodiol for the prevention of gallstone formation following gastric-bypass-induced rapid weight loss. Am J Surg. 1995;169:91–6; discussion 96–7.

33. Schirmer B, Erenoglu C, Miller A. Flexible endoscopy in the management of patients undergoing Roux-en-Y gastric bypass. Obes Surg. 2002;12:634–8.
34. Capella RF, Iannace VA, Capella JF. Bowel obstruction after open and laparoscopic gastric bypass surgery for morbid obesity. J Am Coll Surg. 2006;203:328–35.
35. Zainabadi K, Ramanathan R. Intussusception after laparoscopic Roux-en-Y gastric bypass. Obes Surg. 2007;17:1619–23.
36. Edwards MA, Grinbaum R, Ellsmere J, et al. Intussusception after Roux-en-Y gastric bypass for morbid obesity: case report and literature review of rare complication. Surg Obes Relat Dis. 2006;2:483–9.
37. Moon RC, Teixeira AF, Ducoin C, et al. Comparison of cholecystectomy cases after Roux-en-Y gastric bypass, sleeve gastrectomy, and gastric banding. Surg Obes Relat Dis. 2013;10(1):64–8.
38. Cirignotta F, Manconi M, Mondini S, et al. Wernicke-korsakoff encephalopathy and polyneuropathy after gastroplasty for morbid obesity: report of a case. Arch Neurol. 2000;57:1356–9.
39. O'Donnell KB, Simmons M. Early-onset copper deficiency following Roux-en-Y gastric bypass. Nutr Clin Pract. 2011;26:66–9.
40. Davies DJ, Baxter JM, Baxter JN. Nutritional deficiencies after bariatric surgery. Obes Surg. 2007;17:1150–8.
41. Ukleja A. Dumping syndrome: pathophysiology and treatment. Nutr Clin Pract. 2005;20:517–25.
42. King WC, Chen JY, Mitchell JE, et al. Prevalence of alcohol use disorders before and after bariatric surgery. JAMA. 2012;307:2516–25.
43. Lier HO, Biringer E, Stubhaug B, Tangen T. Prevalence of psychiatric disorders before and 1 year after bariatric surgery: the role of shame in maintenance of psychiatric disorders in patients undergoing bariatric surgery. Nord J Psychiatry. 2013;67:89–96.
44. Tindle HA, Omalu B, Courcoulas A, et al. Risk of suicide after long-term follow-up from bariatric surgery. Am J Med. 2010;123:1036–42.
45. Gabert DL, Majumdar SR, Sharma AM, et al. Prevalence and predictors of self-reported sexual abuse in severely obese patients in a population-based bariatric program. J Obes. 2013;2013:374050.
46. Ikossi DG, Maldonado JR, Hernandez-Boussard T, Eisenberg D. Post-traumatic stress disorder (PTSD) is not a contraindication to gastric bypass in veterans with morbid obesity. Surg Endosc. 2010;24:1892–7.
47. Gumbs A, Duffy A, Bell R. Incidence and management of marginal ulceration after laparoscopic Roux-Y gastric bypass. Surg Obes Relat Dis. 2006;2:460–3.
48. Smith MD, Patterson E, Wahed AS, et al. Thirty-day mortality after bariatric surgery: independently adjudicated causes of death in the longitudinal assessment of bariatric surgery. Obes Surg. 2011;21:1687–92.
49. Schauer PR, Kashyap SR, Wolski K, et al. Bariatric surgery versus intensive medical therapy in obese patients with diabetes. N Engl J Med. 2012;366:1567–76.

Index

© Springer Science+Business Media New York 2015
A. Youdim (ed.), *The Clinician's Guide to the Treatment of Obesity,*
Endocrine Updates, DOI 10.1007/978-1-4939-2146-1

Made in the USA
Charleston, SC
18 June 2016